The Neuroscience
of Animal Intelligence

From the Seahare to the Seahorse

ANIMAL INTELLIGENCE

A Series of Columbia University Press

Herbert S. Terrace, Series Editor

ANIMAL INTELLIGENCE
Herbert S. Terrace, General Editor

This series presents significant research on the cognitive capacities of various animals such as apes, monkeys, dolphins, pigeons, and rats. Each volume provides ample evidence of the realization of a previously unfulfilled promise of the Theory of Evolution—a valuable comparative psychology of intelligence.

Also available in the series:

Nim: A Chimpanzee Who Learned Sign Language
by Herbert S. Terrace

Ape Language: From Conditioned Response to Symbol
by E. Sue Savage-Rumbaugh

The Neuroscience of Animal Intelligence

From the Seahare to the Seahorse

Euan M. Macphail

Columbia University Press
New York

Columbia University Press
New York Chichester, West Sussex

Copyright © 1993 Columbia University Press
All rights reserved

Library of Congress Cataloging-in-Publication Data

Macphail, E. M. (Euan M.)
      The neuroscience of animal intelligence : from the seahare to the
  seahorse / Euan M. Macphail.
            p.   cm.—(Animal intelligence)
      Includes bibliographical references (p.   ) and indexes.
      ISBN 0-231-06144-7
      1. Memory—Physiological aspects.   2. Learning—Physiological
  aspects.   3. Animal intelligence.   I. Title.   II. Series.
  QP406.M3   1993
  156'.3—dc20   92-31167
                                                              CIP

⊗

Casebound editions of
Columbia University Press books
are printed on
permanent and durable
acid-free paper.

Printed in the United States of America

c 10 9 8 7 6 5 4 3 2 1

For my parents,
Malcolm and Janet Macphail

Contents

Foreword

Warren H. Meck

In his book *Animal Intelligence* (1911) Edward L. Thorndike set the stage for behavioral scientists to expand upon his studies of animal behavior in a manner that could relate the nature of intelligence to brain function. The influence of that early contribution was made especially evident in Karl Lashley's book *Brain Mechanisms and Intelligence* (1929) in which the acquisition of knowledge and its relation to the nervous system was made explicit. The connections between cognition and neuroscience were further strengthened by the electrophysiologist E. Roy John who began the preface to his classic book *Mechanisms of Memory* (1967) with the following statement: "Although the brain mediates much of reflex control and homeostatic regulation essential for life, the most important function of the brain is to process information. The brain mechanisms involved in storage and retrieval of memories are of particular interest, because memories are among the ingredients of thought. Understanding these processes will provide a uniquely intimate insight into the material bases of the human experience." This leads us to the current text by Euan M. Macphail, which represents an attempt to integrate theoretical formulations of animal intelligence, while at the same time placing them into a functional perspective that does not require, nor preclude, extensions to the human condition. It contains the essential ingredients for the appreciation of the role that behavioral neuroscience plays in our understanding of animal learning and memory. As such, it makes a central contribution to the Columbia University Press series on animal intelligence.

As already suggested, the question of animal intelligence has long been an important theme in both comparative and physiological psychology; the historical basis of which is pieced together well in this volume. Macphail takes the reader on a journey from the early beginnings of "nonassociative or simple learning processes" as represented by habituation, dishabituation, and sensitization in the gill withdrawal response of *Aplysia* (seahare) through the various expressions of associative learning, to the relational forms of learning as represented by spatial navigation and the possible construction of "cognitive maps" in the mammalian hippocampus (seahorse). The documentation of this odyssey is filled with a level of experimental detail and integration that is all too rare for the rapidly growing field of behavioral neuroscience. The overall goal of the book is to highlight discoveries that have shed light on the neural mechanisms involved in intelligence and other "higher levels" of plasticity. Given our current perspective, it is not surprising that much of this material focuses on the brain. This was not always the case, however, and Macphail does well in his description of the intellectual evolution that scholars have made in this regard.

One of the most significant contributions of this book is to remind neurobiologists and psychologists alike that intelligence and/or memory function is not a unitary process. Not only are there different degrees of memory function as measured in a quantitative sense, there are also different types of memory as indexed in a qualitative manner whose definitions are constantly being refined. The fractionation of memory, as initiated in chapter 8, is a case in point. Here the possible dissociation of working and reference memory processes involved in spatial memory are described, as well as the distinction between the clarity and content of memory as revealed by the study of temporal memory. Problems of the anatomical localization of different types and aspects of memory ultimately arise and are addressed by a discussion of the value of lesion studies. As the field of behavioral neuroscience is forced to expand by the ever-increasing availability of new technologies, we will experience the rapid development of brain imaging techniques needed to improve the precision of lesion placements. In turn, this should lead to an improvement in our methods for behavioral evaluation and data analysis.

The Neuroscience of Animal Intelligence: From the Seahare to the Seahorse not only takes an excellent stock of where we've been on this road, it describes where we currently stand (more or less), while at the same time pointing us in the directions that we should be going. I don't think that one could ask for anything more from a knowledge navigator dealing with comparative cognition and neurology. Although some of the arguments constructed within these pages will undoubtedly require future correction or elaboration, the utility of the integrated perspective provided from the point of view of an experimental psychologist substantially outweighs those inevitable developments.

Preface

The intelligent behavior of nonhuman animals presents to psychologists the problem of generating formal accounts of the properties of the information-processing mechanisms that allow animals to learn, to remember, and to solve problems. Behavioral psychologists have found it formidably difficult to provide satisfactory learning theories (theories that seek to provide formal accounts of animal intelligence), and there are good reasons (laid out in the introductory chapter) to suppose that physiological investigations may yield results that would contribute directly to theoretical issues in animal learning. My object in writing this book has been to provide a critical survey of physiological work concerned with the cognitive activity of animals, and to ask whether the work concerned has provided insights of value to behavioral psychologists.

The physiological psychology of learning and memory has seen the use of a remarkably wide range of physiological and behavioral paradigms, and I have not attempted to discuss them all. I have concentrated instead on those approaches that in my estimation either have provided or are most likely to provide psychological insights; this selectivity has allowed me to discuss chosen topics in sufficient detail to allow a clear understanding both of the nature of the experiments carried out and of their potential psychological import. There is at least a rough correspondence between my selection of topics and the research effort that those topics currently attract. Thus I devote much of two early chapters to discussion of learning mechanisms in *Aplysia* (the seahare of my subtitle), and most of three of the later chapters to consideration of the mammalian hippocampus (the "seahorse"); a cursory perusal of the current literature on the neuroscience of learning will show that these topics are indeed central to current research.

Although the theoretical stance adopted here is a psychological one in the sense that the major goal of the research discussed is seen as the provision of an account of intelligent behavior, I have written the book in the hope that it should be of interest not only to behavioral psychologists but also to neuroscientists in general, including those many neuroscientists who work at the cellular (or subcellular) level. Neurophysiologists have over recent decades achieved a degree of technical sophistication that has led to a remarkably detailed understanding of the properties of individual neurons, and of their modes of interaction at synapses; more recent work (work, in particular, on *Aplysia* and on the hippocampus) has begun to throw light on plasticity, on the ways in which neurons may change their properties as a result of experience. Many neuroscientists are naturally interested in the question how plasticity at the neuronal level might find expression at a behavioral level, and the relationship between neuronal and behavioral plasticity is one that receives frequent attention in this book.

The origins of the book lay in Columbia University Press science editor Herb Terrace's suggestion, made more years ago than I care to remember, that I contribute to CUP's series on Animal Intelligence. An attractive aspect of his invitation was that it enabled me reasonably to discuss the neuroscience of intelligence without including detailed consideration of human neuropsychology. The attraction lay in the fact that at the heart of human cognitive activity there is a system for the acquisition and use of language that is, I believe, wholly absent in nonhumans; thus any discussion of psychological aspects of human neuropsychology must necessarily introduce discussion of topics that find no counterpart in the animal literature. In this book, therefore, reference is made to the human literature only when the work is relevant to a topic in animal intelligence— most frequently, when the possibility of there being multiple memory stores is being discussed.

I am grateful to Herb Terrace not only for his original suggestion but for his encouragement throughout—a delicate balance between the carrot and the stick. Herb read each chapter as it was finished, and provided me with extensive and invaluable comments; the book would have been very much the poorer without his contribution. Individual chapters have been read by Tony Dickinson, Geoffrey Hall, Steve Reilly, and Mark Good, and I have benefited from their comments also, as I have from Dorothy Hourston's insightful remarks. Richard Morris provided detailed comments on the sections concerned with the hippocampus; I am particularly grateful for the effort he put in, and have been glad to use many of his suggestions in revising those sections.

My greatest debt is, of course, to my wife Kate, who has given me endless support, has put setbacks into sensible perspective, and has made working at home such a very attractive proposition.

Acknowledgments

I am grateful to David Whiteley and Gordon Smith of the Photography Department in York for their able assistance in the preparation of the figures. I should also like to thank the following scientists for permission to use material from their publications: J. P. Aggleton; D. L. Alkon; D. G. Amaral; P. Andersen; C. H. Bailey; C. A. Barnes; T. W. Berger; V. P. Bingman; O. Braha; J. W. Byrne; T. J. Carew; R. M. Colwill; M. Davis; D. Gaffan; J. W. Grau; P. M. Groves; R. D. Hawkins; L. E. Jarrard; E. R. Kandel; H. J. Karten; H. Kaye; M. Klein; R. N. Leaton; I. Lederhendler; R. R. Llinás; G. Lynch; D. A. McCormick; B. Milner; M. Mishkin; R. G. M. Morris; R. A. Nicoll; J. O'Keefe; D. S. Olton; D. N. Pandya; R. E. Passingham; M. M. Patterson; R. L. Port; C. Sahley; D. P. Salmon; P. R. Solomon; R. F. Thompson; A. R. Wagner; E. T. Walters; S. Zola-Morgan.

The following organizations have kindly allowed me to reproduce material: Academic Press; the American Association for the Advancement of Science; the American Physiological Society; the American Psychological Association; Cell Press; the Company of Biologists; Elsevier Applied Science Publishing; Elsevier Science Publishers, Bvbiomedical Division; Elsevier, New York; the Experimental Psychology Society; W. H. Freeman and Co.; Gordon and Breach Science Publishers; Johns Hopkins University Press; S. Karger AG; Macmillan Press; MIT Press; the National Academy of Sciences of the U.S.A; Oxford University Press; Plenum Publishing Corporation; the Psychonomic Society; Raven Press; the Royal Society of London; Scientific American; the Society for Neuroscience; Springer-Verlag; Wadsworth Publications.

The Neuroscience
of Animal Intelligence

From the Seahare to the Seahorse

1. The Physiological Analysis of Cognition

Historical Background

The aim of this book will be to survey work carried out using physiological techniques to explore intelligence in animals. Before beginning the survey proper, attention will be directed in this first chapter to the question that necessarily precedes any such discussion—namely, why is the work of interest and what questions does it hope to answer? An initial response would be that intelligence is (in some sense) a product of brain activity, so that it may seem obvious that understanding how the nervous system works should help explain intelligence. Now while this is not a particularly sophisticated answer, it is interesting to notice that however obvious it may seem to us now, the fact that mental life has its origins in the brain was not easily established. The discovery of the basic role and method of function of the nervous system is a story that is not only of historical interest. It also helps to emphasize the necessary interplay of a variety of techniques and disciplines in the attempt to understand the most complex achievement of the body.

Early Notions of Brain Function

Spirits: Natural, Animal, and Vital

Anatomy was the discipline that provided the earliest scientists with a basis for their highly speculative physiological theories. Aristotle, for example, had proposed that the seat of mental life was to be found in the heart, and he believed that nerves originated from the heart. Galen, a native of the city of Pergamum (the modern Bergama, in Western Turkey), placed the mind in the brain, partly because dissection of the bodies of animals had shown him that in fact nerves originated from the brain and not from the heart. The rest of Galen's views on the operation of the nervous system were, however, remarkably inaccurate, all the more remarkably because they achieved almost universal acceptance for thirteen hundred years and more from the time of his death at the end of the second century A.D.

At the center of Galen's account was a misconception of the distinction between veins and arteries, a misconception that led to an erroneous view of the function of the nervous system. Galen taught that food was absorbed by the stomach and intestines and transported, via the portal vein, to the liver, in which it was converted into "natural" spirits, which were distributed, in an ebb-and-flow, to-and-fro manner, throughout the venous system. The arteries, however, absorbed air, both from the lungs and directly, where the arteries were sufficiently close to the body surface. In the left ventricle of the heart, this air was combined with a relatively small amount of blood, which reached the ventricle directly through pores in the septum wall dividing the left and right ventricles. The arteries contained "vital" spirits, and these too were transported throughout the body by the arteries. It was believed that the natural spirits were essential for vegetative functions, and the vital spirits for growth. The vital spirits in turn were converted at the base of the brain into "animal" spirits, which were even more refined than the vital spirits and assumed to be of an ethereal nature. These spirits were stored in the hollow ventricles of the brain and were transported along the nerves (assumed, also, to be hollow) to mediate both sensation and movement.

Although Galen believed that the brain itself could manufacture animal spirits, the principal site for the conversion from vital to animal spirits was believed to be the "rete mirabile," the network of blood vessels that Galen had observed at the base of the brain when dissecting animals' corpses (see figure 1.1).

The Medieval Cell Doctrine

Early medieval writers (St. Augustine, for example, in the fourth century) adopted the majority of Galen's views, but laid more emphasis on the role of the ventricles, which they took to be not simply the site of storage of the animal spirits but the seat of mental life itself. Moreover, the various ventricles were assigned different functions (see figure 1.2). The lateral ventricles were believed to receive sensory input and so to subserve per-

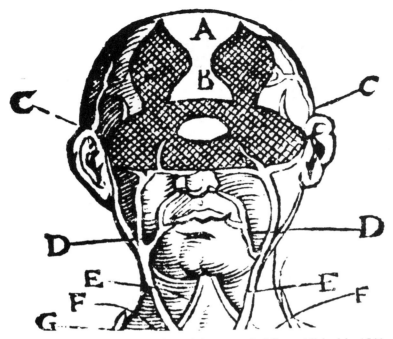

FIGURE 1.1. A representation of the rete mirabile, published in 1541 by Walter Ryff

ception; they were regarded as a single "cell," which communicated with the third ventricle (the second cell), whose function was to reflect on the images it received from the first cell, to think and to reason. The second cell in turn communicated with the third cell (the fourth ventricle), which served the function of memory. There was, of course, no universal agreement on the details of the system (some writers, for example, dividing each cell into more than one component), but there was what seems in retrospect a surprising degree of acceptance of the basic nature of the organization for more than a thousand years. One of the reasons for the longevity of this scheme may be that its psychological aspects seem even now eminently sensible. There is a clear parallel between the psychological stages outlined and stages of processing posited in some modern cognitive theories. Broadbent (1958), for example, has proposed that incoming sensory information is first processed through a perceptual filtering mechanism and then passes on to a decision-making stage (of limited capacity), from which some information passes finally into a long-term memory store.

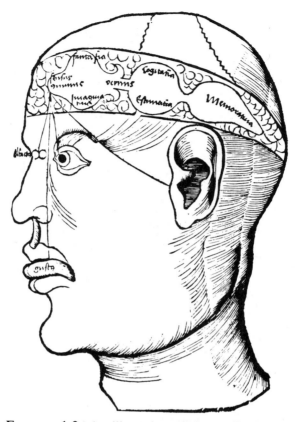

FIGURE 1.2. An illustration of the medieval cell
doctrine, published in 1503 by Gregor Reisch

When Constantinople fell in 1453, Western European scholars redis-
covered the Greek classics, brought to Europe by those fleeing from the
Turks. Reading them stimulated the imagination and curiosity of the men
of the Renaissance and reevoked interest in dissection, in particular; Galen
himself, after all, had laid heavy emphasis on the importance of direct
observation in anatomy, and his writings were made widely accessible
through their translation into Latin in the early fifteenth century.

The Renaissance anatomists soon found important errors in the traditional anatomy. Andreas Vesalius, the most important of them, could find
no evidence for any pores in the interventricular septum, and so, no support for Galen's notion on how the natural spirits might be made available
for conversion into vital spirits. More strikingly, Vesalius could find no

trace of a rete mirabile in the human body. In fact, although such a structure is found in ruminants (animals that Galen frequently used for dissection), it is absent in primates.

The role of the cerebral ventricles, too, was brought into doubt. It was established, for example, that they contained a fluid (the cerebrospinal fluid), and this seemed somewhat too material to form the ethereal substance of the mind. Moreover, Leonardo da Vinci had established the true shape of the ventricles, by taking a wax cast of them in an ox. Their complex shapes were clearly very different from the simple cells so commonly seen in medieval illustrations.

But these anatomical observations did not lead to a full-scale abandonment of Galen's system, largely because they did not suggest alternative functional systems. Descartes, for example, argued in the seventeenth century that the pineal gland was the site of operation of the soul, and that information from sense organs (taking the form of movement or agitation of stringlike nerves) reached it through the ventricular system (still conceived of as containing animal spirits). Bodily response occurred when the pineal gland directed into the hollow motor nerves spirits that entered and expanded the muscles, so causing movement. Descartes, then, abandoned the rete mirabile and the notion that the various ventricles carried out different intellectual functions, but did not assign a role in mental activity to the brain tissue itself. For Descartes, the soul was an indivisible nonmaterial entity, which interacted with the physical body only at the pineal gland.

Thomas Willis finally demolished the notion of a rete mirabile in man by demonstrating the true organization of the blood vessels at the base of the human brain, giving to them the name "the circle of Willis." Willis was among those who supported the notion that the brain tissue itself was the site of mental activity, and he went so far as to assign different functions to different regions of the tissue: the corpus striatum for sensation and perception, the corpus callosum for imagination, the cortex for memory, and the cerebellum for vegetative and involuntary actions. Willis poured scorn on the notion that the ventricles might support mental activity, comparing them instead to sewers, whose function was solely to carry away waste material excreted by brain tissues. But in fact Willis had no more evidence for this organization than had the medieval proponents of the cell theory. Willis, moreover, had not abandoned the notion that nerves activated muscles by infusing them with a spirit of some kind. In Willis's scheme, one type of animal spirit, which he likened to a light, was conveyed in the nerve and met in the blood of the muscle another form of spirit, which he likened to a flame. The resulting explosive processes inflated the muscle.

The sixteenth and seventeenth centuries, then, saw the exposition of many anatomical errors in the schemes that had dominated the preceding thousand years and more. One physiological discovery of major importance was William Harvey's demonstration, in the early sixteenth century, of the circulation of the blood, a discovery that did much to clarify the distinction between the systems of blood vessels and other systems of fluid in the body. Yet it can be seen that very little in the way of positive advance in understanding the nervous system had been achieved (unless it is an advance to go from misunderstanding to no understanding at all). Harvey himself acknowledged that his work threw no light on such questions as whether the heart was not only a pump but might also endow the blood with various spirits; such questions, he observed, must be decided by the use of other techniques.

One simple but powerful physiological experiment was carried out in the seventeenth century by Francis Glisson, of Cambridge. Glisson reasoned that if muscles were activated by the inflow of spirits from nerves, then the volume of a muscle should increase during contraction. This notion was tested by immersing a man's arm in a water-filled glass container and asking the man to contract and relax his arm muscles. Glisson observed that during contraction volume did not increase, but actually decreased. While Glisson's experiment cast much doubt on any account in terms of influx of spirits, it did not, of course, shed positive light on the problem of the activation of muscle. Glisson found that an excised muscle could be made to contract in response to irritant stimulation, and proposed that muscles possessed some sort of intrinsic instability; but he was unable to propose any specific means by which that instability was achieved.

Advances in the Understanding of Nerves

The true nature of the "instability" of muscle (and of nerve) had to await the discovery of electricity and the development of instruments for detecting relatively small electrical events. Luigi Galvani, toward the end of the eighteenth century, found that the muscles of a frog contracted when the frog was either attached to a long wire during a thunderstorm or attached (by brass hooks) to an iron railing (there being no need in this case for atmospheric disturbance). Galvani believed that these results—and particularly the latter finding—demonstrated the existence of electricity intrinsic to the nerves and muscles themselves. He was, however, aware that the type of metal used for attaching the frog to the iron substrate was important in determining the force of the contractions, and Alessandro Volta emphasized that fact in arguing (correctly) that Galvani's preparation reflected a flow of electricity caused by the frog's being a conductor between two dissimilar metals. The controversy between Galvani and Volta led to further experiments. Volta for his part went on to invent the voltaic pile (the first electric battery) and to prove that Galvani's most famous result was indeed due to the stimulation of the muscles by the flow of electrical current between dissimilar metals. Galvani and his supporters provided evidence (however indirect) for their view that there was electrical activity intrinsic to their preparations; such demonstrations consisted in causing muscular contraction by touching a muscle with the severed end of the spinal cord. Both Galvani and Volta were, as we now know, correct: muscles do react to electrical stimulation, but they do also display intrinsic electrical phenomena.

Proof of electrical activity in nerves and muscles was finally provided by Emil du Bois-Reymond, a German of Swiss extraction who worked in Berlin in the mid-nineteenth century. Du Bois-Reymond's achievement was largely technological. He invented a galvanometer far more sensitive than any previously used, and this enabled him to detect not only current flow between cut and intact portions of nerves and muscles but also a wave of potential change that moved along a nerve (in both directions) from the point at which direct stimulation (electrical or mechanical) was applied to the nerve. Du Bois-Reymond's pupil Julius Bernstein went on to propose that the membrane of nerves and muscles showed selective permeability to different ions, and that the resting state was polarized, having relatively more negative ions inside than outside the membrane. He also proposed that the nerve impulse observed by du Bois-Reymond was a self-propagating phenomenon. Bernstein, then, correctly anticipated the essence of the modern theory of nervous conduction. In the early part of the twentieth century, Edgar Adrian proposed the "all-or-nothing" principle for nervous impulses: the amplitude of nerve impulses in individual nerves does not vary with either the quality or the intensity of the triggering event. According to this principle, nerve cells either "fire" or do not fire and can vary only in the rate of their firing, that rate in turn being limited by the absolute and relative refractory periods of the nerve.

The physiological work outlined above, which confirmed the role of electrical phenomena in nervous transmission, was complemented by anatomical work on the structure of the nerves and the nervous system. The critical technical advances concerned were optical and histological. The development through the eighteenth and nineteenth centuries of powerful microscopes that used compound lenses to overcome the problem of chromatic aberration allowed superior visualization of tissue sections. The later nineteenth century saw the emergence of new methods for preserving (fixing) and staining tissue. In 1873, Camillo Golgi reported a technique that stained a small proportion (about 5 percent) of neurons by depositing silver chromate throughout the selected cells. (Even today the selectivity of this procedure is not understood—but it is its most important characteristic. If all cells were stained in their entirety, a stained brain section would simply be impenetrably black.) Golgi's technique allowed anatomists to see for the first time the morphology of individual cells, and to discriminate between cell bodies and their processes and between the long, large axons and the smaller, branching dendrites. In the mid–1880's, Franz Nissl and Karl Weigert reported techniques that stained all neurons, but stained selectively different parts of neurons. Nissl stains allowed visualization of cell bodies, whereas Weigert's technique stained myelin and so revealed the course of axons. These stains led to a much clearer appreciation of the overall architecture of the brain: it was now possible to see the density and organization of cell bodies in different brain regions, and the bundles of nerve fibers coursing between one region and another.

These new techniques were not, however, adequate to show precisely how nerve cells were linked to one another. One school of thought (to which Golgi himself belonged) believed that the nervous system consisted of a collection of nerves whose processes were continuous one with another, so that excitation spread in all directions through the network from a point of stimulation. Opposing this "reticularist" school were those who adopted Theodor Schwann's cell theory of animal structure and held that nerve cells were contiguous, but not continuous, with each other. Support for this latter view, the neuron doctrine, came from the work of the Spaniard Santiago Ramón y Cajal. Cajal, using a modification of Golgi's stain, established that axons touched, but did not merge with, dendrites of other cells, and concluded, from examining sensory nerves (in which the direction of flow of information was known), that transmission in nerves was always unidirectional, being toward the cell body in the dendrites and away from the cell body in the axons. Sir Charles Sherrington dubbed the sites at which nerve cells touch one another "synapses."

The notion that transmission of information across synapses might involve release of chemicals by the presynaptic nerve had its origin in the work of Sir Henry Dale and Otto Loewi in the first two decades of this century. Dale showed that acetylcholine had an inhibitory effect on heart muscle, and Loewi confirmed that stimulation of the vagal nerve of a frog did indeed liberate a substance that inhibited the activity of another heart. The road was clearly open then for the proposal that acetylcholine was the substance released by the vagal nerve, and that acetylcholine, along with other active chemicals such as adrenalin, might act as transmitters at nerve junctions as well.

The modern era has seen a dramatic growth in understanding the details of the operation of single neurons, and of ways in which one neuron may interact with another. No attempt will be made here to outline the progress that has been made, although in subsequent chapters much use will be made of properties of nerves only recently discovered or understood. The purpose now is to set the historical context in which modern work should be viewed. Consideration of modern studies of the properties of nerves will be confined to work that is specifically relevant to the physiological basis of intelligence.

Localization of Function in the Brain

Phrenology

Although the above discussion of anatomical and physiological discoveries in the nineteenth century shows how a grasp was achieved of the basic operating principles of nerves, it does not show how progress was made in assigning mental processes to the brain. How was empirical evidence finally brought to bear on the previously entirely speculative dispute between writers such as Descartes and Willis? The answer to this question may be found in the story of cortical localization, in which real progress began, oddly enough, with the groundless and much-derided claims of phrenology.

Franz Josef Gall, the originator of phrenology, was an anatomist who made important contributions around the end of the eighteenth century to knowledge of central nervous system anatomy. Along with his pupil and collaborator Johann Caspar Spurzheim, Gall established the distinction between gray and white matter throughout the central nervous system, showed that the brain's hemispheres are symmetrical and connected to each other by commissures, and demonstrated the crossing-over of the pyramidal tracts. Not only did Gall distinguish between gray and white matter, he also proposed that the cortex, consisting of gray matter, was of

critical importance in mental life. At this time histology was not sufficiently advanced to allow a demonstration of the fact that gray matter
consisted of nerve cells.

Gall attributed not only intellectual activity but also emotional experience to the brain, so being one of the first to place all mental life unques-
tionably in the brain. The critical step in Gall's localization of functions
within brain tissue (the step that was to lead ultimately to phrenology) was
his adoption of what was in effect a psychological theory. For Gall argued
that the mind consisted of a number of independent faculties, a conclusion
to which he was led by his observation of individual differences in his
fellow human beings. Each faculty, he supposed, must be served by a
different "organ," and those organs were to be found discretely located
within the brain. It required only a small step now to the proposal that
individuals in whom a faculty was well-developed possessed a correspondingly larger organ in the brain. And, since Gall took the cortex to
be the site of these organs, it was not unreasonable to suggest that differential growth of parts of the cortex might be detected by examining the
form of the skull.

These propositions are not necessarily outrageous, and there was—
certainly at the beginning of the nineteenth century—no reason for dis-
carding them outright. What they required, of course, were convincing
demonstrations of the correlation between skull measurements and measurements of mental faculties amongst the population. Now Gall did col-
lect a large number of skulls of persons whose mental capacities were
known to him, along with casts of the heads of living men who excelled
in some talent or other. He claimed, moreover, to have observed the necessary correlations amply demonstrated in the population at large. But
these claims were basically anecdotal in nature, and his data were not only
inadequate statistically but not even systematically collected in any sense.
Despite the absence of real empirical support, Gall and Spurzheim attracted many followers, some of whom contributed to the loss of any
respectability for phrenology. Gall had originally proposed a total of
twenty-seven mental faculties, eight of which (including "mimicry") were
supposed to be peculiar to humans; Spurzheim went on to add eight further faculties (see figure 1.3), and others went on to expand the list of
faculties to well over one hundred, each with a region of the head (including, now, the face) as its seat. It is hardly surprising, then, that phrenology
achieved little prestige among scientists.

The major beneficial effect of phrenology was to direct attention toward
the brain and its involvement in mental activity, if only to disprove Gall's

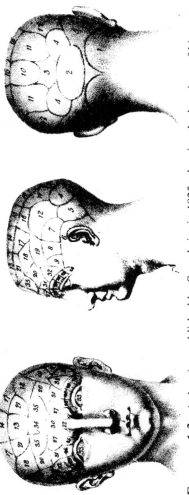

FIGURE 1.3. A drawing published by Spurzheim in 1825, showing the locations of his proposed 35 mental faculties

claims. One of Gall's most trenchant critics was Pierre Flourens, who was the first to use the ablation technique successfully on living animals (others had tried before him but had achieved little since their animals rarely survived long after the operation had been conducted). Early in the nineteenth century, Flourens reported experiments on birds (chickens and pigeons). The findings of most relevance here were, first, that removal of the cerebral hemispheres abolished perception, judging, and remembering, and, second, that cerebellar ablation disrupted motor coordination. Birds without hemispheres were not blind (in the sense that their pupils still constricted in response to light), they could fly when thrown up in the air, and they would swallow food placed in their mouths. But they showed no voluntary initiation of behavior, behaved as though blind and deaf, did not fly unless thrown in the air, and did not eat spontaneously. Birds without the cerebellum, on the other hand, attempted to move—to walk, or to fly—but could not do so adequately, stumbling and falling in their efforts. Flourens showed, then, both that the brain was indeed involved in mental activity (and his was the first wholly convincing demonstration of the truth of that proposition) and that different parts of the brain played different roles. The localization of function was, however, strictly limited. Flourens was unable to find any differentiation within the hemispheres of effects on perception, intelligence, or the will. Progressive removal of layers of the hemispheres resulted in progressive damage to all those capacities, and not in the sparing of one or two at the expense of the others. Flourens used this finding to attack not only Gall's attempts at localization of functions but also Gall's psychological theory of the existence of independent mental faculties. In opposition to Gall, Flourens preferred the Cartesian concept of the indivisible mind, albeit located now within the hemispheres, rather than in (or, at least, operating through) the pineal gland.

In the continuing absence of empirical support for the claims of the phrenologists, Flourens's views were influential. However, one of the major benefits arising from Gall's views was that anatomists in the early nineteenth century began, apparently for the first time, to examine the structure of the cerebral cortex. By the end of the eighteenth century, only one feature of the cerebral surface had been named (the Sylvian fissure, which marks the dorsal boundary of the temporal lobe, and was so named in the seventeenth century). The early nineteenth century saw the introduction of the terms "frontal," "parietal," "temporal," and "occipital" to refer to the major lobes of the hemispheres. It was recognized that the gyri and sulci visible in the hemispheres had, despite some variation between individuals, a consistent pattern, and names were introduced for individual "convolutions." By the end of the nineteenth century, the advance in histological techniques had allowed workers such as Walter Campbell and Korbinian Brodmann to construct detailed cytoarchitectonic maps of the human neocortex (see figure 1.4), maps that indicated the layered structure of cortex, and the variations, from one region to another of the cortex, in the detailed composition of that structure. The gradual emergence of the fact that the microscopic appearance of neocortex varied encouraged, naturally, the view that the neocortex was not functionally identical throughout its extent.

Functional Studies of Cortical Localization

Striking evidence in favor of cortical localization was provided by Paul Broca, who reported cerebral pathology on two patients who had died within a few months of each other, in 1861. Both patients had been unable to speak (although capable of the comprehension of speech), and each

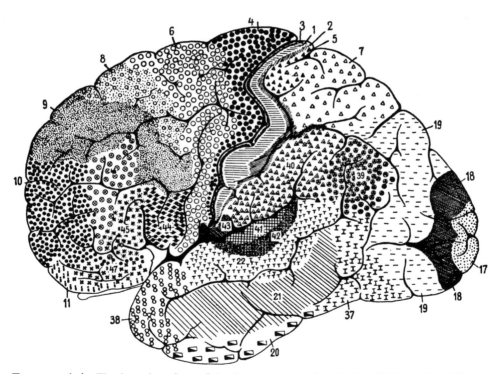

FIGURE 1.4. The lateral surface of the human cortex showing its divisions into different cytoarchitectonic areas, published by Brodmann in 1909

patient showed clear physical damage to the same cortical area, the left third frontal gyrus (a region known ever since then as Broca's area). Further direct evidence of localization of cortical function was provided by a report in 1870, by Gustav Theodor Fritsch and Edvard Hitzig, of movements elicited by localized electrical stimulation of the cortex of dogs. Fritsch and Hitzig found not only that there was localization in the sense that stimulation of certain cortical areas (anteriorly placed) did elicit movements, and that stimulation of others did not, but also that within the effective areas, different sites produced different types of movement. Their work was carried on in England by David Ferrier, who, using both stimulation and ablation techniques with monkeys, found both motor and sensory (vision and hearing) sites in the cortex, the sensory sites being demonstrated primarily through sensory loss following ablation.

Although the work of Broca, of Fritsch and Hitzig, and of Ferrier had indicated that at least some functions could be associated with particular areas of the cortex, there remained the question of the localization of intelligence. Flourens had claimed that all intelligence and memory was lost following cerebral destruction, but had produced no real evidence for that claim. He cited, for example, the fact that birds without hemispheres would bump repeatedly against some object and not learn to turn away from it, or would flutter when struck but would not fly away. Such effects could as easily be explained on the assumption that sensory or motivational systems were impaired (as he acknowledged them to be) as on the assumption that either learning or memory was impaired. Progress in this—the question of most interest here—had to await the development of another new set of techniques, the behavioral techniques that would allow systematic exploration of intellectual capacities. Around 1900, Edward Lee Thorndike introduced puzzle-boxes, and Robert Mearns Yerkes and Willard Stanton Small, mazes, and the study of nonhuman intelligence had begun. It was now possible to use the ablation technique to assess the involvement of cortex in intelligence.

One early proposal made by Paul Fleschig in the late nineteenth century was that the so-called association areas were of particular significance in "higher" mental functions. This notion arose partly by exclusion—the sensory and motor projection areas identified by Ferrier and others already had a function assigned to them, and it was not unreasonable to suppose that the remaining areas might be involved in some integrative activity, using information from more than one modality. There were other grounds also. The association areas were larger in animals that were supposedly of considerable intelligence (e.g., monkeys) than in those of supposedly less intelligence (e.g., dogs), and the association areas, Fleschig found, were the last (in ontogeny) to show myelinization of the fibers leading to and from them, a fact that might explain the graded growth of intelligence in an individual.

The potential role in learning of the frontal lobes, which consisted largely of "association" cortex, was explored by Shepherd Ivory Franz, who used cats and monkeys, testing them in various versions of the puzzle-box. In 1902 he reported that bilateral lesions of the frontal lobes resulted in the loss of recently acquired habits. Old-established habits were not lost, however, and new habits could be acquired in the absence of frontal lobes. This pattern of results led him to the conclusion that there was no strict localization of memory within the cortex: the frontal lobes were involved in the retention of recent learning but were not essential for its acquisition—in their absence, some other area became involved, with equal efficiency. Franz went on to launch a wholesale attack on any form of strict cortical localization—including localization of sensory and motor functions. While that attack is of only historical interest now, it did possess one feature of lasting importance. Franz argued against localization by using not physiological but psychological evidence. He observed that, in escaping from puzzle-boxes, the same cat would use different movements from one trial to the next, but that different cats might use quite different techniques to escape. He argued that if fixed neuronal routes underlay behavior, variability of this kind would not be obtained: particular stimuli would invariably activate the same set of cortical neurons, which would be tightly linked to others leading to the motor neurons. His belief that the brain operates as a whole and not as a set of fixed and independent neuronal circuits was based, then, on psychological at least as much as on physiological considerations. That method of argument is of interest since it hints, as will be shown in a later section, at another of the answers to the question why physiological research should be relevant to psychological issues.

The modern era in physiological analysis of intelligence begins with Karl Spencer Lashley, whose first work in this area was carried out when he was a colleague of Franz. Lashley's work in the second and third decades of the twentieth century led him to two conclusions—first, that retention of "simple" habits was disrupted by lesions of the appropriate sensory projection area and not by damage in any other part of the cortex, and second, that retention of complex habits was disrupted by damage to any cortical region, the severity of disruption correlating with the size (but not the locus) of the lesion. The former conclusion indicated Lashley's acceptance of cortical localization. The latter conclusion led to Lashley's introduction of the two terms ever since associated with his name, "mass action" and "equipotentiality." For complex (but not, it must be emphasized, for simple) learning tasks, the entire cortex was equipotential, since the severity of disruption obtained did not vary with the locus of the cortical damage. The fact that there was a graded rather than an "all-or-none" effect of damage of equipotential regions indicated that each region of cortex must in some way facilitate the others in complex learning, and this is what is meant by "mass action."

With Lashley's compromise between the localization and antilocalization schools, this account has reached what might be called the end of the beginning of the physiological psychology of intelligence. Lashley's work on maze-learning is by no means of only historical interest now, and his results and theoretical stance will be discussed further in the final chapter of this book.

Summary

For fifteen hundred years or so, Western philosophers and scientists totally misunderstood the operation of the nervous system. The sixteenth, seventeenth, and eighteenth centuries saw the slow accumulation of observations that undermined traditional accounts, without providing any acceptable new theory. The nineteenth century brought great advances in both anatomical and physiological techniques (in particular, the development of microscopy and histology, and the growing understanding of electricity), the application of which finally allowed a correct understanding of the basic principles of nervous activity, and of the role of the brain itself, to emerge. The twentieth century saw the use by physiological psychologists of behavioral tests, and the chapters that follow will show how vital the development and variety of those tests have been to progress. A given brain structure may indeed play a critical role in some intellectual capacity, but unless a test is available that selectively taps that capacity, no demonstration of the structure's role will be possible.

The Mind-Body Problem

The historical development of our understanding of brain function has naturally had considerable impact on the philosophical problems associated with the relationship between "mind" and "body." What is quite clear, however, is that physiological research has not yet solved any of these problems, and so has not led to universal acceptance of any one philosophical position. It is probably true, as Sperry has asserted, that most investigators of cerebral function believe that "a complete objective explanation of brain function is possible in principle without any reference to the subjective mental phenomena" (Sperry 1969:533). And most of these scientists would probably agree that descriptions of events in "mental" terms are simply alternative ways of describing events that would be as well described in physical terms (if, that is, we understood fully the nervous events responsible for behavior). According to this view, matter and energy—physical entities—are the only constituents of the universe, and all phenomena are properly to be seen as physical events.

An alternative view, which is certainly widespread in the nonscientific community, is that mental events involve entities that do not consist of matter or energy and that are nonmaterial. Clearly, the first question facing such a proposal is, in what way are events in the physical world related to mental events? If my mind makes the decision to raise my arm, why do motoneurons begin to fire appropriately? One—somewhat extreme—response to this question can be found in Leibniz's version of psychophysical parallelism. Leibniz argued that mental and physical events are, in fact, totally independent. Physical events are subject to the mechanical laws of causality, whereas mental events are governed by rationality. The physical raising of an arm is, then, part of a causal sequence to be analyzed in terms of physiological events; the mental decision to raise an arm is to be analyzed in terms of the reasons that led to the decision. Why, then, do these independent events temporally coincide? Leibniz's answer—that the coincidence between the chain of physical events and that of mental events is due to the miracle of preestablished harmony, a harmony established by God—has never seemed quite satisfactory.

Most philosophers (and scientists) who have assumed a difference between the stuff of the mind and that of the rest of the universe have agreed that the two interact. We have already seen that Descartes took the view that the mind interacted with the body through the pineal gland; what is more pertinent here is that at least some present-day distinguished neuroscientists believe that the mind (assumed by them to be a nonphysical entity) does influence brain activity. Sperry (1969) and Eccles (1977a), Nobel Prize–winners both, agree in such a view, and Eccles goes so far as to suggest that the site of interaction between mind and brain is to be found in the dominant cerebral hemisphere (generally the left hemisphere, in right-handed humans).

Of course, no observation of a modulation of brain activity by mental processes has yet been reported, and it is still not clear what should be looked for. According to Sperry, although conscious forces shape the flow pattern of cerebral excitation, properties of consciousness do not in any way disrupt the physiology of brain cell activity. What he suggests is that in the dynamics of large processes and whole patterns of activity, "the more molar conscious properties are seen to supersede the more elemental physiochemical forces" (Sperry 1969:534). It hardly seems that the modern dualist is much further on than was Descartes.

Whether any experimental work will ever solve these—or any other—philosophical problems may be doubtful. But it is difficult to study brain function without being drawn to speculate on these issues. Philosophical problems have remained problems for centuries precisely because there is no way of resolving them, and the mind-brain problem (what Sperry dubs the "Number 1" problem of brain research) is no exception. It has been suggested here that the proposal that the mind interacts with the brain is still a poorly specified and scarcely comprehensible notion. It should at the same time be pointed out that grave problems face the materialist also.

If "decisions" are the consequence of (or simply a way of describing) causally determined physiological events in the nervous system, is our sense of free will an illusion? Do materialist neuroscientists praise or blame their fellow human beings for behavior that could not in fact have been otherwise? And if conscious activity is no more than the activity of nerve cells, what physicochemical events in those cells constitute pleasure and pain? Is it conceivable that we could discover how to build a device constructed out of the physical constituents of nerve cells which could feel either pleasure or pain?

Current thinking about the mind-body problem has been much influenced by the advent of computers and by the widespread adoption of the computer metaphor for mind. One of the primary goals of artificial intelligence is to devise programs that will successfully simulate human cognitive processes. It has in fact proved to be much more difficult than anticipated to produce such programs, but the attempt has prompted the question: If a computer was programmed to simulate human cognitive processes, would that computer in fact be performing mental activity or would it merely be duplicating the output of a human who really was performing mental acts?

Suppose a computer (hidden behind a screen) was programmed so that a human being could carry on a conversation with it, and that the human could not tell from the contents of the conversation whether he was talking to a fellow human or to a machine. Would that machine be "really" thinking or "simulating" thinking? Would its intelligence, in other words, be real or artificial? The responses of philosophers to this question (known as the Turing test, after British mathematician Alan Turing) have been mixed.

A program that enabled conversation would in effect be a set of rules for the manipulation of symbols, and some philosophers (e.g., Searle 1990) argue that the successful manipulation of symbols does not of itself guarantee understanding. For genuine understanding to occur, symbols must have meaning, and meaning is the critical prerequisite for mental content. The argument may be summarized as the claim that computers may achieve syntax, but not semantics. These philosophers agree that the brain is a computer, but a computer of a special kind having properties that are not to be found in nonbiological systems. It is difficult (e.g., Churchland and Churchland 1990) to establish precisely which properties of biological systems are essential for the occurrence of mental activity, and it is not easy to accept the principle that only our own carbon-based biology could support mental acts. We surely would not want to deny genuine mental life—consciousness—to a creature from some other planet simply on the grounds that its biology was very different from ours. If a natural conversation could be established with such a creature, and if the creature referred freely to mental states and acts and so manifested an understanding of such terms as intention, hope, and pain, we would, I imagine, not hesitate to ascribe mental life to it.

It does not seem likely that the validity of the arguments on one side or the other of the current debate will be proved by logic alone to the satisfaction of all concerned. But the examples used consist primarily of "thought" experiments, and I shall suggest that the dispute might possibly see an end if the thought experiments could be translated into real experiments. This would require considerable progress in artificial intelligence, so that computers might successfully simulate human cognitive processes; progress in artificial intelligence may in turn be stimulated by progress in neuroscience.

Early attempts to model cognitive processes in computers found that, despite using units whose response speeds were many times faster than those of neurons, the time required for complex processing became very long. This outcome cast doubt on the computer metaphor, and indeed the notion that the brain should be conceived as a digital serial processing machine (e.g., Von Neumann 1958) is now being replaced by the proposal that the brain consists of numerous systems that process information simultaneously, in parallel circuits. The computer metaphor therefore now incorporates that notion, and contemporary artificial intelligence is much occupied with the devising of parallel processing models of cognition. But physiological considerations have not only provided impetus for the shift in focus toward parallel processing; physiological research promises also, as we shall see in the following section, to provide insights into the nature of the processes to be simulated—to mark out the properties of at least some of the constituents of the gamut of processes that are human cognition.

Progress in artificial intelligence and in the physiology of cognition may yield two outcomes that could have considerable impact on the philosophy of mind. First, we may be able to achieve empirical versions of the Turing test, to see how humans actually would react when confronted with a conversing machine (it may simply turn out that when actually confronted by such a computer, all humans find it impossible not to accept that they are indeed encountering a being with mental life). Second, the physiological aspects of cognitive processes may become so well understood that the need for any extra (nonphysiological) processes may shrink to the vanishing point. It may be that these ancient philosophical problems will yield not to logical analysis but to empirical demonstrations that mental activity is a particular kind of computing that is routinely carried out in our brains but that may be implemented in quite other "hardware."

Whatever the future may hold for the mind-body problem, it does not currently seem to be an issue that either diminishes the importance of physiological work or influences the ways in which we should proceed. We can all agree that brain events play a critical role in intelligent behavior: whether they are the *only* events of significance in intelligence is a question of enormous intrinsic interest, but of little potential consequence in seeking to understand the ways in which we learn, remember, and solve problems.

Goals of Behavioral Neuroscience

As a final preliminary to the survey of modern experimental work, I shall consider what could in principle be achieved by using physiological techniques.

The ultimate goal of physiological investigations into intellectual activity is to throw light on the nature of that activity. Intelligence is a behavioral capacity, and the analysis of intelligence is therefore a psychological topic. Until recently most physiological work relevant to intelligence fell within the research area known as physiological psychology. That work in general concentrated on mammals and remained relatively distant from work on the physiological properties of single neurons; little could be said, for example, about specific changes at the neuronal level that might be involved in behavioral plasticity. Recently, however, major advances in basic neurophysiology and in the study of simple or reduced preparations (e.g., the mollusk *Aplysia*—see chapters 2 and 4; the hippocampal slice— see chapter 6) have expanded the range of work that is obviously relevant to psychologists. This welcome change has been clearly reflected in the recent history of one of the leading journals in the field, the *Journal of Comparative and Physiological Psychology.* In 1983 that journal was divided into two new journals, one of which—the *Journal of Comparative Psychology*—now covers comparative work, the other of which concerns physiological work. This latter journal is now known not as the *Journal of Physiological Psychology* but as *Behavioral Neuroscience.* The word "neuroscience" reflects the expansion of interest to include basic neuro- physiological work, while "behavioral" preserves the critical emphasis on the psychological aspects of the research.

The fact that the basic goal is to understand behavior implies that so- phisticated behavioral concepts necessarily inform good work in behav- ioral neuroscience. Plasticity observed at the neuronal level need not play a role in behavioral plasticity; moreover, not all forms of behavioral plas- ticity involve learning, and there are (almost certainly) many different types of learning. The true significance of an observed mechanism of syn- aptic plasticity cannot be assessed until its behavioral role is adequately established; to achieve that, sophisticated behavioral techniques will be required. This is an issue that we shall encounter particularly when con- sidering (in chapters 2 and 4) the potential significance for mammals of observations made on what appear to be relatively simple marine inverte- brates.

What, then, can we hope to achieve with the combination of physiolog- ical and behavioral techniques?

Localization of Function

One major objective is to pinpoint the localization of function within the nervous system. This is in effect a continuation of the search that has persisted for the last two millennia. And although we have discussed that search with reference to mammalian brains, it is clear that localization is equally a goal for workers on smaller nervous systems. It is important to know precisely which cells are involved in plasticity, and then to know which sites within cells (e.g., synapses versus cell bodies) are involved. It should be noted, however, that despite the historical emphasis on localization, localization is not—and this is particularly true for studies that involve large nervous systems—an end in itself. It is of interest to know that a given cognitive activity is carried out by a particular brain region, but that does not of itself help us understand that activity. To know that vision is served by posterior rather than anterior cortical regions does not tell us how visual perception proceeds.

Localization of function is nevertheless clearly an important first step; once a function has been localized, more important questions arise: What are the connections of the area? What are its inputs and outputs? What physical events in the area accompany the cognitive activity concerned, and do properties of these events help explain the psychological phenomena?

Localization has one further and more immediate advantage in human neurology. If we understand the relationship between cognitive activity and various brain areas, then it is possible to determine (from an analysis of the nature of a mental disorder in a patient) which brain area is likely to be responsible; one can then look for localized brain abnormality in that region as a preliminary to attempting remedial treatment. Because this book is principally concerned with nonhumans, little will be said about human symptoms of neurological disorder. It is enough here to note that progress in localization does serve a direct medical purpose.

Identification of Physiological Substrates

A second major objective of behavioral neuroscience, one that may be pursued once some measure of localization is achieved, is that of characterizing precisely the physiological events that accompany cognitive activity. The potential psychological value of this endeavor can be understood when we consider learning and memory.

When an animal learns to associate, for example, a bell and food, physical changes are occurring in its nervous system. If we understood the nature of those changes, we might gain valuable insights into some of the characteristics of learning. We might, for example, begin to understand why repetition of an event strengthens memory for the event; and we might find that one contributing cause to forgetting is a physical process of decay in those changes that constitute memories. There are clear potential medical advantages also. If we knew the physical processes underlying intellectual activities, we would be better placed to develop therapies (possibly involving drugs or transplants, for example) that could correct deficits in those activities in human patients with cognitive disorders.

Definition of Cognitive Functions

The goals discussed so far reduce in essence to seeking to establish "where" physical events associated with cognitive activities occur and "what" these events are. In each case it has been suggested that, for all the considerable intrinsic interest of answers to those questions, their value lies ultimately in their capacity to throw light on psychological problems. The discovery that cognitive activity is carried out in the brain rather than in the heart does not of itself help us understand cognitive activity: nor does the discovery that nerve cells communicate with other nerve cells at synapses. The "where" and the "what" of brain activity may lead to psychological insights, but they are not providers in themselves of insights. A third goal of physiological work is more directly concerned with yielding insights of value to psychologists, and these insights concern the organization of cognitive activity.

Localization of function has been discussed without specifying which functions are to be localized; it has tacitly been implied that they are functions that contribute to intellectual activity. But to know the set of functions that constitutes intellectual activity would in effect be to understand the nature and structure of intelligence. Psychologists do not know how intelligence is constituted—what are its constituent processes—and it is for precisely that reason that for insights psychologists look to behavioral neuroscientists. But if we do not know what functions there are, how can we sensibly attempt to localize them?

One answer to this question is that we do at least have a number of plausible hypotheses concerning specific cognitive processes, and behavioral techniques have been developed that are believed selectively to tap those processes. We shall see in chapter 2, for example, that it is widely believed that habituation and sensitization are different learning processes, and one of the topics of interest in chapters 2 and 3 will be the attempt to localize (and then to analyze further) those processes.

A second answer to the question is that one of the goals of the physiological approach is precisely to contribute to the definition and identification of behavioral functions. In general, this may be achieved when physiological phenomena or effects can be seen to be task-specific: to the extent that a set of behavioral tasks appears, on the basis of physiological work, to "belong together," the implication will be that those tasks are served by a common behavioral mechanism. Behavioral analysis of the tasks concerned should then encourage the development of hypotheses concerning the specific cognitive role of that mechanism.

This third goal of behavioral neuroscience is difficult to grasp in the abstract, but a number of concrete examples will emerge in succeeding chapters. In chapter 4, for example, we shall see evidence for the claim that the cellular mechanisms involved in classical conditioning (in *Aplysia*) have much in common with those of sensitization. These observations lead to the suggestion that classical conditioning may be a special case of sensitization. This proposal is, of course, of considerable interest to behavioral psychologists.

Chapters 7 and 8 will concentrate on attempts to establish task-specificity in more complex behavioral environments. Work of this kind poses important conceptual problems that will be introduced briefly here. For the sake of clarity, the discussion will concentrate initially on interpretation of lesion data, but will go on to point out that the arguments involved apply generally to results obtained by other physiological techniques.

Suppose that we damage a brain area and find that, compared to intact animals, the animals with brain lesions are impaired in the performance of one task (task A) but not of another (task B). The immediate implication of this result is that task A poses different intellectual requirements from task B. Now it might be that task B was simply easier than task A, and that the lesions in question caused a general unspecific deterioration of intellectual activity. Alternatively, it might be that task A was solved in a different way from task B and involved quite different learning mechanisms (and if this latter conclusion could be supported, the way would be clear for generating hypotheses of psychological importance concerning the different processes involved in the two tasks).

Suppose, then, that another brain area is damaged and that it emerges that animals with this second lesion are impaired on task B but not on task A—the opposite pattern to that following the first lesion. In this case, the results overall cannot be explained simply as being the result of a general deterioration caused by brain damage. Some degree of specificity of the lesion effects is implied, and this in turn leads to the conclusion that task A is solved in a different way from task B. And, as has been implied above, analysis of the differing demands found by the two tasks may help to understand in psychological terms how each is performed. The set of results described above, in which two lesions have contrasting effects on two tasks, is known as "double dissociation" and is the single most effective way of demonstrating task-specific lesion effects.

Task-specificity may, of course, be demonstrated by techniques other than the lesion technique: one might, for example, seek to establish task-specificity for a particular type of activity recorded from a brain region or for the effect of administering a particular drug. Two general points are being made here: first, care must be taken to show that a particular effect is task-specific (and we have argued that to show its association with one task rather than another is not in itself sufficient to demonstrate specificity); second, the demonstration of task-specificity is important quite independently of which areas have been damaged, what type of activity is being recorded, or what drug is being used. It is in this way that physiological techniques afford a way of seeing which tasks belong together, and which do not. They allow, in other words, a breakdown of behavior according to differences among mechanisms involved, and the establishment of patterns of breakdown allows the psychologist the opportunity to understand the underlying organization of behavior.

To clarify the potential value of behavioral breakdowns, we shall anticipate here work to be more fully discussed in several later chapters, and introduce a classic example of such a breakdown. A patient known as H.M. underwent surgery that involved temporal lobe damage. As a consequence of his operation, H.M. suffered severe anterograde amnesia, so that he could no longer remember events for more than a few seconds (or for as long as he could rehearse them). Since H.M. could recall events that had occurred preoperatively, many have argued that H.M. still possessed and had access to long-term memory; and since H.M. could recall novel events for a brief period, it has been argued that H.M. also had an intact short-term memory to which novel information could gain access. What H.M. could not do, according to this interpretation, was to transfer information into long-term memory. This interpretation provides support for the (controversial) notion that there exist discrete long- and short-term memory stores, and H.M.'s pattern of breakdown thus has contributed significantly to psychological debates about the nature of memory. We shall see in later chapters that H.M.'s disability was (as might be expected) more complicated than at first appeared. But the point made here will not be altered: analyses of patterns of behavioral breakdown promise to make important contributions to psychological accounts of the structure of intelligence.

Although this third goal of behavioral neuroscience is not so easily characterized as the "where" and "what" goals, it is for psychologists the most important goal: behavioral neuroscience consists in doing psychology with the aid of physiological techniques. The questions it seeks to

answer are psychological questions, and the best promise it shows of an-
swering those questions lies in the capacity to expose the organization of
behavior.

On the Organization of This Book

The rationale advanced here for behavioral neuroscience suggests an answer to the problem of how to organize a survey, a difficult problem given
that several principles of organization are available. One could, for example, devote different chapters to discussion of the functions of different
brain areas, or to the results obtained by using certain techniques. But if
physiological psychology (understood here to embrace all behavioral neuroscience) is psychology first, and physiology second, then it is logical
that a survey should be organized around psychological topics, and that is
the major principle selected here; a secondary principle is to progress from
simple to complex. Thus chapter 2 will consider habituation and sensitization (supposedly simpler types of learning) in simple systems (invertebrates and spinal vertebrates), and chapter 3 will consider the role of brain
structures in those types of learning in vertebrates. Chapter 4 will consider
association formation in simple systems, and chapters 5 and 6 will consider the role of brain structures in association formation in vertebrates
(chapter 5 will discuss the role of the cerebellum, and chapter 6 the role
of the hippocampus, a structure whose function appears to be more complex than that of the cerebellum). Chapters 7 and 8 will examine physiological data relevant to the analysis of high-level cognitive processes involved in, respectively, contextual processing and memory. The chosen
method of organization will mean that the discussion of functions of a
particular brain area—the hippocampus, for example—will be distributed
across more than one chapter. But this disadvantage will, it is hoped, be
outweighed by the emphasis that it will then be possible to lay on the
relevance of the work discussed to major issues in the psychology of learning and memory. A final chapter will introduce suggestions for possible
approaches that may help solve some of the problems encountered in earlier chapters, and will return finally to a discussion of the contemporary
status of Lashley's account of cortical involvement in intelligence.

2. "Simple" Learning in "Simple" Systems

Habituation, Dishabituation, and Sensitization

When a stimulus that on its first presentation elicits a response is presented repeatedly, the probability of the response may change. Typically, the probability of response will decline, and this phenomenon is known as "habituation." Under some circumstances, the probability of response will increase, a phenomenon known as "sensitization." A related phenomenon is that of "dishabituation": when a response to a given stimulus has been habituated, it may rapidly be restored to its original level by the presentation of another intense novel stimulus.

These phenomena have been the subject of intense investigation by physiological psychologists, partly because they are, procedurally at least, simple forms of learning. But the very simplicity of the procedures used may sow doubts as to whether the behavioral changes obtained should properly be regarded as instances of learning. A decline in the probability of elicitation of a response could, after all, have a number of different causes, some of which (sensory adaptation and muscular fatigue, for example) would not involve any learning process. Thompson and Spencer (1966) reviewed the effects of presenting trains of identical stimuli to a variety of (intact) vertebrates, and found a number of qualitative similarities between them. The similarities encouraged them to produce a list of characteristics of habituation, some of which provide convincing evidence that habituation is a genuine form of learning. The characteristics may be summarized as follows:

1. The course of habituation generally follows a negatively accelerated curve to asymptote.
2. Spontaneous recovery of habituated responses occurs.
3. Repeated series of habituation training lead to more rapid habituation.
4. The rate of development of habituation is directly proportional to stimulus frequency.
5. The rate of development of habituation is inversely proportional to stimulus intensity.
6. Once a response has been habituated to asymptotic level, further stimulus presentations will postpone recovery of the response (below-zero habituation).
7. Habituation shows a degree of generalization, so that stimuli similar to an habituated stimulus are less likely to elicit a response than dissimilar stimuli.
8. Dishabituation of an habituated response may occur in response to an intense stimulus.
9. Repeated presentations of an intense stimulus result in progressively less effective dishabituation (dishabituation habituates).

Several of the characteristics listed above argue against any simple peripheralist account of habituation—for example, in terms of fatigue of either sensory input or motor output. Such an account would not expect stronger stimuli to obtain less rapid habituation and cannot readily account for the phenomenon of dishabituation: how could a fatigued nerve be restored by the delivery of an intense stimulus?

Most workers in the field now accept that habituation is a central process—a type of learning—and accept also the set of characteristics drawn up by Thompson and Spencer as a criterion for the demonstration of genuine habituation in a preparation. Any two preparations that show all the characteristics listed may be assumed to be demonstrating closely comparable learning processes, however different the gross neuronal organization of those preparations may be.

As the procedures used do not involve the explicit pairing of stimuli, these types of learning are generally regarded as nonassociative. Despite the apparent simplicity of habituation and sensitization there is controversy among behavioral psychologists over their proper analysis, and at least one theoretical account supposes in fact that habituation is a form of associative learning. Physiological work has made major contributions to theories of habituation and sensitization, and the work on simple systems (invertebrates and spinal vertebrates) that we shall review in this chapter will be discussed within the framework of a behavioral theory (the two-process, or dual-process, theory) to which they are particularly relevant. Chapter 3 will consider vertebrate brain mechanisms of habituation and sensitization, and that work will be considered against a framework of a number of rival theories.

In discussing the relevance of physiological findings to theories of habituation, the reciprocal relationship of behavioral and physiological research should be borne in mind. To the extent that physiological mechanisms are uncovered whose characteristics resemble those anticipated on the basis of a behavioral theory, that theory will be strengthened. When physiological work points to a mechanism with properties that appear to be at variance with those anticipated by a behavioral theory, behavioral findings should be reexamined or extended to see whether the theory has difficulty with behavioral phenomena in a way that might now be anticipated on the basis of the physiological results. But if a behavioral theory does comfortably accommodate all the behavioral data, seemingly discordant physiological data will not overthrow that theory since it is the explanation of behavior that is the paramount goal. In practice, of course, any clash between a successful behavioral theory and physiological data would stimulate research into the source of the disparity. That research would presumably throw up new behavioral data against which the theory would be further tested, and new physiological data that might in themselves resolve the conflict. Physiological data must ultimately be interpreted within a framework of behavioral theory; but physiological research must also be expected to impinge on behavioral theory, to throw up new ideas, and to contribute to the plausibility of one theory as against another. We shall in this chapter see a number of examples of the interplay of physiology and behavioral theory and, in particular, instances of behavioral experiments carried out in the light of unexpected physiological results.

Dual-Process Theory

The final two characteristics in the list produced by Thompson and Spencer (1966) refer to dishabituation. Thompson and Spencer went on to suggest that dishabituation reflected not the disruption of habituation but the superimposition of an independent facilitatory process of sensitization. This notion was further developed by Groves and Thompson (1970), who proposed that any stimulus activates two independent processes, one decremental (habituation) and one incremental (sensitization) and that the behavioral response elicited is a consequence of the summated activity of the two processes.

A brief introduction to some of the behavioral support for the dual-process view may be given here by describing two phenomena that give good support to the theory. Figure 2.1 shows the course of habituation of the acoustic startle response to a tone stimulus in the intact rat and the effect on the habituated response of the delivery of a novel flashing light stimulus (a fuller account of the acoustic startle response may be found in chapter 3). The figure shows an initial "hump" in the curve, with the second and third stimuli being more effective in obtaining a response than the initial stimulus. Such humps are commonly obtained in a variety of preparations (Groves and Thompson 1970) and are readily accounted for by dual-process theory. The explanation according to that theory is that the stimulus concerned is sufficiently intense to cause sensitization. Sensitization is a short-lived effect, and the ability of a stimulus to obtain sensitization habituates (one of the nine characteristics of Thompson and Spencer, 1966). Thus the initial one or two stimulus presentations sensitize the organism, and the (waning) effect of the first presentation summates with that of the second to obtain a larger response to the second presentation; as the sensitizing effect of the stimulus habituates, the decremental (habituating) effect of the stimulus presentations comes to predominate.

It is evident from figure 2.1 that the flashing light dishabituated the response. The figure also shows that the effect of the novel stimulus waned rapidly, so that the response to the next test stimulus was again at the habituated level. This in turn argues that the response was in effect not truly dishabituated, but rather, that an additional excitatory process had been superimposed. The result provides good evidence for the proposition that habituation and sensitization are independent processes, and that dishabituation is a special case of the latter.

The dual-process theory of Groves and Thompson supposes that the systems concerned have distinct anatomical substrates. Habituation is supposed to occur in the stimulus-response (S-R) pathway, defined as "the most direct route through the central nervous system from stimulus to response" (Groves and Thompson 1970:421), whereas sensitization is taken to reflect an increase in activation of state—state being defined as "the collection of pathways, systems and regions that determines the general level of responsiveness of the organism" (ibid.). Thus habituation can be obtained only by presentations of the to-be-habituated stimulus,

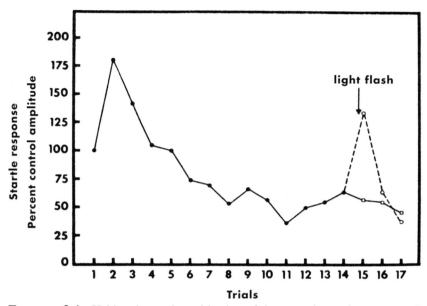

FIGURE 2.1. Habituation and sensitization of the acoustic startle response. A 2-sec tone stimulus was presented at 1-min intervals to intact rats. Following habituation one group (broken line) received a novel flashing light stimulus prior to trial 15, the other group (solid line) did not. Note that although the experimental group showed dishabituation to the tone stimulus on trial 15, response amplitude had decayed to approximately the level of the controls within one minute. (*From* Groves and Thompson 1970)

whereas sensitization (including dishabituation) may be obtained by presentations of any suitably intense stimulus. Direct physiological support for these propositions from studies on vertebrate spinal preparations will be discussed in a later part of this chapter. First, however, we shall see how appropriate the dual-process model is to the analysis of habituation and related phenomena in an invertebrate.

Analysis of "Simple" Systems

The vertebrate nervous system is, and this hardly need be said, one of redoubtable complexity. The human central nervous system, for example, contains some 10^{12} neurons, and a single neuron may have several thousand synaptic contacts (Nauta and Feirtag 1986). Psychologists have therefore explored the possibility that there might be nervous systems of greatly reduced complexity which nevertheless display learning phenomena, in the expectation that principles relating nervous activity to learning will generalize from the simpler system to the more complex.

Two principal methods of obtaining simpler nervous systems have been used. The first is to use a "reduced" version of a vertebrate nervous system by investigating learning in spinal animals, animals in which the great mass of the central nervous system has been segregated by a cut from the spinal systems that control limb movements. Despite the removal of the brain, the spinal animal remains a distinctly complicated system, containing many millions of cells, many of them extremely small and so not readily amenable to physiological analysis. We shall nevertheless consider them here as "simple" systems and discuss them after considering what may be more genuinely simple preparations.

A second method for obtaining simple systems is to use an invertebrate animal having a nervous system that contains far fewer neurons than any vertebrate. Work is currently in progress on the physiological and behavioral analysis of learning in a number of invertebrate species, and the most detailed information we now possess concerns a few of the 35,000 extant gastropod mollusks (snails and their relatives). In this chapter and in chapter 4 we shall concentrate on one of those preparations, the sea slug *Aplysia californica;* this is partly to avoid repetition and partly because of the somewhat arbitrary impression that work on this preparation has progressed further than work on the others toward the eventual goal of providing a comprehensive physiological account of the changes that occur during learning in *any* animal.

Advantages of *Aplysia*

There are some thirty-five species of the large marine snail genus *Aplysia,* sometimes known as the "seahare" on account of the earlike appearance of the posterior tentacles, the rhinophores (see figure 2.2). All of these animals live on seaweed and occupy shore regions. Some may grow extremely large: *Aplysia californica,* for example, which is the animal most frequently used in work of interest here, may grow up to 1 m in length and weigh up to 7 kg (Kandel 1979).

The nervous system of *Aplysia* possesses many features that facilitate neurobiological investigation when compared to vertebrate nervous systems. There are about 20,000 nerve cells in its central nervous system, and these are arranged in nine ganglia. The ganglia are relatively well spaced, so it is not difficult to cut the nerve bundles that connect one ganglion to another. The cell bodies of the neurons in ganglia are arranged around the outside of the ganglia, and the central core of ganglia consists of neuropil—a dense network of nerve filaments—in which synaptic contacts are made (as is generally the case with invertebrate nerve cells, there are very few synaptic contacts on the cell bodies themselves). Nevertheless, because the regions of synaptic contact are close to the cell bodies, it is possible to record from electrodes located in the cell bodies potentials generated in axons and dendrites and derived from activity at synapses.

Eight of the nine ganglia in the *Aplysia* central nervous system are arranged in four symmetrical pairs. The ninth (abdominal) ganglion is asymmetrical and in fact represents the fusion of a number of discrete ganglionic masses. The abdominal ganglion is of particular interest here since much of the work on habituation and sensitization has been concentrated upon it. The nerve cells in the abdominal ganglion are extremely large—up to 1 mm in diameter—and, in striking contrast to nerve cells in vertebrate nervous systems, some fifty of the cells are readily recognizable in all individuals on the basis of position, size, and color. As a consequence, many individual cells have been given "names" such as L10 and R14. Moreover, it has been established that specific cells also make the same connections with other specific cells in all individuals, and that the functional type of those connections (e.g., excitatory, inhibitory) is also invariant. Besides individually recognizable cells, there are also iden-

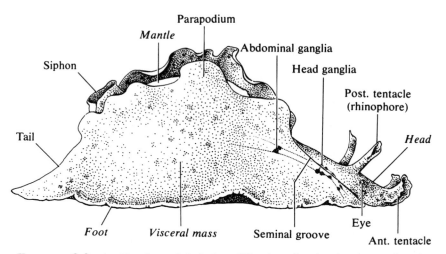

FIGURE 2.2. A side view of *Aplysia californica*, showing head, mantle, visceral mass, and foot. The major ganglia of the nervous system are superimposed in the relative position they occupy inside the animal. (*From* Kandel 1976)

tifiable cell clusters, the cells of which belong to the same functional system (e.g., heart excitation; siphon motor neurons). Some 50 per cent of the cells in the abdominal ganglion belong to identifiable clusters (see figure 2.3).

Habituation in *Aplysia*

There are not only anatomical and physiological advantages for neuroscientists in using *Aplysia; Aplysia* has also proved to be an efficient performer in nonassociative (and, as we shall see, in associative) tasks. This work has concentrated on the gill and siphon-withdrawal reflex.

Aplysia use movements of the parapodia and the gill to create a current of water between them. The current leaves the mantle cavity through the siphon, a structure formed from the posterior edges of the mantle. Tactile stimulation of the gill or the siphon causes defensive withdrawal contractions of both structures (see figure 2.4). The siphon withdraws between the parapodia, and the gill withdraws under the mantle shelf.

When tactile stimulation of the siphon (e.g., by a jet from a Water Pik) is repeated at relatively short interstimulus intervals (from 30 sec to 3 min), the withdrawal response shows a marked decline (habituates). The effect is short-lived, and the response shows spontaneous recovery within an hour or two. When habituation training sessions are repeated on a number of different days, long-term habituation that persists for at least 21 days may be seen. This long-term effect is due to the spacing out of sessions and not to an increase in the total number of trials: Carew, Pinsker, and Kandel (1972) found retention of habituation over a 21-day interval following four daily sessions of ten trials each; but forty trials given on one day provided no evidence of retention of habituation over intervals of either one or 21 days. Figure 2.5 summarizes the results of their experiment and illustrates both short- and long-term habituation, and spontaneous recovery.

All of the nine characteristics of habituation drawn up by Thompson and Spencer (1966) have been demonstrated in *Aplysia* (Kandel 1976; Goldberg and Lukowiak 1984). Let us therefore assume here that habituation in *Aplysia* is a process that corresponds behaviorally to habituation in vertebrate preparations, and assume also that the invertebrate work is relevant to dual-process theory, a theory that was developed largely on the basis of vertebrate data. The general question of the relevance of invertebrate work to vertebrates will be taken up in more detail in chapter 4, in which we shall find reason to question whether all (or any) of the phenom-

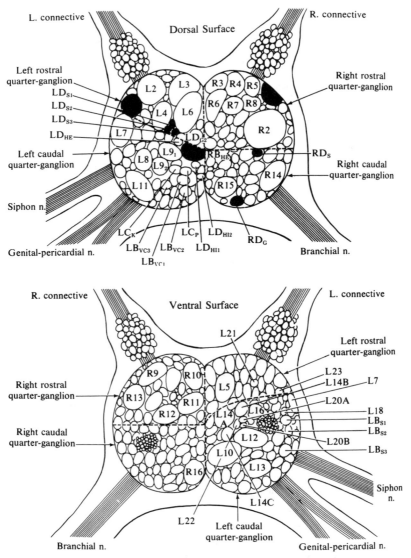

FIGURE 2.3. Map of identified cells in the abdominal ganglion of *Aplysia* indicating positions of these cells, which are labeled L or R (left or right hemiganglion) and assigned a number. Cells that are members of clusters are identified by the cluster name and a subscript identifying the behavioral function of the cell (e.g., LD_{HI1} and LD_{HI2}, two heart inhibitors belonging to the same cluster). (*From* Kandel 1976; *adapted from* Frazier et al. 1967)

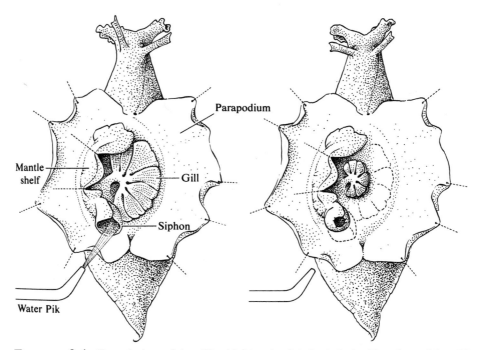

FIGURE 2.4. Dorsal view of the gill-withdrawal reflex in *Aplysia*. The view of the gill is normally obscured by the parapodia and mantle shelf, which have been retracted to allow direct observation. The left half of the figure shows the relaxed position. The withdrawal reflex to a weak tactile stimulus to the siphon (a jet of seawater delivering an effective pressure of 250 g/cm^2) is shown in the right half of the figure, in which the relaxed position of the gill is indicated by dotted lines. (*From* Kandel 1976)

ena described as instances of conditioning in invertebrates should in fact be assumed to reflect the operation of processes comparable to those involved in vertebrate conditioning.

The physiological analysis of these effects has involved the use of a variety of preparations. In most of these, gill responses rather than siphon responses are measured. The basic neuronal circuits that are concerned in the gill- and siphon-withdrawal reflex are reasonably well established (and this is particularly true for the gill component, which is most widely mentioned in the physiological work). When working with free-moving intact animals, only the siphon component is readily seen, so that it is most commonly the target response when unrestricted *Aplysia* are used; it appears, however, that both components invariably co-occur so that results obtained with either component may be generalized to the whole withdrawal system.

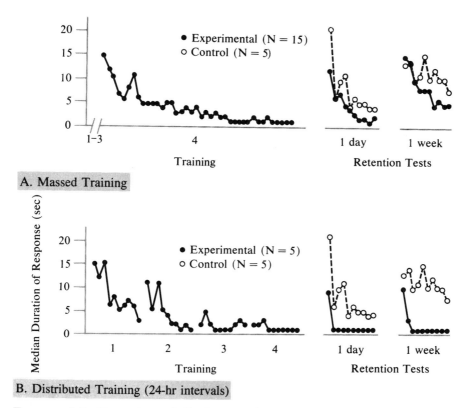

FIGURE 2.5. Comparison of effectiveness of massed versus distributed training on retention of habituation of the siphon-withdrawal reflex in *Aplysia*. Fig. 2.5A shows the effect of massed training. Experimental animals received no stimulation for the first three days, followed by forty stimuli (jets of seawater administered at 30-sec intervals) on Day 4. Control animals received no training. Retention was tested one day and one week after training, and there were no significant differences between control and experimental animals on either retention test. Fig. 2.5B shows the effect of distributed training with a 24-hour interval between training sessions, in each of which ten stimuli were delivered (with a 30-sec intertrial interval). The experimental animals in this condition showed significantly shorter siphon-withdrawal responses than controls in the retention tests conducted at both the one-day and the one-week retention intervals. (*From* Kandel 1976; *adapted from* Carew, Pinsker, and Kandel 1972)

The skin of the siphon is served by some 24 sensory neurons, and movements of the gill are controlled by 6 motor neurons. The cell bodies of both the sensory and the motor neurons lie in the abdominal ganglion. The siphon sensory neurons make direct synaptic contact with the gill motoneurons; they also make contact with interneurons which in turn connect with the gill motoneurons. Kupfermann et al. (1970) have shown that habituation of the gill withdrawal response proceeds normally in animals in which the connections between the abdominal ganglion and other ganglia have been severed: the search for the physiological basis of habituation may therefore be restricted to the abdominal ganglion and its sensory inputs and motor outputs.

We have seen that both short-term and long-term habituation may be demonstrated in *Aplysia*. There is physiological evidence that somewhat different mechanisms are engaged in these two processes, so these will be considered in separate sections. Throughout this discussion the major issue of theoretical interest will be whether, as anticipated by dual-process theory, habituation involves a conduction decrement that is restricted to the S-R pathway. I shall then go on to discuss sensitization with a view to seeing whether, as dual-process theory would expect, the physiological analysis points to a general facilitation by intense stimuli of transmission in multiple S-R pathways.

Short-Term Habituation

Mediation by Homosynaptic Depression

A first step in the physiological analysis of a response decrement is to ask whether the phenomenon might be of peripheral origin, the result of either sensory adaptation or neuromuscular fatigue. There are, in the case of the gill-withdrawal reflex, good reasons for rejecting both possibilities. When recordings are taken from sensory neurons innervating the siphon skin, it is found that their response to stimulation does not change over the course of short-term habituation; moreover, when the sensory nerve is electrically stimulated to bypass peripheral adaptation, habituation to repeated stimulation occurs just as to external tactile stimuli (Kupfermann et al. 1970). Neuromuscular fatigue can be ruled out also since repeated direct stimulation of gill motor neurons (at rates comparable to those used to obtain habituation) produces a withdrawal response of constant magnitude. Further, once habituation has occurred, "spontaneous" gill contractions (part of centrally controlled pumping movements) continue to occur (Pinsker et al. 1970). These spontaneous contractions are controlled by the same motor neurons that are involved in the withdrawal reflex.

It appears, then, that the excitability of neither the sensory cell nor the motor unit changes during habituation; the capacity of the sensory cell to activate the motor cell must therefore decline. Direct evidence for this conclusion was provided by Kupfermann et al. (1970), who recorded from one of the gill motoneurons (labeled L7) of a restrained *Aplysia* during the course of habituation, and established that the excitatory postsynaptic potentials (EPSPs) obtained by stimulation of the siphon reduced in magnitude as habituation proceeded. The reduction in EPSP could have been due either to an increase in inhibitory input to L7 or to a change in the efficiency of the synapse mediating the siphon sensory input to L7.

The EPSP recorded in L7 following sensory stimulation of the siphon is complex in the sense that it represents the net effect of a number of EPSPs elicited by the various fibers within the siphon nerve. The complex EPSP could also reflect the influence of inhibitory postsynaptic potentials (IPSPs) lost in the overall excitatory result. Could habituation be caused by an increase in the magnitude of IPSPs? Castellucci et al. (1970) explored this possibility in an experiment that employed the isolated abdominal ganglion preparation (see figure 2.6). Castellucci et al. hyperpolarized the motor neuron L7 to a level well below the reversal potential of IPSPs: in such a preparation, any increase in release of the inhibitory transmitter would contribute to the net depolarization of the cell. But when the siphon nerve was stimulated repeatedly, the complex EPSP showed a decline, indicative of habituation. It appears, then, that habituation is not due to an increase in IPSPs.

An alternative possibility is that presynaptic inhibition might be involved. Siphon nerve stimulation might recruit interneurons that make contact with the terminals of the siphon nerve (at synapses with the motor neurons), and obtain presynaptic inhibition. Castellucci and Kandel (1974) have ruled out this possibility. An isolated abdominal ganglion was bathed in a solution containing a high concentration of divalent cations (Mg^{2+} and Ca^{2+}), a solution that would markedly elevate the firing threshold of neurons and would therefore minimize the likelihood of the effective recruitment of interneurons. Castellucci and Kandel identified sensory neurons that were monosynaptically connected with the motoneuron L7 and measured the (unitary) EPSP obtained in L7 when a single spike was elicited by direct electrical stimulation of a sensory neuron. Figure 2.7 summarizes their experiment and shows that EPSPs declined when a train of spikes was elicited. A cellular analogue of habituation was, then, obtained in a preparation in which the activity of interneurons had been suppressed.

If an increase in inhibition is ruled out, the implication is that the decline in synaptic efficiency is in some way intrinsic to the synapse itself. A decrease in magnitude of EPSPs could be the result of a change in the input resistance of the postsynaptic membrane. Castellucci et al. (1970)

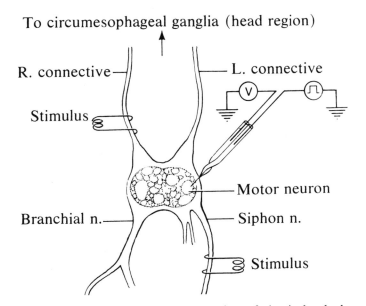

FIGURE 2.6. Schematic representation of the isolated abdominal ganglion test system. The ganglion, along with its major associated nerves, is dissected out and maintained in a chamber perfused with seawater. The figure shows an arrangement that would allow direct stimulation of either the siphon nerve or the right connective, and intracellular recording from motoneuron L7. Stimulation of the siphon nerve, which contains axons of primary sensory neurons serving siphon skin, elicits monosynaptic EPSPs in L7. Stimulation of the right connective, which carries nerves from the head region, may be used to obtain facilitation of synaptic transmission between the siphon nerve and L7. (*From* Kandel 1976)

reported that repetitive stimulation of the siphon nerve obtained a depression of the complex EPSP elicited in L7 but had no effect on the electrotonic potential produced by a brief constant-current hyperpolarizing pulse to the L7 soma. This indicates that synaptic depression is not associated with a change in input resistance at the soma and so is not due to a gross change in L7's resistance. Direct measurement of input resistance in the synaptic region of the cell is not yet possible, but there is indirect evidence for absence of change in input resistance in the synaptic region: Carew, Castellucci, and Kandel (1971), for example, have shown that depression of the complex EPSP obtained by repetitive siphon nerve stimulation has

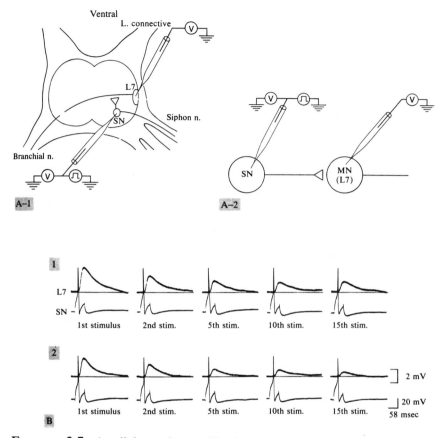

FIGURE 2.7. A cellular analogue of habituation. Fig. 2.7A–1 shows the general position of the stimulating and recording electrodes. Fig. 2.7A–2 shows schematically the monosynaptic connection between the sensory neuron and the L7 motoneuron. Fig. 2.7B–1 shows the progressive decline in the EPSP evoked in L7 as a result of a series of stimulations using an interstimulus interval of 10 sec. Fig. 2.7B–2 shows that a second series of stimulations delivered after a 15-min interval obtains a more profound depression. (*From* Kandel 1976; *adapted from* Castellucci and Kandel 1974)

no effect on the magnitude of the EPSP obtained by branchial nerve stimulation.

The work discussed thus far indicates that as habituation proceeds, an action potential in the sensory nerve becomes less effective in obtaining an action potential in the motor nerve, and that this is due to a reduction in size of the EPSP evoked by sensory nerve activity. The reduction is not due to a change in the membrane properties of the motor nerve, nor to an increase in inhibition, either pre- or postsynaptic. Other nerves (interneurons) are not necessary for the effect, and it is therefore known as "homosynaptic depression." Repeated direct stimulation of the motor nerve does not cause any reduction in the effectiveness of sensory input to the nerve, and synaptic depression is obtained when the motor nerve is hyperpolarized to prevent spike activity. The conclusion appears to be that repeated activation of the sensory nerve reduces the capacity of presynaptic action potentials to obtain EPSPs.

Mechanisms of Homosynaptic Depression

Reduction of an Inward Calcium Current. Direct light was thrown on the mechanism responsible for the reduction in EPSPs by Castellucci and Kandel (1974). Transmission between siphon sensory nerves and gill motor nerves is mediated by a chemical neurotransmitter (the identity of which is currently unknown). Castellucci and Kandel analyzed the frequency distribution of amplitudes of EPSPs evoked in L7 by a single action potential in a sensory neuron. The analysis supported the notion that the EPSPs were generated by the quantal release of transmitter, since the distribution was not continuous but organized into relatively discrete peaks. Quantal release is mediated by the all-or-none release of the contents of presynaptic vesicles. The peaks in the distribution of the EPSP amplitudes would, then, reflect the release of the contents of one, two, or more vesicles. Analysis of EPSPs generated during the course of repeated stimulation of the sensory nerve indicated that quantal size remained constant, but that the number of quanta released declined. This argues that the sensitivity of the postsynaptic membrane to the neurotransmitter had not altered, further confirming the conclusion that the site of habituation is to be found in the presynaptic membrane.

What causes the depression in transmitter release when a sensory cell is stimulated repeatedly? The full details are not yet known, but the effect appears to be due to a reduction in the calcium current obtained by action potentials. There is an inflow of calcium ions during an action potential, and these ions are critical for the release of packets of transmitter; they play a role in the binding of vesicles to the presynaptic membrane, a precursor to the release of transmitter across the synapse. Klein, Shapiro, and Kandel (1980) showed that the calcium current (measured at the cell body, not in the terminals themselves) declined as the effectiveness of synaptic transmission declined in response to repeated stimulation. The parallel between their time courses (shown in figure 2.8) encouraged the view that short-term habituation of the withdrawal reflex was due to a decline in calcium current caused by repeated stimulation of sensory neurons.

Reduction of Readily Releasable Transmitter. There is evidence for another change, besides the decline in calcium current, that is associated with short-term habituation in *Aplysia*. Bailey and Chen (1988a) microscopically examined individual varicosities (presynaptic terminals) of neurons taken from animals that had previously been subjected to homosynaptic depression. The varicosities were of individual mechanoreceptor sensory neurons, and depression was induced (in an isolated abdominal ganglion preparation) by evoking in the cells a series of spikes (35 or 250) using a brief (30s or 10s) interstimulus interval. The course of depression was monitored by measuring the EPSPs in motoneurons with which the cells made synaptic contact. Chemical activity in the ganglion was halted by perfusion with a fixative solution immediately following the final stimulus of the depression series.

High resolution microscopy allowed the visualization within the varicosities of "active zones," modified regions of the presynaptic membrane at which neurotransmitter is released. Bailey and Chen compared the active zones of cells that had been subjected to the depression treatment with those of control cells that had experienced no treatment. They found no differences between depressed and control cells in the number or size of active zones, nor in the total number of synaptic vesicles observed in the vicinity of active zones (vesicles observed within a vertical distance of 240 nm above the active zone, a distance that corresponds to approximately three vesicles stacked one on top of another). There was, however, an interesting shift in the distribution of vesicles. Vesicles observed within 30 nm of the presynaptic active zone membrane were classified as being members of "readily releasable" pools; vesicles observed between 30 and 240 nm above the membrane were classified as belonging to storage pools. There were significantly more vesicles in readily releasable pools in the cells that had not undergone synaptic depression: whereas some 28 percent of active zone vesicles of nondepressed cells were readily releasable, only 11 percent of those of depressed cells were similarly classified. Short-term habituation leads, then, to a decline in readily releasable transmitter at the presynaptic membrane.

Summary

Homosynaptic depression constitutes the physiological basis for short-term habituation in *Aplysia*. The mechanisms responsible for this depression are, first, a decline in calcium current, and second, a decline in the

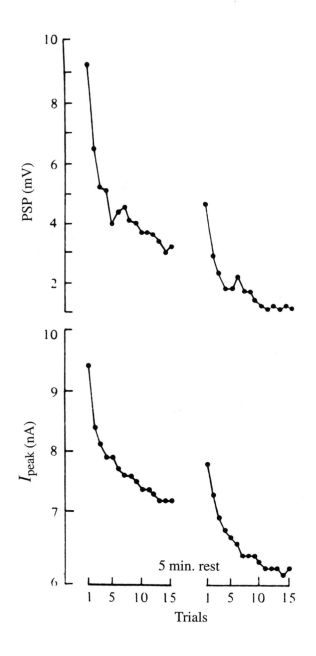

amount of readily releasable transmitter at presynaptic active zones. Each of these (presynaptic) mechanisms may be presumed to contribute to a decline in the number of quanta released in response to a spike in a pre-synaptic cell. This account of habituation gives good support to the dual-process model since it supposes that habituation is indeed specific to the S-R pathway activated by a to-be-habituated stimulus.

Long-Term Habituation

Mediation by Homosynaptic Depression

As in short-term habituation, homosynaptic depression also mediates long-term habituation. It will be recalled that where a number of sessions of habituation training are administered on successive days, habituation persists for three weeks and more. Castellucci, Carew, and Kandel (1978) explored the cellular basis of long-term habituation by examining the efficiency of sensorimotor synapses following habituation training. *Aplysia* were first given long-term habituation training in which the siphon skin was stimulated ten times each day for a minimum of five days. After either one day, one week (eight to ten days), or three weeks (24 to 32 days), sensorimotor connections in the isolated abdominal ganglion were monitored by recording EPSPs from the gill motor neuron L7 while eliciting a single action potential in a sensory neuron serving the siphon skin. In control animals, a single sensory neuron spike elicited a detectable EPSP in L7 on 89 percent of occasions. Habituated animals showed a significantly reduced probability of obtaining detectable EPSPs: one day and one week following training, sensory neuron spikes obtained EPSPs on 30 and 28 percent of occasions only, and three weeks following training, the success rate was still only 58 percent. In other words, long-term habituation (like short-term habituation) training reduces the efficacy of the monosynaptic connection between sensory and motor neurons.

FIGURE 2.8. Correlation of the magnitude of the monosynaptic EPSPs produced in a follower cell by repeated depolarizations of a sensory neuron and magnitude of presynaptic inward (Ca^{2+}) currents in the neuron. The top part of the figure shows the magnitude of the EPSP elicited in an L7 cell by 50 msec depolarizing pulses delivered every 10 sec to the sensory neuron. Two consecutive habituation training sessions were separated by a 5-min rest period. The sensory neurons were voltage clamped in artificial seawater containing Na^+ and K^+ current blockers. The lower part of the figure shows the peak presynaptic inward current evoked by the depolarizing pulses; with Na^+ current blocked, inward current is due to Ca^{2+}. (*From* Klein, Shapiro, and Kandel 1980)

Mechanisms of Long-Term Homosynaptic Depression

Morphological Changes. Less is known of the detailed physiological mechanisms involved in long-term (as compared to short-term) habituation. There is, however, evidence that, as in the short-term phenomenon, the locus of the effect is presynaptic. Bailey and Chen (1983, 1988b) examined varicosities in *Aplysia* that had previously been subjected to long-term habituation training (ten habituation sessions per day for ten days). The varicosities were of identified mechanoreceptor sensory neurons serving siphon skin. Bailey and Chen (1983) found, first, that the probability of there being an active zone found in a varicosity was lower in animals subjected to long-term habituation than in control animals having received no training: whereas 41 percent of varicosities of control cells had an active zone, only 12 percent of varicosities of cells from trained animals possessed one; second, that the mean area of active zones was smaller in habituated animals; third, that the number of readily releasable vesicles associated with active zones was smaller in habituated animals (no count of vesicles in storage pools was made in this 1983 study). Finally, Bailey and Chen (1988b) found that the total number of varicosities per neuron was lower in habituated than in control *Aplysia*. These findings indicate that extensive morphological changes occur as a consequence of long-term habituation training, changes that result in a decline in the efficiency of synaptic transmission by the neuron.

In the light of the morphological changes observed (changes that presumably require some time to reverse), it is important to note that both the behavioral and the physiological consequences of long-term habituation may rapidly be counteracted by a dishabituating stimulus. Carew, Castellucci, and Kandel (1979) found that a single powerful shock to the neck region delivered two hours after a fifth daily session of habituation training resulted in the abolition of the effect of habituation training when the withdrawal reflex was tested two hours later: the dishabituated animals showed significantly higher levels of response when compared to habituated animals that had not received shock, and the dishabituated animals showed the same level of response when tested following the shock as they had shown on original exposure to the test stimulus (a water jet on the siphon skin).

Carew, Castellucci, and Kandel (1979) went on to measure the capacity of action potentials in siphon sensory nerves to obtain EPSPs in L7 in habituated animals, and in dishabituated animals that had received habituation training and the strong shock: detectable EPSPs were found in 9 percent of tests on habituated animals but in 68 percent of tests on dishabituated animals. Given the evidence discussed above on the morphological changes accompanying long-term habituation, the effectiveness of a dishabituating shock clearly raises questions concerning the mechanisms of dishabituation, and it is to that issue that we shall turn after the following section.

Summary

Long-term habituation, like short-term habituation, is mediated by homosynaptic depression and so is compatible with the dual-process theory of habituation and sensitization. The mechanisms of long-term depression, however, differ. Whereas short-term habituation involves decreases in calcium current, long-term habituation involves major morphological changes: decreases in the number of presynaptic terminals, and in the number and size of active zones within terminals. But long-term habituation, like short-term habituation, does involve decrements in the availability of readily releasable transmitter.

Sensitization in *Aplysia*

The discussion of nonassociative learning in *Aplysia* will now consider the phenomena of sensitization and dishabituation. Dual-process theory supposes that dishabituation is a special case of sensitization, and that proposition will therefore form one focus of the survey. A second issue will be whether the mechanisms uncovered in *Aplysia* are consonant with the view that sensitizing stimuli activate a general, statelike system that modulates the performance of all S-R pathways.

Before discussing the physiological data, we shall introduce some behavioral data that show, first, that sensitization and dishabituation are, at the least, closely related phenomena in *Aplysia,* and second, that both short-term and long-term sensitization may be obtained.

Pinsker et al. (1970) reported that a strong tactile stimulus to the neck dishabituated the withdrawal reflex to stimulation of the mantle shelf. They also noted that occasionally the dishabituated response was larger than the response obtained at the outset of habituation training—indicating that the dishabituating stimulus had done more than simply to remove the effects of habituation.

Further pertinent evidence was provided by Carew, Castellucci, and Kandel (1971). The gill withdrawal reflex may be obtained by stimulating a number of skin regions. Habituation to stimulation of one region does not generalize to relatively distant skin regions, which remain effective elicitors of the reflex. Carew and his associates habituated the reflex to stimulation of either (in some animals) the siphon or (in others) the purple gland, and then delivered a sensitizing stimulus (a strong neck stimulus). The sensitizing stimulus not only dishabituated the previously habituated (siphon or purple gland) stimulus: it also facilitated response to stimulation of the nonhabituated stimulus. There is, then, behavioral support for the notion that dishabituation in *Aplysia* may be a special case of sensitization, a process that facilitates responding irrespective of the state of habituation.

Pinsker et al. (1970) reported that the dishabituating effect of a single strong stimulus dissipated rapidly, over the course of a few minutes. They also reported that the dishabituating effect of a stimulus declined with repeated presentations. Both these phenomena have been seen in mammalian preparations (Thompson and Spencer 1966). But long-term sensitization to repeated stimuli has also been reported. Pinsker et al. (1973) delivered four strong shocks to the neck four times per day on four consecutive days; when the withdrawal reflex to tactile stimulation of the siphon was tested—one day, one week, and three weeks later—sensitization of the response was observed, the degree of sensitization growing smaller as the interval increased. This finding parallels the phenomenon of long-term habituation: long-term retention is seen when training sessions are spaced over a number of days. Since there is evidence (as there was for habituation) that the mechanisms for short-term and long-term effects differ, we shall consider them in separate sections.

Short-Term Sensitization

Mediation by Heterosynaptic Facilitation

By using procedures similar to those used in the investigation of habituation, it has been shown that sensitizing stimuli produce effects that go in the opposite direction to the effects of habituation. Sensitizing stimulation increases the magnitude of the complex EPSP in gill motor neuron L7 elicited by stimulation of the siphon skin; it also increases the magnitude of the unitary EPSP elicited by intracellular stimulation of a single mechanoreceptor neuron (Castellucci et al. 1970). Both of these effects occur without there being any alteration of the resistance of the motoneuron (Carew, Castellucci, and Kandel 1971).

Repetitive firing of the L7 motoneuron does not result in facilitation of the EPSP elicited by sensory stimulation (Castellucci et al. 1970); therefore, although sensitizing stimuli themselves activate the motoneurons involved in the withdrawal reflex, motoneuron activity cannot be the cause of the facilitation. The implication is that the sensitizing stimulus directly affects the synaptic effectiveness of activity in sensory neurons. Dishabituation may be obtained by stimuli that do not elicit action potentials in the sensory neuron whose synaptic efficiency is facilitated: the mechanism of facilitation is, therefore, not posttetanic potentiation (a facilitation of synapses obtained in a variety of preparations following a train of action potentials in the presynaptic neuron).

Castellucci and Kandel (1976) showed that a sensitizing stimulus (electrical stimulation of the connective between the head and the abdominal ganglion) obtained an increase in the number of quanta released by an individual mechanoreceptor cell serving the siphon skin in response to an action potential elicited in that cell. The mechanism of sensitization appears, then, to be the precise reverse to that of habituation. Facilitation is, however, obtained as a consequence of activity at a synapse or synapses other than that which is being facilitated, and is therefore known as "heterosynaptic facilitation." Castellucci and Kandel (1976) proposed that the effect is mediated by synapses of facilitatory interneurons upon the terminals of the sensory cells: activity at these synapses facilitates transmitter release, and the effect is known as "presynaptic facilitation." A schematic model of that proposal is shown in figure 2.9.

Mechanisms of Heterosynaptic Facilitation

The sensitizing effect of intense stimuli is mediated by interneurons, some of which have been identified. A group of abdominal ganglion neurons labeled L29 show direct anatomical contacts with mechanoreceptor neurons and are activated by cutaneous stimuli that obtain sensitization in intact *Aplysia* (Hawkins and Schacher 1989). Stimulation of an L29 neuron produces facilitation of the unitary EPSP in the L7 gill motor neuron obtained by a spike in a siphon sensory neuron (Hawkins, Castellucci, and Kandel 1981). Two further facilitator interneurons have been identified in the B cluster of the left and right cerebral ganglia (the LCB1 and RCB1 cells). These cells also project to the abdominal ganglion, and their activation obtains facilitation of siphon sensory neurons (Mackey, Kandel, and Hawkins 1989)

The LCB1 and RCB1 cells are known to be serotonergic (Hawkins 1989); the transmitter used by the L29 neurons is unknown, although it may be closely related to serotonin. Other, as yet unidentified, facilitatory neurons use two related peptides—SCP[A] and SCP[B] (small cardioactive peptides, one eleven, the other nine amino acids in length, each derived

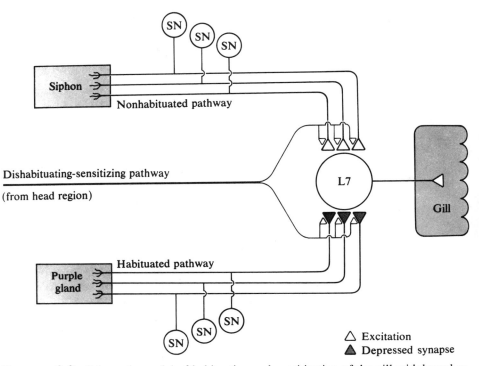

FIGURE 2.9. Schematic model of habituation and sensitization of the gill-withdrawal reflex. Following stimulation of either the purple gland or the siphon, only the stimulated pathway is habituated: the figure shows that after stimulation of the purple gland, there is homosynaptic depression of the synapses between the purple gland sensory neurons (SN) and the motoneuron L7. By contrast, a strong stimulus from the head sensitizes both habituated and nonhabituated pathways due to presynaptic facilitation of all the synapses made by primary sensory neurons on L7. (*From* Kandel 1976; *adapted from* Carew, Castellucci, and Kandel 1971)

from the same precursor). The role of serotonin as a facilitatory transmitter is currently best documented, and some of the supporting evidence is summarized below. (Excellent reviews of work on biochemical correlates of facilitation are available, and for further details, along with extensive references to primary sources, see Carew 1984 and Castellucci et al. 1986.)

The abdominal ganglion is rich in serotonin, and, as we have seen, serotonergic processes that make contact with sensory cells have been identified anatomically. Bathing the abdominal ganglion in a solution rich in serotonin facilitates sensorimotor synapses; solutions rich in other amine transmitters do not obtain facilitation. The serotonin receptor antagonist cinanserin has the opposite effect, blocking the normal facilitatory effect of stimulation of connections (Brunelli, Castellucci, and Kandel 1976). And when serotonin is depleted by administration of a serotonergic neurotoxin, both behavioral sensitization and heterosynaptic facilitation are reduced (Glanzman et al. 1989).

The delivery of serotonin onto presynaptic terminals appears to facilitate the release of transmitter from those terminals by two routes, each of which will now be considered.

Reduction of an Outward Potassium Current. Klein and Kandel (1980) showed that the inward Ca^{2+} current during an action potential is increased in sensory neurons by stimuli that sensitize those neurons. This modulation of the calcium current would lead to an increase in transmitter release and so contribute to presynaptic facilitation. But Klein and Kandel also showed that at least part of the modulation is indirect: facilitatory stimulation prolongs the duration of an action potential by reducing the delayed outward K^+ current, which forms a part of the normal process of repolarization. It is the broadening of the action potential that results in the prolonged Ca^{2+} current.

There has been much progress in the biochemical analysis of the events that mediate the reduction in the K^+ outward current obtained by the release of serotonin from facilitatory interneurons. Since, as we shall see in chapter 4, Kandel and his colleagues believe that the process of sensitization is critically involved in associative learning in *Aplysia,* an understanding of the biochemistry of sensitization is of general significance to our understanding of learning in *Aplysia.* It is also one of the most detailed biochemical analyses of learning available in *any* species, so that is worth going into in some detail.

During the repolarization of a neuron following an action potential, potassium ions flow out of the neuron through a number of separate channels. Klein, Camardo, and Kandel (1982) showed that the channel that is sensitive to serotonin release is different from any of the previously identified channels (four in all); and Siegelbaum, Camardo, and Kandel (1982) showed that the effect of serotonin is to close individual potassium channels (or gates). Serotonin therefore reduces the total number of open potassium gates by closing a subset of them, so that the outward current flow of potassium is retarded.

The effect of serotonin on potassium channels is mediated by an increase in cyclic adenosine monophosphate (cAMP), which acts as a "second messenger" (as it does in a number of nonneural cells). The increase in cAMP in turn activates an enzyme, a protein kinase, which consists of two regulatory subunits and two catalytic subunits. The protein kinase is activated by the binding of cAMP to the regulatory subunits, which dissociates them from the catalytic subunits. The catalytic subunits phosphorylate (add phosphates to) a membrane protein, which either is or is associated with the potassium channel, and phosphorylation of the protein constitutes a closing of the gate.

Direct support for the "cascade" of events outlined above is provided the following observations: first, both bathing of the abdominal ganglion in serotonin and stimulation of the connections to the ganglion increase cAMP in the ganglion; second, intracellular injections of either cAMP or the catalytic subunits of cAMP-dependent protein kinase obtain both decreases in potassium current and increases in transmitter release in sensory cells. Finally, intracellular injection of a molecule that inhibits protein kinase activity both prevents and (when injected subsequently) disrupts the facilitation obtained by serotonin. The fact that facilitation may be disrupted supports the notion that the short-term, temporary, effect of a sensitizing stimulus is mediated by the temporary increase in cAMP (which persists and decays with a time course that parallels that of facilitation).

Mobilization of Vesicles. A series of experiments reported by Hochner et al. (1986) has shown that serotonin engages a second facilitatory process, independent of spike-broadening. There is reason to suppose that this process involves mobilization of vesicles held in storage pools. Both these points may be given empirical support by considering one experiment in the Hochner et al. series, an experiment that concerned a preparation even more reduced than the isolated ganglion. Hochner et al. dissected out one or two sensory cells from the LE cluster of the abdominal ganglion, along with the gill motoneuron L7. These cells were then maintained for several days in culture medium, where they spontaneously developed synaptic sensorimotor connections, so that when a sensory and a motor cell were impaled by electrodes, an action potential in the sensory cell (elicited by a depolarizing pulse) obtained an EPSP in the motor cell (hyperpolarized to prevent the generation of action potentials that would obscure the EPSP).

Hochner et al. voltage-clamped the sensory cell and delivered depolarizing pulses of varying durations. They first confirmed that longer pulses (analogues of broadened spikes) obtained larger EPSPs from the motor cell. They then subjected the sensory cell to repeated activation so that the synapse was depressed, and now found that lengthening the duration of depolarizing pulses had virtually no effect on the EPSPs elicited. However, when serotonin was applied to the depressed synapse, a large facilitation of EPSPs was observed.

The implication of this work is that the facilitatory effect of serotonin at depressed synapses is not due to spike-broadening. Given the fact that synaptic depression involves loss of readily releasable transmitter, a reasonable possibility is that serotonin somehow mobilizes transmitter from storage pools to active zones.

This second facilitatory process, like spike-broadening, appears to be mediated, at least in part, by a rise in intracellular cAMP. Hochner et al. confirmed that the rise in cAMP obtained by serotonin is, as would be expected, independent of spike-broadening, and Braha et al. (1990) have shown that cAMP, like serotonin, obtains enhanced transmitter release from depressed synapses. There is, however, evidence of a contribution to this second process that is engaged by serotonin but is independent of cAMP. Sacktor and Schwartz (1990) have reported that both behavioral sensitization and the administration of serotonin to isolated ganglia result in the mobilization from the cytoplasm to the membrane of a protein kinase (PKC) whose activity is independent of cAMP. A similar effect was obtained when phorbol esters (activators of PKC) were applied to the ganglia. These findings imply that mobilization of PKC may play a role in the second process of sensitization.

Braha et al. (1990) provided concrete support for this possibility by showing that administration of phorbol esters enhanced transmitter release at depressed synapses of cultured neuron pairs; the enhancement of transmitter release was obtained with no accompanying change in potassium currents. Figure 2.10 summarizes current views on the pathways activated by facilitatory neurotransmitters.

The notion that facilitation in *Aplysia* involves two processes suggests that there is a distinction in *Aplysia* between sensitization and dishabituation. For although spike-broadening has little effect on depressed synapses (in which readily releasable transmitter is reduced), it does have a marked effect on nondepressed synapses (synapses that have not been subjected to repeated activations). Thus Hochner et al. (1986) suggest that sensitization is largely attributable to the spike-broadening effect of serotonin whereas dishabituation is largely attributable to its transmitter mobilization effect. These physiological findings have prompted renewed interest in the relationship between dishabituation and sensitization in intact *Aply-*

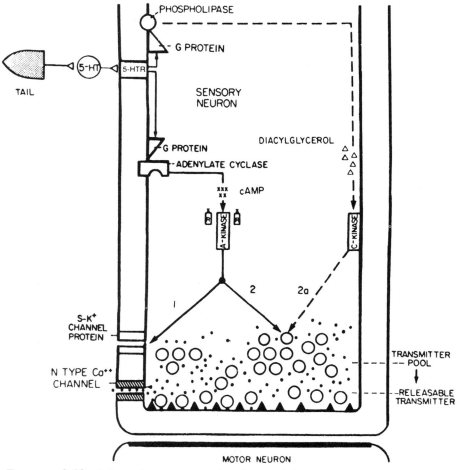

FIGURE 2.10. Schematic summary of pathways believed to be involved in pre-synaptic facilitation. Sensitizing stimulation of the tail (upper left) causes release of a facilitatory neurotransmitter; the transmitter shown here is serotonin (5-hydroxytryptamine, commonly abbreviated to 5-HT). Serotonin activates membrane serotonin receptors (5-HTR) that lead (through a process mediated by coupling G-proteins) to activation of adenylate cyclases that in turn obtain synthesis of cAMP and dissociation of regulatory (R) from catalytic subunits of the cAMP-dependent protein kinase (A-kinase). The cAMP pathway leads to two detectable effects (arrows 1 and 2) that contribute to an increase in transmitter release: (1) an effect on the serotonin-sensitive K^+ (S-K^+) channel, leading to its closure; (2) an effect of transmitter mobilization. In addition, activation of serotonin receptors may lead to a sequence of events (broken lines) that obtain the activation of PKC, which may influence mobilization of transmitter but does not affect the S-K^+ channel. (*From* Braha et al. 1990)

sia, and we shall consider recent behavioral data that support a distinction between these processes in a subsequent section, following our discussion of long-term sensitization.

Does Heterosynaptic Facilitation Modulate All S-R Pathways?

Dual-process theory supposes that sensitization involves the activation of a general "state" system so that all responses are facilitated by a sensitizing stimulus. That theory would therefore predict that sensitizing stimuli would obtain presynaptic facilitation at all sensorimotor synapses. There is, however, physiological evidence that this is not the case, that facilitation may be "branch-specific" within a neuron.

Clark and Kandel (1984) used a preparation consisting of an isolated abdominal ganglion having an intact connection via the siphon nerve with a piece of siphon skin. Individual siphon sensory neurons were sought in the abdominal ganglion that showed (by electrophysiological criteria) monosynaptic connections with both a central neuron (a motoneuron or an interneuron in the abdominal ganglion) and a peripheral motoneuron (in the siphon skin). They then delivered strong shocks to the (severed) pleurobranchial connective. These shocks are known to drive L29 cells (facilitator interneurons), and the effect of the shock was, as anticipated, to obtain enhanced transmission at the synapse between the sensory neuron and the central neuron. However, that same stimulation did not facilitate transmission at the peripheral sensorimotor synapse, indicating that there is at least some specificity in presynaptic facilitation. This finding (like the dissociation seen between the physiological mechanisms for sensitization and dishabituation) raises the question whether there is behavioral evidence for response specificity in the effects of sensitizing stimuli in *Aplysia,* and that too is an issue that will be considered in a later section.

Summary

Short-term sensitization is mediated by presynaptic facilitation, a phenomenon that reflects the cooperation of two processes. The first process involves spike-broadening and is particularly important in sensitization. The second process may involve mobilization of transmitter and is particularly important in dishabituation. The distinction implied between the processes of dishabituation and of sensitization poses problems for dual-process theory. That theory finds difficulty also with the fact that presynaptic facilitation can show response specificity, a finding that suggests that sensitizing stimuli may not affect globally the reactive state of the animal.

Long-Term Sensitization

Mediation by Heterosynaptic Facilitation

Long-term sensitization is also mediated by heterosynaptic facilitation. We have seen that distributed training sessions may obtain sensitization that persists for three weeks and more. There is evidence that the locus of this sensitization is the same as that for short-term sensitization, since the strength of synaptic connections is increased (Frost et al. 1985). Further indications of parallels between short-term and long-term facilitation are provided by studies using cultured neuron pairs. Montarolo et al. (1986) showed that bathing the cell culture in serotonin for five minutes produced an immediate strengthening of the synaptic contact between two cultured cells (EPSP amplitudes were increased), and that this facilitation lasted for some five minutes following the washing out of the serotonin. However, if serotonin was applied five times (with a 15-min interval between applications), a long-term facilitatory effect was obtained: when the synaptic strength was assessed 24 hours later, the mean evoked EPSP amplitude was increased by more than 70 percent. Dale, Schacher, and Kandel (1988) found that multiple applications of serotonin resulted in increases in the number of quanta released by sensory cells in response to depolarizing pulses; increases were seen both immediately after the serotonin applications and 24 hours later. Quantal size (of both spontaneous miniature EPSPs and evoked EPSPs) did not change following the sensitization treatment.

Mechanisms of Long-Term Facilitation

Reduction of an Outward Potassium Current. There is evidence (e.g., Scholz and Byrne 1987) that long-term sensitization training leads to a reduction in the serotonin-sensitive outward potassium current (the S-current), and evidence also that both serotonin and its associated second messenger, cAMP, are involved in triggering the processes that obtain the long-term changes. Dale, Kandel, and Schacher (1987), for example, found that four applications of serotonin to cultured single presynaptic sensory neurons obtained, 24 hours later, increases in the excitability of the cells; these increases are presumed to reflect reductions in the S-current. Dale and colleagues' 1987 report is of particular interest since it implies that at least one of the processes involved in long-term facilitation may be engaged in the absence of the motoneurons that normally form the postsynaptic target cells for sensory neuronal activity. And Scholz and Byrne (1988) showed that intracellular injections of cAMP obtained reductions in the S-current measured 24 hours after injection. It will be recalled that sensitizing stimuli also activate PKC: however, Schacher, Castellucci, and Kandel (1988) found that (unlike cAMP) phorbol esters, which activate PKC and obtain short-term facilitation, did not obtain long-term facilitation in cultured neuron pairs.

The elevation of cAMP elicited by serotonin is short-lived: how could a temporary elevation of cAMP bring about long-term changes? One possibility (Kandel and Schwartz 1982) is that the long-term effects involve the formation of new proteins, as a consequence of novel gene expression. We shall consider that suggestion after introducing evidence of morphological changes accompanying long-term facilitation, changes that also imply the formation of new proteins.

Morphological Changes. Morphological changes accompany the induction of long-term sensitization. Bailey and Chen (1983) reported that long-term sensitization training (either two shocks to the neck region per day for ten days or four stronger shocks per day for four days) resulted in increases (in mechanoreceptor sensory cells) in the probability of there being an active zone associated with a varicosity, in the area of synaptic active zones, and in the number of readily releasable vesicles associated with each zone. In a subsequent report, Bailey and Chen (1988b) found that long-term sensitization training also led to increases in the total number of varicosities per cell and in the arborization of the terminals of those varicosities. Such findings imply that sensitized neurons increase the total number of synapses made by them onto associated motoneurons, and Bailey and Chen (1988c) have confirmed that long-term sensitization does indeed increase the number of presynaptic contacts observed on the motoneuron L7. Figure 2.11 summarizes the morphological changes that are believed to accompany long-term habituation and long-term sensitization.

Morphological changes may also be obtained in response to both serotonin and cAMP. Glanzman, Kandel, and Schacher (1990) have reported that repeated application of serotonin to cultured pairs of sensory and motor neurons obtains increases in the number of varicosities per cell. Interestingly, these changes could not (in contrast to the changes in excitability described in the preceding section) be obtained in sensory neurons that were cultured in the absence of motor neurons. Similarly, an increase in varicosity number has been reported by Nazif, Byrne, and Cleary (1991) 24 hours after a 15-min iontophoretic injection of cAMP into *Aplysia* tail sensory neurons (whose cell bodies are located in the pleural ganglion).

The series of findings reported by Bailey and Chen referred to measurements taken on *Aplysia* that were killed within 48 hours of the end of

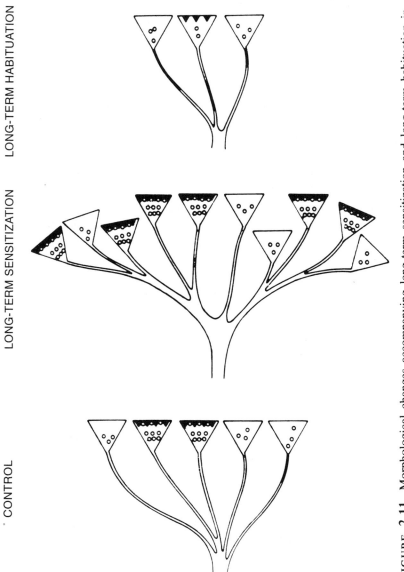

CONTROL   LONG-TERM SENSITIZATION   LONG-TERM HABITUATION

FIGURE 2.11. Morphological changes accompanying long-term sensitization and long-term habituation in *Aplysia*. Long-term sensitization (center) is accompanied by increases in the number of sensory neuron varicosities, in the number of active zones (solid triangles) per varicosity, and in the amount of readily releasable transmitter (synaptic vesicles are shown as open circles). Long-term habituation (right) is accompanied by decreases in those same three morphological features. (*From* Bailey and Chen 1988b)

sensitization training. Since long-term sensitization may persist for three weeks, it is of interest to know whether all those changes persist over periods longer than 48 hours. This question was explored by Bailey and Chen (1989), who found only two morphological changes that persisted as long as one week. There were no significant differences between sensory cells from control and sensitized *Aplysia* in either active zone area or in readily releasable vesicle numbers one week after training; sensitized *Aplysia* did, however, show (relative to controls) more varicosities per cell, and more active zones per varicosity when measured one week after training.

Protein Synthesis Is Necessary for Long-Term Sensitization

Support for the general proposition that synthesis of new proteins is involved in long-term (but not short-term) sensitization is provided by Montarolo et al. (1986). Their study explored the effects of protein synthesis–inhibiting drugs on the short-term and long-term facilitation obtained by either single or multiple applications of serotonin to cultured neuron pairs. The drugs had no effect on short-term facilitation (and no effect, either, on short-term habituation); but protein-synthesis inhibition blocked long-term facilitation. By varying the times at which protein synthesis was inhibited, Montarolo et al. showed that there was a relatively brief time window for its effectiveness: protein-synthesis inhibition for the period during and immediately after the facilitation treatment blocked long-term facilitation; inhibition of synthesis prior or subsequent to the serotonin application was without effect. A subsequent report (Schacher, Castellucci, and Kandel 1988) found that the long-term (but not the short-term) facilitatory effect of intracellular cAMP release was, similarly, blocked by protein-synthesis inhibitors. The implication of these reports is, then, that some short-term process initiated by serotonin and mediated by cAMP activates a gene so as to produce a protein that is essential for long-term sensitization.

Both short-term and long-term sensitization involve a reduction in the S-current, a reduction that is believed to be mediated by the phosphorylation of a membrane protein. Direct evidence that the same membrane protein may be involved in each case has been provided by Sweatt and Kandel (1989), who assessed protein phosphorylation following administration of serotonin to clusters of sensory neurons in the pleural ganglia. A single pulse (2 min) of serotonin obtained phosphorylation of (at least) seventeen proteins; this phosphorylation was not affected by protein-synthesis inhibitors. Five pulses of serotonin (sufficient to obtain long-term facilitation) obtained phosphorylation of the same seventeen proteins when assessed 24 hours later; this phosphorylation was disrupted by protein-synthesis inhibitors. Precisely similar results were obtained from brief or prolonged application of cAMP. These findings suggest, then, that both short-term and long-term sensitization are mediated by phosphorylation of the same protein or proteins that are in turn concerned in the closure of the serotonin-sensitive potassium gate. The fact that the long-term effect was disrupted by protein-synthesis inhibition suggests that long-term phosphorylation is mediated by proteins that are newly formed as a consequence of training.

Much current research is focused on the nature of the proteins responsible for long-term phosphorylation of the membrane proteins. Barzilai et al. (1989) explored protein synthesis in sensory neurons at various times after applications of serotonin sufficient to obtain long-term facilitation. They found two surges of protein synthesis, one at one hour and a second at three hours after serotonin application. This work supports the possibility that there may be an intermediate process that mediates retention over a period between the decay of the short-term process and the full expression of the long-term process; such a possibility is also suggested by the differences seen among the time courses of the morphological changes associated with long-term sensitization (Bailey and Chen 1989).

Barzilai et al. (1989) suggested that the early proteins induced by serotonin might contain a transient protease that degraded the regulatory units of the cAMP-dependent protein kinase. Selective degradation of the regulatory units would lead to an increase in phosphorylation in response to relatively low levels of cAMP (such as might be obtained by weak stimuli). This proposal receives support from the finding (Greenberg et al. 1987) that long-term sensitization training did indeed lead to a reduction in the ratio of regulatory to catalytic subunits of cAMP-dependent protein kinase, measured 24 hours later; short-term sensitization training did not affect that ratio. However, Greenberg et al. also reported that the change in ratio was not dependent on protein synthesis, so that although the early proteins identified by Barzilai et al. may contribute to the change in ratio, they are not wholly responsible for it.

Little can yet be said of the nature of the later proteins identified by Barzilai et al. Some of these proteins might be regulators that would operate on genes responsible for the longer-term changes. These changes would, presumably, involve morphological changes and the formation of proteins that might serve to enhance permanently the ability of relatively low levels of cAMP to stimulate phosphorylation. Kandel and Schwartz

(1982) suggested that such proteins might be either proteases that could permanently alter the ratio of regulatory to catalytic subunits of the cAMP-dependent protein kinase, or novel regulatory subunits of the kinase that were particularly sensitive to cAMP. Recent work tends to support the former proposal. Bergold et al. (1990), for example, have reported that 24 hours after a two-hour exposure to serotonin, *Aplysia* sensory neurons (from the pleural ganglion) showed a reduced ratio of regulatory to catalytic subunits, and that that reduction was blocked by application of a protein-synthesis inhibitor during (but not after) application of serotonin.

Summary

Long-term sensitization, like short-term sensitization, is mediated by heterosynaptic facilitation. That facilitation is mediated partly by a reduction in the S-current and partly by morphological changes that include long-term increases in numbers both of presynaptic terminals and of active zones in those terminals. Unlike short-term sensitization, long-term sensitization is dependent upon protein synthesis and may involve the formation of novel proteins, some of which presumably contribute to the long-term phosphorylation of membrane proteins that form the serotonin-sensitive potassium gates.

From Physiology to Behavior

This review of the physiological bases of nonassociative learning in *Aplysia* has thrown up three findings that were not predicted by dual-process theory. The first is that there are major differences between the short- and the long-term processes responsible for habituation and sensitization. Although not predicted by dual-process theory, this is not a finding that seems to pose problems for that theory. Both short- and long-term habituation involve homosynaptic depression, and both short- and long-term sensitization involve heterosynaptic facilitation. We have seen no reason why there should not be behaviorally a seamless transition from one (short-term) set of mechanisms to the other (long-term) set, and no reason why these distinctions should concern the major tenets of dual-process theory—namely, that habituation involves the S-R pathway, and that sensitization/dishabituation involves a state system. These tenets are, however, challenged by the other two unpredicted findings, first, that dishabituation and sensitization are mediated by distinguishable mechanisms and, second, that heterosynaptic facilitation—the mechanism of sensitization—does not invariably modulate all S-R pathways. These findings suggest that closer examination of *Aplysia* behavior might reveal corresponding behavioral difficulties for dual-process theory.

Behavioral Distinctions Between Sensitization and Dishabituation

Turning first to the distinction noted physiologically between dishabituation and sensitization, we find that there are indeed now demonstrations of behavioral distinctions also. The first comes from a series of studies of the ontogeny of nonassociative learning in juvenile *Aplysia*. The development of *Aplysia* is conventionally taken to pass through thirteen stages, Stage 13 being the adult *Aplysia*. Carew and his colleagues have studied siphon withdrawal in juvenile *Aplysia*. They found that habituation was first observed in Stage 9 *Aplysia*, a stage at which neither dishabituation nor sensitization was observed. This is a result that poses no difficulty for dual-process theory, since that theory supposes precisely that the anatomical substrate for habituation differs from that for dishabituation/sensitization. But Rankin and Carew (1988) found that whereas dishabituation could be demonstrated in Stage 11 *Aplysia* (at which stage, the animals would be some 1.5 to 3 mm in length), sensitization could not be obtained until late in Stage 12 (animals of 5 to 8 mm in length).

Marcus et al. (1988) have confirmed that a distinction between dishabituation and sensitization can be demonstrated in adult *Aplysia* also. Their report found that the dishabituating effect of a (single) tail stimulus (on an habituated siphon withdrawal response) could be observed 90 sec after its delivery, but that this dishabituating effect dissipated rapidly, and was not detectable either 10 or 20 min after a tail stimulus. A range of tail-stimulus intensities was used and only the three weakest (of five) stimuli were successful in obtaining dishabituation. However, the sensitizing effects of the same tail stimuli showed quite a different pattern: the stronger stimuli were more effective in obtaining sensitization (of a non-habituated siphon-withdrawal response), and the sensitizing effects were most marked after long post-stimulus intervals: no sensitization was observed in tests carried out 90 sec or 10 min after the tail stimulus, but sensitization could be seen in 20- and 30-minute tests.

There is, then, evidence from the behavior of intact *Aplysia* that dishabituation and sensitization are not the same process, and this is a conclusion that is clearly at variance with dual-process theory.

Sensitization Training May Obtain Pseudoconditioning

The third unexpected physiological finding was that branch-specific heterosynaptic facilitation may be obtained. This prompted the question whether, as dual-process theory would expect, sensitizing stimuli modulate equally all S-R pathways: there is now behavioral evidence that they do not.

The (unconditioned) responses made by *Aplysia* to different types of noxious stimulation show qualitative variations according to the locus at which the stimulation is delivered (Walters and Erickson 1986). Confining our attention here to siphon responses, three different types of response may be seen to head, tail, or midbody stimulation: head stimuli cause constriction and forward rotation of the siphon; tail stimuli cause flaring and backward rotation; midbody stimuli cause partial constriction, and longitudinal contraction. Erickson and Walters (1988) explored the effects of noxious stimuli (trains of strong electric shocks) delivered to either the head or the tail on responses to midbody test stimuli (a mild tactile stim-

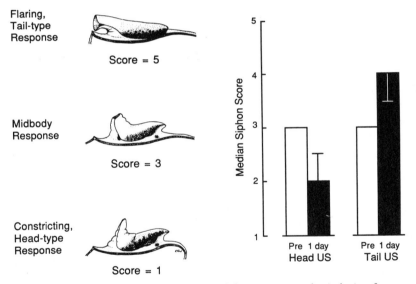

FIGURE 2.12. Contrasting effects on siphon responses in *Aplysia* of a sensitization training procedure using a strong shock to the head and a procedure using a strong shock to the tail. On the left of the figure are shown responses that correspond to the extremes and to the midpoint of the siphon-scoring scale used; scores of 4 and 2 were given to responses that were, respectively, clearly taillike or headlike but were not as pronounced as those shown for scores of 5 or 1. On the right of the figure are shown median siphon scores (with interquartile ranges indicated) to midbody test stimulation before and 24 hours after training with either a head or a tail stimulus. (*From* Erickson and Walters 1988)

ulus or a weak electric shock) delivered 24 hours after the noxious stimulation. They used, in other words, a standard long-term sensitization training procedure. Their results (see figure 2.12) were clear-cut: *Aplysia* that
had received head shocks now tended to show head-type (rather than
midbody-type) responses to the midbody test stimulus, and animals that
had received tail shocks showed tail-type responses.

Although Erickson and Walters used procedures appropriate to sensitization training, the phenomena obtained are properly regarded as instances of pseudoconditioning rather than sensitization. Pseudoconditioning refers by definition to the elicitation by a test stimulus of a response
that resembles the unconditioned response (UCR) to an unconditioned
stimulus (UCS) that has been previously presented but has not been paired
with the test stimulus. Sensitization strictly refers only to the enhancement
by a UCS of a response initially elicited by a test stimulus, when the
enhanced response differs in intensity only and not in quality from that
originally elicited.

It is clear, then, that sensitizing stimuli do not enhance equally all S-R
pathways, and this is a result that might have been expected, given the
Clark and Kandel (1984) demonstration of branch-specific heterosynaptic
facilitation. It is, however, not yet clear that the mechanism of pseudoconditioning should be assumed to be branch-specific facilitation: Erickson
and Walters (1988) note a number of alternative possibilities (such as, for
example, an enhanced excitability of the motoneurons involved in the response to the noxious stimulation), and further work on the physiology of
pseudoconditioning will be required before its mechanism can safely be
determined.

Aplysia: Not Such a Simple System

Work on nonassociative learning in *Aplysia* exemplifies well the technical
capacity of contemporary neuroscience to delve deep into the physiology
and biochemistry of behavior. It has also provided excellent examples of
the reciprocal relationship between physiological and psychological work,
principally by pointing to discrepancies between the physiological data
and dual-process theory, discrepancies that are now backed by behavioral
data that confirm that dual-process theory cannot account adequately for
nonassociative learning in *Aplysia*.

Despite the progress that has been made, much remains to be uncovered before anything approaching a full account of the physiological bases
of nonassociative learning in *Aplysia* will be possible. We have looked in

some detail at the mechanisms involved, but there have even so been simplifications and omissions in this account. It may be salutary before moving on to consider the complexities of studying vertebrates (even spinal vertebrates), to note at least some of the complicating issues that have been avoided.

First, although the gill and siphon do typically withdraw simultaneously, this is far from universally the case, and both the gill and the siphon response may be subdivided into further discrete responses under relatively independent neural control (Leonard, Edstrom, and Lukowiak 1989). Second, both habituation and sensitization of the siphon-withdrawal response can take place in the absence of the abdominal ganglion (or any other part of the central nervous system; Lukowiak and Jacklet 1972): these processes can be mediated by the peripheral nervous system, and a full account of nonassociative learning will have to take into account the contribution of the peripheral system. Finally, there is now good evidence that a process of inhibition (which may be mediated by heterosynaptic inhibition) is engaged alongside the processes of habituation, dishabituation, and sensitization (Mackey et al. 1987; Marcus et al. 1988); and in fact Frost, Clark, and Kandel (1988) were able to cite three further processes that may contribute to the output seen in response to stimuli presented in nonassociative paradigms.

It may well be that it will turn out to be simpler to provide a full account of learning for *Aplysia* than for any vertebrate. But that does not mean that it will be simple to understand *Aplysia: Aplysia* may be simpler than a vertebrate, but simple it is not.

Analyses of Spinal Vertebrate Preparations

We move now from the fine-grained analysis of habituation and sensitization in *Aplysia* to a consideration of those phenomena in a quite different "simple" system, the spinal vertebrate. The discussion will continue to be cast within the framework of dual-process theory, with a view to seeing to what extent the physiological data are congruent with that theory. But we shall, of course, also be interested in somewhat more specific questions that derive from the *Aplysia* survey, questions such as the following: Are habituation and sensitization caused by alterations in the efficacy of specific synapses rather than by a decline in excitability of whole cells? Is any alteration in synaptic efficacy caused by changes in the presynaptic rather than in the postsynaptic cell? Is habituation a homosynaptic, and sensitization a heterosynaptic, process? Do both habituation and sensitization reflect alterations in the quantity of transmitter released?

Frog Spinal Cord

Habituation

The simplest vertebrate preparation studied to date has concerned the habituation of a monosynaptic response in the isolated spinal cord of the bullfrog, *Rana catesbeiana*. A large part of the spinal cord (sections 3 to 11) is removed from a frog and maintained in a functional condition in an oxygenated solution. Direct stimulation of axons in the lateral column (LC) elicits monosynaptic activation of motoneurons, whose activity can be monitored by recording the ventral root response (VRR). When LC stimulation runs at a slow rate (for example, one stimulus per second or less), the VRR declines steadily, showing eight of the nine characteristics of habituation listed by Thompson and Spencer (1966; Farel, Glanzman, and Thompson 1973). The solitary exception is that generalization of habituation has not yet been demonstrated, and this is probably because there has been a substantial difference between the type of stimulus used to obtain habituation (LC stimulation) and that used to test for generalization (stimulation of dorsal root fibers, which also obtains, via a polysynaptic pathway, a VRR). Recovery from habituation, which is retarded after longer trains of habituating stimuli, takes approximately 14 min following a train of stimuli at a rate of one stimulus per second. We are, then, considering an example of short-term habituation.

Habituation Is Mediated by Homosynaptic Depression. Evidence has accumulated to support the view that the habituation observed in this preparation is caused by homosynaptic depression; this evidence basically takes the form of ruling out alternative accounts. There is no evidence, for example, of a decline in excitability of LC cells as training proceeds: the LC response to antidromic stimulation does not alter (Farel, Glanzman, and Thompson 1973), and the (presynaptic) effect of LC stimulation, recorded in the motoneuron pool where the LC axon terminals make their synapses, does not decline with repeated stimulation (Glanzman and Thompson 1979). LC stimulation might become less effective because of inhibition mediated by interneurons, either presynaptically (onto LC terminals) or postsynaptically. A role for presynaptic inhibition is unlikely since presynaptic inhibition in the spinal cord involves a depolarization of terminals, which not only reduces transmitter release in response to invasion by a spike but also increases terminal excitability: if terminal excitability was increased, one would expect an increased response to antidromic stimulation after habituation training, but no change is observed. Moreover, treatment with pentobarbital, which should reduce recruitment of interneurons, does not affect the rate of habituation (Farel, Glanzman, and Thompson 1973), a finding that argues against the involvement of interneurons, and so, against a role for either pre- or postsynaptic inhibition.

Habituation does not result if the motoneurons are stimulated antidromically via the ventral root, and, as has already been noted, the VRR to dorsal root stimulation is not affected by habituation treatment via LC fibers. These observations indicate that habituation is not a consequence of fatigue or reduced excitability of motoneurons. More direct evidence on motoneuron excitability is provided by Glanzman and Thompson (1980), who placed intracellular electrodes in individual motoneurons in the cord of both bullfrogs and leopard frogs (*Rana pipiens*). They recorded "spontaneous" minipotentials (minis) both before and after a series of habituating stimuli to LC fibers. They found that although the habituating train obtained an overall increase in minis, there was no change in the amplitude of "singlet" minis—minis that appeared to be due to the release of single packets or quanta of transmitter from the presynaptic fibers (many of which were taken to be LC fibers). This finding argues against the possibility of a decline in sensitivity of the postsynaptic receptor sites on the motoneurons as habituation proceeds. The increase in minis also suggests that any decrease in synaptic efficiency is unlikely to be due to a depletion of neurotransmitter in the presynaptic terminals, a conclusion reinforced by Rogers and Levy (1978), who varied the concentration of divalent ions in which the cord was bathed. The addition of Mg^{2+}, which reduces calcium inflow, reduced the overall level of response of the LC-VRR preparation, but did not affect the (relative) rate of habituation; addition of Ca^{2+} increased the response level, but again, did not affect rate of habituation. In other words, manipulation of the amount of transmitter released on each trial had no effect on rate of habituation, a finding that appears to rule out transmitter depletion as the mechanism of habituation.

All the evidence cited above points to the conclusion that the locus of habituation in the LC-VRR preparation is to be found at the synapse between the LC fibers and the motoneurons, and probably (given the evidence for unchanged postsynaptic receptor sensitivity) in the presynaptic terminals. Thompson and Glanzman (1976) cite unpublished work that has found that the number (but not the size) of quanta released in response to stimulation of an LC fiber decreases with habituation training. This finding points to a parallel with the mechanisms of short-term habituation in *Aplysia*. There is, however, no direct evidence from the frog preparation for a decline in calcium inflow in response to spikes in LC axons, and no evidence of a loss of readily releasable vesicles (indeed the fact that minipotentials increase following habituation training points to quite the opposite conclusion). Thus, although habituation in this preparation does appear to involve homosynaptic depression, it is not yet known whether the mechanisms of that depression are comparable in *Aplysia* and in this spinal frog preparation.

Sensitization

Farel (1974a) has reported that potentiation of VRR may be obtained by a brief (500 msec) train of high frequency LC stimulation (500 per sec); the effect is relatively long-lasting and may persist for two hours or more. Farel (1974b) reported an ingenious experiment designed to test whether sensitization and habituation are independent processes in this preparation. Different groups of frogs were given an habituating train of either high- or low-intensity stimuli; the low-intensity train was presented either alone or eight minutes after tetanic stimulation. Frogs given the habituation train alone showed, as would be expected, more rapid habituation to the low- than to the high-intensity stimuli. Following sensitization treatment, the animals given low-intensity stimuli showed initial response levels of comparable amplitude to those shown by animals given high-intensity stimuli without preceding sensitization. But despite starting at the same response levels, the groups showed very different rates of habituation: the frogs given low-intensity stimuli following tetanus showed more rapid habituation than those given high-intensity stimuli alone. The rate at which habituation proceeded was, then, independent of the manipulation of overall response level brought about by sensitization. This result supports the view that sensitization affects the intensity of responding but does not influence the process of habituation.

Farel's report (1974a) showed that sensitization was not accompanied by changes in excitability of either LC fibers or motoneurons, and that the process of sensitization was not mediated by the recruitment of more neurons. These findings encouraged Farel to argue that the same synapses that mediate habituation also mediate facilitation. The relevance of this conclusion to the position adopted by Groves and Thompson (1970) will become clear in the subsequent discussion of "plastic" interneurons in cat spinal cord. At present it will be sufficient to note that Farel's conclusion could imply that the mechanisms of both habituation and sensitization coexist in the same neurons (so that both the depression and the facilitation effect should be regarded as homosynaptic); but the data currently available on facilitation in this preparation are equally amenable to interpretation in terms of presynaptic facilitation by interneurons of LC terminals. The fact that we cannot decide between these two significantly different alternatives serves to bring home clearly the fact that work on this, the simplest vertebrate preparation, has not achieved the detailed analysis attained in *Aplysia*.

It may be appropriate to inject a note of caution concerning the LC-VRR preparation: despite the impressive correspondence between the characteristics of habituation in this preparation and those listed by Thompson and Spencer, the fact remains that there is currently no evidence that the LC-motoneuron synapses are involved in habituation (or sensitization) in the intact animal, and no way of knowing which (if any) specific reflexes in intact frogs show a plasticity that reflects the plasticity seen at the LC-VR synapses. These problems reflect the difficulties inevitable in working with vertebrates. Other well-explored vertebrate preparations have involved polysynaptic pathways mediating specific reflexes seen in intact animals. But in these cases, as we shall see, dispute is possible over the identity of the interneurons involved, so that neurophysiological analysis has become more complicated.

Cat Spinal Cord

The Flexor Reflex

Habituation. A second vertebrate preparation that has been extensively explored is the (polysynaptic) flexor reflex in the spinal cat. The spinal cord is sectioned at T12, the stimulus is an electric shock to the skin of a hind paw, and the response is activity of the tibialis anterior muscle of the left hind limb (associated with flexion or withdrawal of the limb). Thompson and Spencer (1966) report that this preparation shows all nine parametric features of habituation. As in the case of the frog LC-VRR preparation, habituation is relatively short-lived, persisting for a maximum of two hours or so.

Spencer, Thompson, and Neilson (1966) recorded intracellularly from spinal motoneurons that showed marked habituation—a reduction in postsynaptic potential—in the course of a train of cutaneous stimuli. Those same motoneurons showed no change in excitability (in threshold or in PSP magnitude) to occasional stimuli delivered to the peroneal nerve, which makes monosynaptic connections with the motoneurons. The general excitability of motoneurons does not, therefore, alter with habituation training.

Stimulation of the afferent terminals of the cutaneous nerve elicits a constant antidromic response from the nerve, indicating that terminal excitability does not alter during habituation training (Groves et al.1970). This finding argues against the possibility of presynaptic inhibition operating on the afferent terminals, a conclusion supported by the observation that picrotoxin, which blocks presynaptic inhibition, does not prevent habituation in this preparation (Spencer, Thompson, and Neilson 1966). The possibility that postsynaptic inhibition might be responsible for habituation (Wickelgren 1967), has received little support: strychnine, which blocks postsynaptic inhibition, does not prevent habituation and, as we shall see, no interneurons have yet been found that increase their rate of firing as habituation proceeds (such an increase would be expected if an increase in postsynaptic inhibition was taking place).

It is, however, technically extremely difficult to pinpoint with any confidence the locus of habituation in this preparation. A major problem is that the flexor reflex is polysynaptic, and the locations of the interneurons concerned are not known. Interneurons have been found whose activity shows correspondence with the overt response, but the precise role of those interneurons is not clear. The response properties of interneurons will be discussed following a brief discussion of dishabituation in the spinal cat.

Sensitization. Figure 2.13 shows the course of habituation of the flexor reflex and the effect on the habituated response of the delivery of a brief shock train to an area of skin close to that used for the habituating stimulus. The figure shows the same initial "hump" that was seen in the data gathered on habituation of the acoustic startle response in the intact rat (see figure 2.1). It is evident from figure 2.13 that the shock train dishabituated the response. The figure also shows that the effect of the shock train waned over time, and that the "recovery of habituation" shown on figure 2.13A was not due to the continuation of the train of habituating stimuli. This result also parallels the data on dishabituation obtained from intact rats (see figure 2.1). The correspondence between the results from the intact and the spinal animals is striking and confirms that the spinal cord does contain mechanisms that are sufficient to generate the phenom-

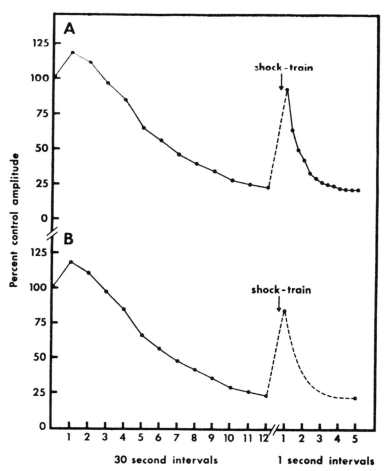

FIGURE 2.13. Habituation and sensitization of the hind limb flexor reflex in the spinal cat. Fig. 2.13A shows the effect of single shocks delivered at a rate of 2 per sec until pronounced habituation had developed. A brief sensitizing shock train was then delivered to nearby skin electrodes, and the habituation stimulus was continued at a rate of 1 per sec. Fig. 2.13B shows the outcome of an identical procedure with the exception that the habituation stimulus was discontinued after the sensitizing shock train. A single test shock delivered after 5 sec showed that response amplitude had decayed spontaneously to its previously habituated level. Note the similarity of these results to those shown in fig. 2.1, obtained with intact rats. (*From* Groves and Thompson 1970)

ena seen in intact animals. A successful analysis of those spinal mechanisms would therefore be expected to throw considerable light on those
processes in intact as well as spinal animals.

The excitability of sensory afferent terminals (assessed by the antidromic response to terminal stimulation) does not change as a result of
sensitization treatment (Spencer, Thompson, and Neilson 1966): this suggests that presynaptic facilitation of afferent terminals is not the mechanism of sensitization. But other mechanisms are less easily ruled out. Excitability of motoneurons does increase following sensitization (ibid.,
1966), but whether this is due to change intrinsic to the motoneurons cannot yet be determined. The difficulty is, as noted previously, that the interneurons involved in this reflex have not been identified, and it is to a
consideration of interneuron activity that we shall now turn.

Two Types of Plastic Interneuron. Groves and Thompson (1970) described experiments on intracellular recording from neurons in the dorsal
horn of spinal cats during the course of habituation treatment, and identified three principal classes of response. One group of cells (nonplastic
interneurons) showed no systematic change in response as training proceeded. A second group of cells showed only response decrement as training proceeded (these cells at no stage showed an increment in response,
even when the overt muscular response is incremented). The cells of this
group were labeled plastic interneuron type H cells. The third group of
cells showed an initial increment in response, followed by a decrement—
paralleling the muscular response—and these were labeled type S cells.
Type H cells typically showed shorter latencies than type S cells and were
located in the more dorsal (peripheral) layers of the horn (Rexed's layers
1-V). Type S cells were more ventrally located (in layers 5–7), and
showed marked increases in tonic activity during sensitization treatments.

Groves and Thompson (1970) suggested that these findings supported
the view that habituation and sensitization are processes that are mediated
by different anatomical routes. Specifically, they proposed that habituation
is mediated by interneurons that lie in the stimulus-response (S-R) pathway, and that sensitization is mediated by interneurons that contribute to
the excitation of the state of the organism: a schematic diagram of their
proposal is shown in figure 2.14. The short latency of the type H cells
suggests that they could form part of the S-R pathway; the more central
location of the type S cells would be suitable for their making extensive
connection with the spinal fiber systems that convey information to and
from other segments of the spinal cord, and beyond into the brain. There

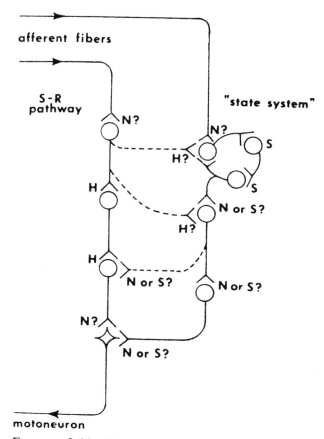

FIGURE 2.14. Schematic diagram of the Groves and Thompson (1970) proposals concerning possible neuronal substrates of habituation and sensitization. N = non-plastic synapses; H = habituating synapses; S = sensitizing synapses. (*From* Groves and Thompson 1970)

is, then, a general agreement between the data and the theory. But the proposal remains speculative, given the difficulty of deriving and testing specific predictions: it is not possible, for example, to damage selectively either type H or type S neurons to see whether, as a result, habituation or sensitization would fail to appear. And it is not yet possible to trace the S-R pathway with sufficient accuracy to enable us to determine whether type H cells *do* form part of that pathway and, in particular, to determine whether the activity of type H cells has any effect on the activity of motoneurons.

The Plantar Cushion Reflex

Doubts over the roles of type H and type S cells are strengthened by a consideration of results obtained using another spinal reflex in cats, a reflex whose pathway is very much better understood than that for the flexor reflex. Stimulation of the central pad of the hind paw of the cat obtains reflex activation of the hind limb (the plantar cushion reflex). The reflex is trisynaptic (possibly even disynaptic) and involves at most two dorsal horn interneurons; and although the work to be described here concerns anesthetized cats, the reflex seen in these animals is similar to that seen in spinal cats (Egger and Wall 1971). The plantar cushion reflex can be elicited in intact but anesthetized and immobilized cats by stimuli of sufficiently low intensity that only the largest-diameter cutaneous afferents are activated, an intensity well below that required for elicitation of the flexor reflex in this preparation (Egger, Bishop, and Cone 1976).

Egger (1978) explored cells in the dorsal horn during sensitization and habituation of the plantar cushion reflex, finding two groups of cells, in layers 3 and 4, that showed short-latency responses to pad stimulation. One group showed decreases in response rate to pad stimulation with repetition of the stimulus; the second group showed an initial increase followed by a gradual decrease in response, a pattern that paralleled the response monitored in the ventral root. These groups have similarities to Groves and Thompson's type H and type S cells, with the one potentially important distinction that both types were found in the same (peripheral) layers of the dorsal horn. More significantly, however, the cells had characteristically different thresholds, those of the decrementing cells being lower than those of the incrementing-then-decrementing cells. The thresholds of the decrementing cells were in fact considerably lower than the threshold for obtaining the behavioral reflex; whereas those of the incrementing-then-decrementing cells closely matched the behavioral threshold. In other words, the cells most likely to be involved in the direct S-R pathway showed both "sensitization" and "habituation," and cells that showed "habituation" only seemed unlikely to be involved in the reflex.

Egger's (1978) report casts doubt on the notion that, at least in the dorsal horn, separate neurons mediate sensitization and habituation; it will be recalled that Farel (1974a) claimed that both effects occurred at the same synapse in the frog LC-VRR preparation. It should, however, be noted that to conclude that the same synapses mediate both habituation and sensitization does not necessarily imply dismissal of dual-process theory. The same synapses, after all, mediate both habituation and sensitization in *Aplysia*. But the existence of a network of facilitatory interneurons whose function it is to alter the efficacy of synapses of other cells provides a perfectly good example of a system that (in that respect, at least) conforms to dual-process theory in showing a different anatomical basis for sensitization as opposed to habituation.

Spinal Vertebrates: Not Simple Systems

This brief survey of work on spinal vertebrates points to one clear conclusion, namely, that work on these preparations has shown very much less progress than has corresponding work on *Aplysia*. One major reason for this has been the fact that work on polysynaptic reflexes is severely hindered by the difficulty of establishing precisely which interneurons mediate the reflex—that is, of establishing what is in Groves and Thompson's (1970) terms the S-R pathway.

The evidence currently available simply does not allow us to decide whether there are major differences between the mechanisms employed by spinal vertebrates and those employed by *Aplysia*. There are suggestions of some differences: we saw that short-term habituation of the frog LC-VRR preparation may not involve depletion of readily releasable vesicles, and that sensitization of the cat flexor reflex does obtain increases in excitability of motoneurons. But in no case was there sufficient evidence for a firm conclusion about the mechanisms involved in the vertebrate preparation so that confident comparisons with the *Aplysia* data are not yet possible.

The very difficulty of making progress with spinal vertebrates emphasizes that although *Aplysia* are not simple they are more amenable to analysis than any vertebrate system: their introduction as a central preparation in neuroscience has been amply justified.

Nonassociative Learning: Not Simple Processes

This chapter has used the dual-process theory of habituation and sensitization as a conceptual framework within which to interpret the physiological findings. We have seen good support for one central tenet of that theory, namely, that habituation occurs as a result of processes intrinsic to the S-R pathway. But difficulties have arisen, particularly in the *Aplysia* data, for the account of sensitization proposed in dual-process theory.

The difficulties that have arisen suggest that the admirably parsimonious dual-process theory has oversimplified nonassociative learning. Both physiological and behavioral data point, for example, to the conclusion that dishabituation is not the same as sensitization (although those processes do have much in common), and that sensitization does not influence a monolithic statelike system that modulates all S-R pathways equally. We have, moreover, seen that yet another process, one of inhibition, may be engaged by the simple presentation of a stimulus. It seems, then, that nonassociative learning is more complicated than dual-process theory allows. This is a conclusion that is of importance to behavioral psychologists, but the fact is that behavioral theorists have had very little to say about either the process of sensitization or that of (nonassociative) inhibition. The physiological data reviewed in this chapter have therefore served to emphasize a lacuna concerning those processes in current behavioral theories. Behavioral psychologists have, however, been much interested in the process of habituation (and, to a lesser extent, in dishabituation), and we shall consider in chapter 3 theories of habituation that were developed with reference to vertebrate supraspinal reflexes, theories that challenge the dual-process account of habituation. The question whether a general account of habituation can be provided without the introduction of mechanisms extrinsic to the S-R pathway will be considered further at the end of chapter 3.

3. Habituation in Vertebrates

Extrinsic Theories of Habituation

The vertebrate reflexes discussed in chapter 2 were spinally mediated and so avoided the complications occasioned by the involvement of the brain. This chapter will consider nonassociative learning of supraspinal reflexes and will concentrate almost entirely upon habituation since this is the process to which most research effort has been directed. Before discussing the physiological data, three further theories of habituation will be introduced, theories that were generated with explicit reference to habituation of supraspinal reflexes. The three theories all have in common the notion that habituation occurs as a result of an inhibitory effect upon the S-R pathway (defined as in Groves and Thompson 1970) mediated by a mechanism extrinsic to that pathway. They all therefore directly challenge a central tenet of Groves and Thompson's two-process theory, namely, that the process of habituation is intrinsic to the S-R pathway.

Afferent Neuronal Inhibition

An early physiological account of habituation was proposed by Hernandez-Péon (e.g., 1960), whose view was that habituation was mediated by a reduction in effectiveness of transmission in the sensory pathway of the stimulus concerned. The reduction in effectiveness was accomplished through inhibition of peripheral sensory relays by centrifugal efferents from the reticular formation. The principal evidence for this theory came from observations of reductions in activity recorded at peripheral sensory nuclei with repetition of stimuli. An interesting feature of this physiological theory is that it clearly faces immediate difficulties with behavioral data: if, for example, transmission is inhibited, how could the organism detect a novel stimulus from that modality? There were problems also with the physiological support for the theory, and those problems will be discussed after introducing two further extrinsic theories.

Neuronal Models

A second account of habituation, which specifically concerns only the orienting reflex, was proposed by Sokolov (e.g., Sokolov 1960). The orienting reflex consists of a set of reactions to a change in stimulus conditions, independent of the modality of the stimulus. In mammals, such changes include desynchronization of EEG, arrest of movement, reduction of respiration and heart rate, and peripheral vasoconstriction accompanied by cephalic vasodilation. The object of the various components of the orienting reflex is to channel resources toward the cortical analyzers responsible for forming models of novel stimuli. Sokolov has proposed that in order for habituation of orienting to occur, neuronal models of stimuli are formed. Incoming stimuli are scanned to see whether they correspond to any preexisting model: if no match is found, an orienting reflex is elicited.

Sokolov and his colleagues (e.g., Vinogradova 1975) have suggested that the neuronal model for a stimulus is both elaborated and stored in sensory neocortex, and that the hippocampus serves as a "comparator" which determines whether a match exists between an incoming stimulus and an existing cortical model. A mismatch results in activation of the reticular formation by the hippocampus, and that activation elicits the orienting reflex. (The hippocampus will form a central focus of interest in chapters 6, 7, and 8, and a discussion of its basic anatomy and physiology may be found in chapter 6, which also contains an introduction to the major functional subdivisions of neocortex.)

One of Sokolov's principal reasons for supposing that the hippocampus may act as comparator derives from the work of Vinogradova (e.g., 1970), who recorded from single units in rabbit hippocampus during the presentation of trains of repeated stimuli: Vinogradova reported that about 90 percent of dorsal hippocampal cells showed systematic changes in response to novel stimuli, irrespective of their modality. Of these cells, some 60 percent (type I cells) showed progressive increases in activity as a stimulus was repeated, and 30–40 percent (type A cells) showed decreases. Sokolov and Vinogradova suppose that the type I cells, which are inhibited by the presentation of a novel stimulus, have an inhibiting effect on the reticular formation, so that an orienting reflex is obtained when type I cells are inhibited; they further suppose that the type A cells, which are activated by novel stimuli, serve in turn to activate the neocortex directly, facilitating the forming of a new neuronal model. The interpretation of these data will be discussed following one further account of habituation, an account that has much in common with Sokolov's view.

Priming Theory

The third theory to be introduced here has no specific physiological proposals associated with it but does possess features that are of considerable relevance to the interpretation of physiological work. The theory is due to Wagner (e.g., 1976), and forms part of a larger body of theory concerning the processing of stimuli in learning tasks. Wagner assumes a distinction between short-term memory and long-term memory, and proposes that the degree of representation of a stimulus in short-term memory directly determines its effectiveness in eliciting any response (learned or unlearned) associated with it.

In the present context, Wagner's key proposal is that the effectiveness of a stimulus in gaining access to short-term memory is reduced if it is already represented there. Such prerepresentation could arise in two ways: either through a recent occurrence of the stimulus, which obtained a representation that has not yet decayed (self-generated priming), or through a representation having been elicited as a consequence of the occurrence of another stimulus that is associated with the target stimulus (retrieval-generated priming). Short-term habituation may be accounted for, therefore, by supposing that the interstimulus interval is sufficiently brief that a representation of the preceding stimulus still exists in short-term memory when a stimulus is delivered; that representation prevents efficient access to short-term memory by the current stimulus, so that the response elicited is reduced. Wagner's explanation of long-term habituation requires a further assumption—namely, that an association is formed between stimuli and the context in which they are presented. So that where an animal is replaced in a context in which a stimulus has been delivered, a representation of the stimulus is elicited in short-term memory, mediated now by the association, stored in long-term memory, between context and stimulus. Two features of Wagner's account that will prove of particular interest in later sections are, first, that short-term habituation and long-term habituation involve different processes and, second, that long-term habituation depends upon associative learning and is context-specific.

Evidence from Recording Studies

Difficulties in Establishing Causal Relationships

The physiological aspects of two of the theories discussed above (those of Hernandez-Péon and of Sokolov) relied heavily upon evidence drawn from studies in which recordings were taken of electrical activity while trains of identical stimuli were being presented. But there is a difficulty in interpreting changes in responsiveness of cells with stimulus repetition. To put the problem in an oversimplified way: are these systematic response changes the cause of habituation, or are they caused by a process of habituation that occurs elsewhere?

Consider first Hernandez-Péon's proposal that centrifugal inhibition of peripheral sensory relays is the cause of habituation. We may observe, first, that many of the early experiments had a number of serious weaknesses (see, for example, Buchwald and Humphrey 1973). There was the problem of artifact; for example, reduction in evoked responses at, say, the cochlear nucleus, to trains of clicks could be caused by changes in activity of the middle ear muscles, or by changes in an animal's orientation. There was also the problem that many studies failed to record habituation behaviorally, so that there was no clear link between the recordings and anything else that might be regarded as habituation. A further problem was that evidence accumulated to show that electrical activity was reduced in stations of one modality by stimuli delivered to another modality. But overriding all these problems is the difficulty of demonstrating a causal link: how can one decide whether a change in activity in any site is causally involved in the development of habituation? One answer to that question is to employ the lesion technique. The argument can best be illustrated by considering an interesting study of a change in electrical activity with repeated stimulation.

Willott, Schnerson, and Urban (1979) compared the effects of varying certain parameters of a tone stimulus (frequency, intensity, rise time, and interstimulus interval) on both behavioral habituation of the startle response to the tone and unit activity of single cells in various divisions of the inferior colliculus of the mouse. They found very good agreement between activity in two divisions of the inferior colliculus (the pericentral nucleus and the external nucleus) and behavioral responding: in particular, when the level of behavioral responding fell with repetition of stimuli, so did unit activity in these divisions. Units in a third region, the ventrolateral division of the central nucleus of the inferior colliculus, showed no systematic decline in activity as stimuli were repeated. These units, unlike those of the pericentral and external nucleus, and unlike the startle response, were not affected by changes in rise time, or by changes in interstimulus interval. The cells of the central nucleus, which belongs to the classical auditory lemniscal system, reflected consistently the physical parameters of the stimulus; the cells of the other two divisions, which belong to what some (e.g., Graybiel 1973) have called the "extralemniscal" or lemniscal adjunct system, were modified by the animal's experience of the stimuli and reflected also (in their sensitivity to rise time) the behavioral effectiveness of the stimulus. The distinction between lemniscal and nonlemniscal auditory pathways is of considerable interest and will be encountered again in chapter 5: but the question here is whether we should suppose that the nonlemniscal cells of the inferior colliculus contribute to the process of habituation, or simply reflect that process (just as muscles do).

A relevant lesion study was reported by Jordan and Leaton (1983), who investigated habituation of acoustic startle in rats with lesions of the inferior colliculus: long-term habituation was unaffected by the lesions (which did, however, reduce initial responsiveness somewhat). Short-term habituation was also unaffected, except that the lesioned rats could not attain as low an asymptote as controls when high-intensity stimuli and a short interstimulus interval were used, a result that could equally well be due to a minor change in either sensitization or habituation. Lesions to the brachium of the inferior colliculus, which severed auditory input to medial geniculate body and auditory cortex, had no effect on short-term habituation or long-term habituation of either acoustic or tactile startle (although such lesions did increase initial responsiveness to both auditory and tactile stimuli) (Jordan and Leaton 1982a). These data indicate that although changes in activity in inferior colliculus cells may parallel changes in behavioral responsiveness, they do not cause those changes and must be presumed to be reflecting changes that occur elsewhere.

Hernandez-Péon's "afferent neuronal inhibition" theory of habituation was introduced here largely to help illustrate the problems associated with data from recordings. It will not be further considered because of the conceptual problems referred to previously. One of the standard characteristics (e.g., Thompson and Spencer 1966) of habituation is stimulus generalization—that is, habituation to a given stimulus will obtain a reduced response to other stimuli, the degree of reduction varying with the similarity of the stimuli. In other words, habituation to, say, a tone of one frequency will have relatively little effect on response to a tone of a very different frequency. This selectivity, which is basic to habituation, cannot be accounted for by afferent neuronal inhibition, which may therefore be rejected as an account of habituation.

There are serious doubts also about the interpretation of the recording data provided by Vinogradova. The problem is that she took no behavioral measures of responsiveness during presentation of stimuli, during which rabbits were restrained in a dimly lit box. O'Keefe and Nadel (1978) have suggested that the rabbits tended to fall asleep in the box, and that the alterations in unit activity reflected the effect on unit activity of overall arousal differences, rather than any specific orienting reflex. As we shall see in chapters 6 and 7, Vinogradova's account of unit activity in the rabbit differs markedly from accounts derived from recordings taken from alert animals in more stimulating environments. More particularly, Thompson and his colleagues (e.g., Berger and Thompson 1978) have reported activity of cells in the hippocampus of the rabbit both before and during conditioning. Prior to conditioning, the animals experienced, as a sensitization control, repeated unpaired presentation of the conditioned stimulus (CS, a tone) and the unconditional stimulus (UCS, an airpuff directed at the cornea). During this procedure, which would presumably obtain a fairly constant level of arousal, Thompson failed to observe systematic changes in the response of hippocampal cells to tone presentations, and in particular, did not find systematic *increases* in firing with repetitions of the tone. It will be recalled that Vinogradova claimed that 60 percent of hippocampal cells showed progressive increases in response rate to repetitions of initially novel stimuli. Thompson's data are particularly convincing since he did find systematic increases in hippocampal cells responding to the tone when it was paired with the airpuff, and served as a CS.

Given the problems of interpretation associated with the recording techniques, the remainder of this chapter will concentrate on results obtained using lesions. The response systems to be considered will be, first, the startle reflex in rats and, second, the constellation of responses that constitute the orienting reflex. In the following sections we shall concentrate first on reporting relevant physiological findings for the two reflexes, then consider their broader behavioral implications in a subsequent section.

Habituation of the Startle Reflex

The startle reflex of the rat consists of a pattern of muscular responses elicited throughout the whole body by the presentation of an intense sensory stimulus with an abrupt onset; the response results in a characteristic crouchlike posture. Although the reflex may be elicited by stimuli from other modalities, it is the acoustically elicited reflex which has been most widely studied. One preliminary point is that the repeated elicitation of the acoustic startle response does result in a pattern of habituation that conforms to the nine characteristic parameters set out by Thompson and Spencer (1966). There is, moreover, evidence for the independence of habituation and sensitization in the system also: it will be recalled, for example, that figure 2.1 showed that a "dishabituating" stimulus does not directly influence the process of habituation.

The minimal (or S-R) pathway for the acoustic startle reflex has been established by Davis et al. (1982) and is summarized on figure 3.1. Auditory nerve fibers synapse onto the first station of the pathway, the ventral cochlear nucleus. From this nucleus, fibers travel via the ventral acoustic stria to the second station, the ventral nucleus of the lateral lemniscus. From the ventral nucleus, fibers travel to a nucleus of the bulbopontine reticular formation, the nucleus reticularis pontis caudalis. Fibers from this third station travel in the reticulospinal tract to synapse directly onto motoneurons in the spinal cord that obtain limb movements, and probably onto spinal interneurons also. There may, moreover, be direct spinal projections from the ventral nucleus of the lateral lemniscus, so that the minimal pathway may contain only some three to five synapses. Davis et al. (1982) have shown that direct electrical stimulation of any of the proposed stations of this pathway elicit the startle response, and that lesions at any point within it abolish the response.

We may now ask the question, is the process of habituation intrinsic to the S-R pathway, as expected in the Groves and Thompson (1970) model? We can begin to answer this question by describing an experiment that shows, first, that short-term habituation and long-term habituation involve different mechanisms and, second, that the mechanisms of long-term habituation are extrinsic to the S-R pathway. Leaton, Cassella, and Borszcz (1985) investigated habituation of the acoustic startle response in chronic decerebrate rats (animals having transections of the brainstem at a level that effectively eliminated any influences on the response of mid- and forebrain structures). The decerebrate animals showed (compared with controls) normal within-session habituation, but no evidence of any between-day habituation; interestingly, the decerebrates did show evidence of retention of habituation between two sessions of one day, when those sessions were separated by forty minutes.

Since short-term habituation and long-term habituation are physiologically dissociable, we shall consider them in separate sections.

Short-Term Habituation

The fact that decerebrate animals show short-term habituation encourages the notion that short-term habituation does take place within the S-R path-

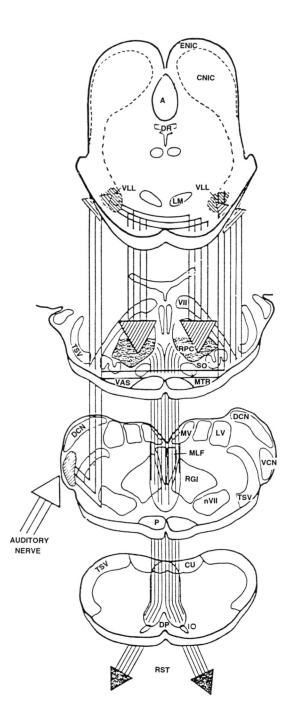

way, and Davis and File (1984) provided an answer to the question where, within the S-R pathway, does short-term habituation take place? Direct stimulation of the ventral cochlear nucleus elicits the startle response, and repeated stimulation resulted in habituation at a rate comparable to that obtained using sound stimuli. But repeated stimulation of the nucleus reticularis pontis caudalis, which also obtains the response, did not result in habituation. The implication is that the site of short-term habituation is to be found in the afferent limb of the pathway, between the ventral cochlear nucleus and the nucleus reticularis pontis caudalis.

Sensitization

Before going on to consider the mechanisms involved in long-term habituation, I should interject here a brief discussion of the little that is known of the mechanisms of sensitization of the startle reflex. In general, it is not possible to distinguish between short- and long-term sensitization because sensitization effects in normal animals typically dissipate within 24 hours (Davis 1972). Fear-inducing stimuli do, however, sensitize the startle reflex, so that long-term sensitizing effects may be seen when the test apparatus or cues within it have become fear-inducing as a consequence of some conditioning procedure (e.g., Borszcz, Cranney, and Leaton 1989). Since it is an associative effect, this type of long-term sensitization will not be considered further here. It may be worth digressing to note that the long-term sensitization effects seen in *Aplysia* could similarly be mediated by fear induced by an association of the context with the (aversive) sensitizing UCS. We shall see in chapter 4 that *Aplysia* do exhibit fear conditioning and conditioning to contextual cues. But the physiological analysis of long-term sensitization advanced in chapter 2 envisaged a nonassocia-

---

FIGURE 3.1. Schematic diagram of the minimal (or S-R) pathway of the acoustic startle response. A = aqueduct; DCN = dorsal cochlear nucleus; VCN = ventral cochlear nucleus; CNIC = central nucleus of the inferior colliculus; CU = cuneate nucleus; DP = decussation of pyramids; ENIC = external nucleus of the inferior colliculus; IO = inferior olive; LL = lateral lemniscus; VLL = ventral nucleus of the lateral lemniscus; LM = medial lemniscus; MLF = medial longitudinal fasciculus; MTB = medial nucleus of the trapezoid body; NVII = nucleus of the seventh nerve; SO = superior olive; P = pyramids; RGI = nucleus reticularis gigantocellularis; RPC = nucleus reticularis pontis caudalis; RST = reticulospinal tract; TSV = spinal tract of the fifth nerve; VAS = ventral acoustic stria; VII = seventh nerve; LV = lateral vestibular nucleus; MV = medial vestibular nucleus. (*Adapted from* Davis et al. 1982)

tive process, and current physiological accounts of learning in *Aplysia* in fact, as we shall see, find difficulty in accounting for context learning.

The question whether stimuli that sensitize acoustic startle also sensitize other response systems (and, in particular, response systems that are engaged by nonaversive stimuli) has attracted little behavioral investigation, so that it is not possible to say whether sensitizing stimuli in fact activate a general statelike system.

Davis and File (1984) sought the locus of (short-term) sensitization effects by eliciting the startle response by direct stimulation at various points on the S-R pathway, and asking whether there were sites at which the elicited response would *not* be affected by a sensitizing stimulus (in this case, an elevation in background noise). No such sites were found: the response to direct spinal stimulation was, for example, enhanced in the presence of increased noise. The implication is that sensitization is a process that enhances the effectiveness of spinal motoneuron activation and, of course, that it is a process anatomically distinct from habituation. It is of interest to add that Leaton, Cassella, and Borszcz's decerebrate rats showed signs of an enhanced susceptibility to sensitizing effects of stimuli, and evidence too of between-days retention of sensitization: these findings are difficult to interpret since in that experiment controls showed no overt evidence of any sensitization. Currently, little is known of the structures involved in the sensitization of the startle response, but it is evident that mid- and forebrain structures are not necessary for sensitization, and at least possible that long-term retention of sensitization may be obtained in the absence of those structures.

Long-Term Habituation

The most dramatic effect to date of a brain lesion on long-term habituation of the startle reflex involves the cerebellar vermis (the medial cerebellar region, excluding the deep nuclei; for further details of the anatomy and physiology of the cerebellum, see chapter 5). Leaton and Supple (1986) reported that vermal aspiration, while having no effect on either initial response level or within-sessions habituation, virtually abolished long-term habituation (measured after one or five days) of the acoustic startle response in rats; their results are summarized in figure 3.2. In view of the involvement of the cerebellum in classical conditioning (to be discussed in chapter 5), it is important to note that cerebellar areas that appear to be critical for acquisition of skeletal conditioned responses were not damaged in this study: in particular the cerebellar hemispheres received little damage, and the dentate and interpositus nuclei were intact.

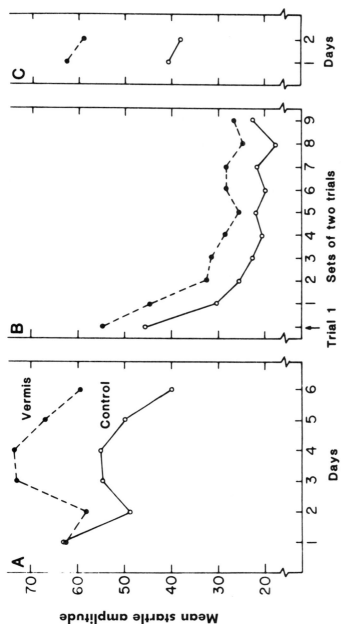

FIGURE 3.2. Effects of vermal aspiration on habituation of the acoustic startle response in rats. Fig. 3.2A shows performance over 6 days, each of which contained three presentations of a 1-sec loud white-noise stimulus, separated by 1-hr intervals. Initial startle amplitude was similar in controls and in rats having lesions of the vermis, but long-term (between-day) habituation was not observed in the vermis group. Fig. 3.2B summarizes performance over the next 3 days, each of which contained eighteen presentations of the white-noise stimulus, separated by a 20-sec interval; the first trial of the session is shown separately, followed by sets of two trials. Short-term habituation developed normally in the vermis group. Fig. 3.2C shows performance on a retest of long-term habituation that took place 5 days after the testing summarized on fig. 3.2B. For 2 days the rats were again tested with three white-noise presentations each day, separated by a 1-hr interval. The vermis group showed no evidence of long-term habituation. (*From* Leaton and Supple 1986)

Involvement of the cerebellum is surprising, given the fact that the decerebrate rats of the Leaton, Cassella, and Borszcz report (1985), with an intact cerebellum, showed no long-term habituation: since the vermis is apparently not sufficient for the occurrence of long-term habituation, it may be assumed to form part of a circuit components of which lie rostrally in mid- and forebrain regions. This conclusion is strengthened by the finding that although the vermis is essential for the development of long-term habituation, it is not essential for the maintenance of preoperatively established long-term habituation (Lopiano, De'Sperati, and Montarolo 1990). It appears, then, that the cerebellar vermis may be necessary for the induction of the changes in conductivity that mediate long-term habituation, but that those changes actually occur in some other structure. There is, however, very little information available on what that structure might be.

Jordan and Leaton (1982b, 1983) found that long-term habituation (but not short-term habituation) of acoustic startle was attenuated by lesions of mesencephalic reticular formation; since these lesions were sited rostrally to the level of decerebration in the Leaton, Cassella, and Borszcz report, it may be that decerebration disrupts long-term habituation because of the loss of these mesencephalic structures. The attenuation of long-term habituation that resulted from reticular lesions was much less marked than that following vermal lesions, and appeared only when control response levels had been driven to a low asymptote by, for example, using brief interstimulus intervals during within-session training.

Subsequent research (Jordan 1989) has found that the mesencephalic reticular formation (unlike the vermis) is essential for retention of preoperatively established long-term habituation of the acoustic startle response. This report provides further confirmation that the structures that mediate long-term habituation are extrinsic to the S-R pathway. It could have been the case that structures outside the pathway (the vermis, for example) were necessary for the induction of changes within the S-R pathway, changes that would then be independent of extrinsic structures. Jordan's (1989) report shows that an extrinsic structure (or structures) modulates conduction through the S-R pathway during both the development and the maintenance of long-term habituation.

The work discussed in this section has concerned only the acoustic startle response. We do not know whether vermal lesions disrupt long-term habituation of any other response system, but there is evidence that the effects of reticular formation (RF) lesions are specific to acoustic startle: Jordan and Leaton (1982b) also assessed habituation to the same auditory stimulus using a second measure, lick suppression (the duration of the interruption by a stimulus of licking of a water tube by thirsty rats). Mesencephalic RF lesions had no effect on either short-term habituation or long-term habituation of lick suppression to an auditory stimulus. There is, then, no evidence for a general role in habituation of either the cerebellar vermis or the mesencephalic reticular formation.

Summary and Conclusions

The basic conclusions of this survey of work on the acoustic startle reflex may be summarized rapidly: short-term habituation of acoustic startle does appear to be intrinsic to the S-R pathway, but long-term habituation involves extrinsic mechanisms that include the cerebellar vermis (essential for development but not for maintenance of long-term habituation) and the mesencephalic reticular formation (involved in both development and maintenance). Before leaving the startle reflex, one negative result should be noted in view of the general importance in learning of the hippocampus and of Sokolov's proposal that the hippocampus plays a critical role in the habituation of the orienting reflex: Leaton (1981) has shown that hippocampal lesions have no effect on either short- or long-term habituation of the acoustic startle reflex.

Habituation of the Orienting Reflex

The orienting reflex, or at least components of the reflex, conforms to the basic parameters of habituation set out by Thompson and Spencer (e.g., 1966; Megela and Teyler 1979). Two major physiological issues arise from Sokolov's physiological speculations: first, what is the role of the neocortex in habituation; second, what is the role of the hippocampus? The discussion of hippocampal involvement will lead to the introduction of the topic of exploration, behavior that is closely related to orienting but is distinct from the orienting reflex proper (which involves behavioral arrest).

Neocortex and Habituation of Orienting Reflexes

One classic early study was reported by Sharpless and Jasper (1956). These authors presented auditory stimuli to sleeping cats and measured arousal, as measured by desynchronization of the EEG. They found that extensive lesions of primary and secondary auditory cortex were without effect on either short-term or long-term habituation of the arousal response. The only effect of their cortical lesions was found when they tested for the "pattern specificity" of habituation by presenting modulated tones that fell (or rose) during their 4-sec duration from 500 to 200 Hz (or vice versa). Whereas control animals, having habituated to a falling tone, were (usually) aroused by a rising tone, efforts to find pattern specificity in control subjects were "generally unsuccessful." Such a finding would support the view that cortical processing is necessary for the analysis of certain "higher order" properties of stimuli, but does not indicate for the cortex any specific role in habituation per se.

Thompson and Welker (1963) investigated the effects of large auditory cortex lesions on habituation of behavioral orienting reflexes (head turning) to brief bursts of white noise presented either to the left or to the right of waking cats. They found that these lesions decreased both the number of overt orientations and their directional accuracy. There was, however, no effect of these lesions on short-term habituation to the noise bursts, although, unlike controls, the cortical animals showed no long-term habituation. A difficulty in interpreting these findings arises from the fact that the baseline level of responding to noise bursts was lower in the cortical animals, with the result that although they did not show between-days habituation their level of response was nevertheless lower at the end of training than that of controls.

The above reports show that cortical sensory areas, while involved in the processing of stimuli, are not essential for short-term habituation, and may not be for long-term habituation either. We may now look briefly at the question whether total absence of all neocortex influences habituation.

It seems clear that no neocortex is required for short-term habituation of (at least some components of) orienting reflexes: Yeo and Oakley (1983) removed more than 95 percent of neocortex from rats, and then trained them to push a door for a food reward, delivered after every tenth response. They then presented tone stimuli (four per day) and measured the duration of the interruption of responding. They found in rats without neocortex normal short-term habituation of this arrest response, and substantial between-day retention of habituation also. Once again, it is difficult to compare data directly with controls, since the neocortical rats showed lower baseline rates of response.

Klosterhalfen and Klosterhalfen (1985) used the spreading-depression technique to obtain total (but reversible) cessation of neocortical activity, and explored habituation of an (accelerating) heart-rate response to an auditory stimulus (a bell). They found normal short-term habituation, but no evidence for long-term habituation after a 24-hour interval; they did, however, find successful retention of habituation over a 30-min interval in their functionally decorticate rats, an effect they refer to as "medium-term" habituation.

The findings reviewed in this section may be summarized as follows: the neocortex is not necessary for short- (or medium-) term habituation. Long-term habituation is also possible in the absence of neocortex, although it may be attenuated or abolished under certain conditions.

Hippocampus and Orienting Reflexes

The literature on the effects of hippocampal lesions on habituation of the various components of orienting is confusing and frequently appears contradictory. Consider, for example, studies of behavioral "arrest," studies that measure the duration of interruption of some ongoing behavioral pattern by a distractor. Leaton (1981) measured the duration of interruption of licking at a water spout by thirsty rats induced by presentation of auditory or visual stimuli and found that both short-term habituation and long-term habituation of lick suppression proceeded normally in hippocampal animals. In Leaton's study, the absolute level of lick suppression was similar in hippocampal and normal rats. But in many other studies, the magnitude of the initial arrest reaction in hippocampal animals is much reduced compared to controls (e.g., Crowne and Riddell 1969; Riddell, Rothblat, and Wilson 1969; Gustafson and Koenig 1979), with the consequence that a smaller (absolute) decrease in magnitude of the reaction is seen in hippocampals as compared to controls when the distractor is presented repeatedly. Some authors (e.g., Gustafson and Koenig 1979) have interpreted such results as indicating a disruption of habituation in hippocampal rats. But an alternative interpretation, which supposes that hippocampals display a smaller change as habituation proceeds simply because of a floor effect, and not because of any defect in habituation, is entirely plausible and is well supported by Leaton's result.

Studies of autonomic indices of orienting also give general support to the view that hippocampal lesions do not impair habituation although, once again, interpretation is somewhat obscured by the fact that the response to initial presentation of stimuli may differ between hippocampals and controls. Bagshaw, Kimble, and Pribram (1965) measured the galvanic skin response (GSR) in monkeys to a series of presentation of a tone and found no differences between normals and hippocampals in either the size of the response to initial tone presentation, or the rate of short-term habituation. Studies of habituation of heart-rate changes have reached a broadly similar conclusion. Jarrard and Korn (1969), for example, found no differences between hippocampal and normal rats in either the absolute level of heart rate or the progressive decline when naive animals were placed in a novel experimental chamber. Crowne and Riddell (1969) found no differences between control and hippocampal rats in either initial level or within-session habituation of a decelerative cardiac orienting reflex to presentations of a salient auditory and visual stimulus to satiated rats in a familiar environment. But Crowne and Riddell also found that thirsty hippocampal rats working for a water reward showed (unlike controls) no cardiac orienting reflex to the first presentation of that same stimulus; the hippocampal rats did, however, show orienting reflexes to subsequent presentations, and the orienting reflex then habituated at a rate comparable to that of controls.

Hippocampus and Exploration

The studies described in the preceding section indicate that orienting reflexes, while they may be less likely to occur in hippocampal subjects, do habituate normally when they occur. The arrest reaction, the GSR, and cardiac orienting reflexes are indices of orienting, but it is important to note that they may be quite independent of behavioral orienting (such as, for example, moving toward a sound source). Remarkably little work has been carried out on such specific behavioral orienting in hippocampal subjects, although much has been done on general environmental exploration. But when either specific or general exploration is studied, the effects of hippocampal lesions are clear: they slow its decline and raise the question whether hippocampal lesions impair the habituation of exploration.

Kaye and Pearce (1987) investigated the behavioral reactions of hippocampal rats to presentations of a light stimulus in a familiar test chamber. They scored orienting reflexes, which they defined as touching the light bulb, rearing in front of it, or standing with the tip of the snout almost touching the bulb. It can be seen that these responses involve more than a simple orientation toward the bulb and constitute in effect active investigative or exploratory responses. Kaye and Pearce (see figure 3.3) found that these investigative responses, which began at a level similar to that seen in controls, showed a very much reduced decline over a series of daily sessions.

The Kaye and Pearce report may be considered along with a large number of reports that indicate that hippocampal animals show exaggerated persistence of exploratory behavior when exposed to novel environments (for a review, see O'Keefe and Nadel 1978). One way of describing these

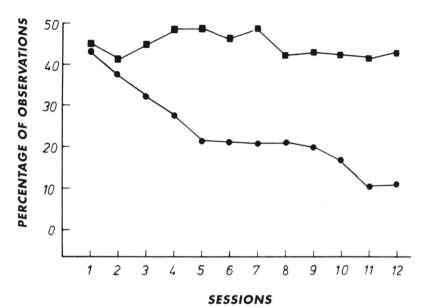

FIGURE 3.3. Effect of hippocampal lesions on repeatedly elicited orienting reflexes. A 10-sec light stimulus was presented 6 times on each of 12 sessions with an interstimulus interval of 6 min, and rats were observed twice during each light presentation (once 4 sec after light onset, and once 5 sec later). The graph shows the percentage of observations that comprised an orienting reflex in rats having hippocampal lesions (squares) and in sham-operated control rats (circles). (*From* Kaye and Pearce 1987)

results is to conclude that hippocampal lesions disrupt the habituation of exploratory behavior. But we have already seen that the hippocampus plays no general role in habituation; there is virtually no support for the view that the hippocampus disrupts habituation of any response other than exploratory responding. Could the effect on exploration be described in a way that does not suppose a response-specific disruption of habituation?

O'Keefe and Nadel (1978) have proposed that the hippocampus contains a spatial map which in normal animals serves to detect novelty, by which is meant a novel environment, a novel stimulus in a familiar environment, or a familiar stimulus in a novel place within an environment. Novelty, according to this view, is a context-specific property, and an animal without knowledge of a context (obtained through the spatial mapping system) would neither detect novelty nor be stimulated by novelty to engage in exploratory behavior. Their argument, then, is that hippocampal animals do not explore and that the behavior seen in novel environments in hippocampal subjects is not in reality exploratory at all, but rather a generalized increase in reactivity to stimuli of all kinds. They also make the very reasonable logical point that to call behavior "exploratory" when it in fact shows no (or very little) progressive decline amounts to a contradiction in terms.

The spatial map theory of hippocampal function will be discussed more fully in chapter 7, and we shall concentrate here on the claim that the "exploratory" behavior of hippocampal animals is a symptom of generalized hyperreactivity. Applied to reports of "exploration" of novel environments, this is not an unreasonable account, since the reports concerned in fact record the gross amount of ambulation within the apparatus, or some fairly direct correlate of ambulation. But it does not seem to apply to the Kaye and Pearce (1987) data, which specifically concerned exploratory responses, responses that could not simply be regarded as general activity but that showed active investigation of the novel stimulus. Since Kaye and Pearce reported a pattern of results very similar to those obtained in studies on general activity in novel environments, it is more economical to conclude that hippocampal lesions do not obliterate exploratory behavior but that, on the contrary, they prolong it. Why should this be?

An alternative proposal is that the hippocampus is involved in recognition memory. Exploratory behavior is initiated when a stimulus or an environment is not recognized. Given that hippocampal subjects have severely impaired recognition capacity, they will accordingly show enhanced and prolonged exploratory behavior. But where a stimulus does not elicit exploratory behavior from hippocampal animals, habituation of the behavior that *is* elicited will proceed normally.

The notion that the hippocampus is involved in recognition memory will be discussed more fully in chapter 8, but it is important to note here that the term "recognition" is being used in a somewhat specialized sense. The fact that habituation can proceed normally in hippocampal animals implies that the difference between novel and previously experienced stimuli is detected normally without the aid of the hippocampus. The suggestion under consideration here is that some low-level system is involved in habituation and allows discrimination between novel and familiar stimuli, but that that system operates independently of a higher-level cognitive system of recognition intimately involved in, for example, the initiation of voluntary activity, such as exploration; the notion is derived in part from human data (to be discussed in chapter 8), which indicate that humans with hippocampal damage may learn to respond appropriately to stimuli they do not consciously recognize. The stimuli are, then, clearly familiar in the sense that they elicit the appropriate response; but they are, nevertheless, not consciously recognized.

This interpretation of hippocampal function may also explain the perplexing fact that distractors sometimes obtain increased disruption in hippocampals, and sometimes no disruption. In general, distractors are less effective (or even wholly ineffective) in hippocampals when they are presented while animals are engaged in some other motivated behavior, such as lever pressing for food, but more effective when not presented in competition with another behavior (for a review, see O'Keefe and Nadel 1978). According to the recognition memory account, since no environment is fully recognized as familiar by hippocampal subjects, the presentation in an environment of a novel stimulus will be a less salient event— merely one more novel stimulus in a background of (relatively) novel stimuli; so, interruption of motivated behavior will be less likely. But given that the stimulus does initiate investigation, which it is more likely to do in a noncompetitive situation, that investigation will indeed be prolonged in hippocampal subjects.

In summary, the data may be accommodated by the proposal that the hippocampus does not play any role in habituation but that, as a consequence of the role of the hippocampus in recognition, exploratory behavior is both less likely to be initiated and slower to be terminated in hippocampal animals. The application of this notion may further be illustrated by considering some data reported by Gustafson and Koenig (1979). Hungry rats were trained to press for food on a schedule yielding one reward for every eighth response. A novel stimulus (intermittent interruption of the background white noise and of the houselight) was presented twice each session for a number of sessions. They reported that hippocampals and normals both showed a brief arrest reaction to initial presentations of the stimulus; normals, however, initially showed extensive exploration of the test chamber following the initial orienting, and this response was not seen in hippocampals. Habituation of the arrest reaction proceeded rapidly in hippocampals, and this implies that the (brief) orienting reflex habituated normally. In this experiment, then, exploration was not elicited in hippocampals and there was no deficit in habituation of the response that *was* elicited.

It can hardly be claimed that the interpretation offered here will accommodate all the available data without some strain. For example, Leaton (1981) found comparable absolute durations of arrest reactions in hippocampal and normal rats (and comparable rates of habituation). According to the present view, the absence of disruption in hippocampals indicates that no exploratory responding was involved (in either group). But the arrest reactions to the initial presentations of distractors were fairly prolonged, well over a minute in duration: it might seem surprising that such lengthy interruption occurred without initiating any active investigatory behavior. But precisely what the subjects were doing while not licking was not recorded, and this same difficulty applies to many other reports of distraction. The explanation offered here provides an economical account of the data, and a more extended discussion of the potential role of the hippocampus in recognition will be presented in chapter 8.

Summary and Conclusions

This survey of lesion data has found no support for the physiological aspects of Sokolov's theorizing. Various components of the orienting reflex show normal short-term habituation in the absence of neocortex, and there is evidence that long-term habituation is also possible for at least some components in the absence of neocortex. It does not, then, seem that the neocortex is necessary for the elaboration of a "neuronal model" of a stimulus. Similarly, there is little encouragement for the view that the hippocampus functions as a "comparator." Although damage to the hippocampus does exaggerate exploratory responding (once initiated), Sokolov distinguishes between such responding and the orienting reflex proper. And there is clear evidence that components of the orienting reflex, such as arrest reactions and autonomic changes, may habituate normally in hippocampal subjects. Since we have also seen reason to doubt the interpretation of the electrophysiological recording data that had been supposed to support Sokolov's account, we may now reject Sokolov's physiological speculations.

The hippocampus is critically involved in exploratory behavior, and that involvement can be accommodated by the notion that the hippocampus plays a role in recognition memory. That conclusion in turn suggests that more than one system must be involved in distinguishing between novel and familiar stimuli, and this is a point to which we shall return at the end of the chapter.

Extrinsic Versus Intrinsic Theories of Habituation

Priming Theory

Two of the three extrinsic theories introduced at the beginning of this chapter have now been rejected. The third, Wagner's priming theory, remains, however, a coherent alternative to the intrinsic account of habituation, and we should now consider the relevance of physiological work to that theory.

The Distinction Between Short-Term Habituation and Long-Term Habituation

It might seem at first sight that the distinction established physiologically between short-term habituation and long-term habituation provides good support for Wagner's contention that two separate processes are responsible for the prerepresentation of stimuli in short-term memory. But the properties of short-term habituation seem to be similar in spinal animals to those in intact animals, and the notion that spinal animals possess a limited capacity short-term memory seems considerably less plausible than the proposal that short-term habituation is due to homosynaptic depression within the S-R pathway. It is also the case that the time constants of the processes of habituation revealed by certain lesions do not seem to correspond to those one would expect of either short-term memory or long-term memory. Both Leaton, Cassella, and Borszcz (1985), who used decerebrate rats, and Klosterhalfen and Klosterhalfen (1985), who used functionally decorticate rats, reported that although no between-day retention of habituation was observed, between-session retention was found, using intersession intervals of approximately 30 min. Self-generated priming would be expected to decay in very much less than 30 min (e.g., Whitlow 1975), and if retrieval-generated priming was effective after 30 min, it is not clear why it should not also have been effective after 24 hours.

Habituation and Latent Inhibition

One further difficulty for Wagner's theory concerns a phenomenon closely related to habituation. If a CS is presented to animals on a number of occasions prior to subsequent pairings with a UCS in a conditioning paradigm, then the rate of conditioning is typically retarded as compared to that seen in a group for which the CS is novel when pairings commence. This effect is known as latent inhibition, and a number of reports have shown that latent inhibition is attenuated or abolished by hippocampal lesions (e.g., Ackil et al. 1969; Solomon and Moore 1975; Kaye and Pearce 1987). Wagner's account of latent inhibition is the same as his account of long-term habituation: the prior presentations of the CS result in an association between the context and the CS. The context therefore elicits from long-term memory a representation of the CS in short-term memory: this prevents the CS from full representation in short-term memory and so reduces the amount of coprocessing of the CS and UCS. Since the amount of coprocessing determines the strength of the association formed, prior exposure of a CS leads to a reduced rate of association formation.

We have seen that hippocampal lesions do not in general attenuate the rate of habituation, although they do disrupt latent inhibition. While this would appear to contradict Wagner's account of the phenomenon, it will be recalled that Kaye and Pearce (1987) found that "habituation" of investigatory "orienting reflexes" *was* disrupted in their experiment: could Wagner's theory of habituation be modified so as to apply only to investigatory responses? This does not seem likely, first, because there is no obvious rationale for any such restrictions, and second, because Wagner (e.g., Wagner 1976) has used in support of his account data drawn from studies using a wide range of response measures, none of which involved investigatory responses. In particular, Wagner cites studies of the acoustic startle response, and it is quite clear that hippocampal lesions have no effect on habituation of acoustic startle (Leaton 1981). There are, moreover, behavioral studies that show major differences between latent inhibition and habituation: Hall and Channell (1985) have, for example, shown that whereas latent inhibition is abolished by a change in context (as Wagner would predict), habituation is not. This study is of particular relevance since the response used for assessment of habituation was in fact an active investigatory response similar to that scored by Kaye and Pearce (1987).

Dual-Process Theory

Relevance of Work on Simpler Systems

Chapter 2 found good support in work on simple systems for the notion that habituation (both short-term and long-term) is a process intrinsic to the S-R pathway. The work reviewed in this chapter provides further support for an intrinsic account of short-term habituation, and this measure of agreement encourages the notion that work on invertebrate and spinal vertebrate preparations does promise to yield physiological insights that will be relevant to vertebrate brain systems.

The behavioral parallels between habituation in *Aplysia* and habituation in intact vertebrates are sufficiently striking that we may surely conclude that the processes involved are either closely similar or identical. But correspondence between processes whose similarity may well have emerged through quite different evolutionary stages—a correspondence that may reflect evolutionary convergence—does not necessarily imply correspondence between the neural implementation of those processes. It could have been that an understanding of the neuronal bases of habituation in *Aplysia* would have thrown no light on its mechanisms in vertebrates. Similarly, of course, it could have been the case that mechanisms uncovered in spinal vertebrates would have had little relevance to the physiology of processes seen in supraspinal reflexes of intact vertebrates. The general agreement in all these preparations that short-term habituation, at least, involves mechanisms that are intrinsic to the S-R pathway argues that detailed analysis of processes in simpler systems may be directly relevant to those processes in intact vertebrates.

Long-Term Habituation Involves Extrinsic Mechanisms

A major modification of two-process theory is required as a result of demonstrations that long-term habituation of supraspinal reflexes does involve mechanisms extrinsic to the S-R pathway. Little is known of those mechanisms, although we have seen evidence for a role of both the cerebellar vermis and the midbrain reticular formation. It is not yet clear what the behavioral implications of that distinction may be: we have seen that Wagner's priming theory, the only theory that predicts an important distinction between short-term habituation and long-term habituation, did not succeed in providing a good overall account of the data. The physiological distinction between short-term habituation and long-term habituation does not necessarily imply, for example, that long-term habituation involves the storage (outside the S-R pathway) of a representation of a stimulus; the distinction is equally compatible with the basic psychological notion at the heart of the intrinsic account, namely that the repeated elicitation by a stimulus of a response leads in a straightforward and relatively simple way to the reduced effectiveness of that stimulus. But this account of habituation should not be accepted without some consideration of its broader implications.

Implications of an Intrinsic Account of Habituation

One very reasonable view of habituation is that it provides a mechanism through which an organism may learn to ignore unimportant stimuli. It is this view that provides a rationale for "extrinsic" theories of habituation such as those of Sokolov and Wagner. Extrinsic theories allow an organism first to recognize a previously presented stimulus and then either to ignore it, if it has had no significant consequence associated with it, or to respond to it appropriately according to some associated consequence of significance. But "intrinsic" theories suppose that the very use of a synapse in an S-R pathway leads to a decline in its subsequent efficiency. Such theories have a problem in dealing with the case in which a stimulus—as in a conditioning paradigm—is associated with an important consequence. If homosynaptic depression is an inevitable consequence of synapse use, how can information about stimuli that signal important events continue to be transmitted efficiently? One way to approach this issue is to consider the neurophysiological correlates of conditioning, and the processing of conditioned stimuli in particular. This will be one of the central topics of interest in chapters 4 and 5.

This review of the physiological bases of habituation has led to a view of habituation in intact animals that conflicts with a common sense view involving recognition as a critical step. The interpretation preferred here supposes that habituation is a process that is independent of recognition, and that relies on different neuronal mechanisms. A recent review of behavioral data on habituation and related topics has also concluded that habituation and recognition are independent processes (Mackintosh 1987). The congruence that has emerged between behavioral and physiological analyses constitutes a convincing case for the distinction proposed. But Mackintosh (1987) also argues that there is no substantive difference between short-term habituation and long-term habituation, and no difference either between sensitization and dishabituation; in each case, Mackintosh provides alternative accounts of behavioral data that might seem to support the distinctions. The physiological evidence of a real difference between short-term habituation and long-term habituation is strong, and this should encourage psychologists to seek more solid evidence than is currently available of major behavioral differences between short-term habituation and long-term habituation. Similarly, the case for a real distinction between sensitization and dishabituation is supported in *Aplysia* by both physiological and behavioral data. To the extent that we accept the case of the relevance of invertebrate data to vertebrates, this should again promote interest in a search for differences between sensitization and dishabituation in vertebrates. What is clear from both the agreement and the disagreement between behavioral and physiological analyses is that physiological psychology does make important and relevant contributions to theories of cognitive activity in intact organisms.

4. Association Formation in Simple Systems

The Physiological Analysis of Conditioning

In this chapter we begin consideration of the physiology of association formation, the topic that has traditionally been at the center of behavioral learning theory. The behavioral procedures used in experiments on association formation are generally fairly simple, but this should not obscure either the fact that it has proved exceedingly difficult for psychologists to produce convincing theoretical accounts of the phenomena concerned or the possibility that association formation may constitute the major component of nonhuman intelligence (Macphail 1987). Any contribution that physiological techniques can provide to our understanding of association formation will therefore be valuable and potentially of very general relevance.

This major part of this chapter will focus on conditioning in two invertebrate species. Work is proceeding using other invertebrates (Mpitsos and Lukowiak 1985), but the most complete accounts of the physiology of conditioning have been obtained from the species to be described here. The many advantages of using invertebrates have been previously outlined (in chapter 2), and here again we look to the relative simplicity and ease of access of their nervous systems for a better opportunity of understanding the basic physiological events associated with conditioning. The chapter will go on finally to discuss conditioning in spinal vertebrates, and will reencounter there some of the difficulties in analyzing those preparations that were encountered in chapter 2.

Two Types of Conditioning Procedure

The procedures used for exploring association formation fall into two general classes: classical (or Pavlovian) procedures and instrumental procedures. In classical procedures, the experimenter arranges a contingency between two stimuli so that one stimulus, the CS, reliably signals the imminent occurrence of another stimulus, usually of biological significance (the UCS). The behavior of the animal is irrelevant to the occurrence of either stimulus, but the typical outcome is that the subject comes to respond to the CS in a way that closely resembles the response elicited by the UCS. Thus if a bell signals the delivery of food to a hungry dog, the dog comes eventually to salivate to the bell.

In instrumental procedures, a contingency is arranged between some response made by an animal and the delivery (or nondelivery) of a UCS; thus food may be delivered for pressing a lever, or shock may be avoided by jumping over a hurdle. In this case, the animal's response is instrumental in obtaining (or avoiding) the UCS, and the form of the conditioned response (CR) does not normally resemble the UCR to the UCS employed.

Experiments on simple systems have concentrated almost exclusively on classical training procedures, which have the advantage that the experimenter has complete control over the series of events involved in training the animals; when instrumental procedures are used, the delivery of UCSs depends upon the behavior of the animal, and this may result in problems in preparations that show low levels of "spontaneous" responding (in, for example, species whose demeanor is regarded as "sluggish").

Psychologists use simple conditioning paradigms to explore questions about the formation of associations. When, for example, a dog begins to salivate in response to a bell that regularly precedes food, we may conclude that an association has been formed. But we may not be certain about what events have been associated. The bell (or an internal representation of it) may now be associated with the food (and activation of the representation of food elicits salivation), or it might be associated directly with the response of salivation itself (since that response was as regularly preceded by the bell as was the food). One way in which the true nature of the association might be revealed would be to track the changes in neuronal activity that accompany association formation, to follow the path from sensory input to motor output. We shall see, for example, that much of the physiological work adopting this strategy for simple systems has suggested that conditioning involves the strengthening of preexisting excitatory connections between a stimulus and a response—a proposal that runs counter to much current behavioral theorizing. One goal of this work is, then, to establish *where* modifications occur as a consequence of conditioning.

If the first question to be pursued is, where do conditioning-related changes occur, the second is, what is the nature of the changes that do occur? The sorts of question likely to be of interest here have been foreshadowed in chapters 2 and 3: do the changes involve alterations in the excitability of whole neurons or of specific synapses in neurons? Are the changes presynaptic, postsynaptic, or both? And are there distinguishable changes associated with short-term and long-term retention of associations?

One major new question will also arise. Associations involve the contingent pairings of stimuli, and associations are not formed when two stimuli are presented independently of each other in, for example, a random sequence. What mechanism could obtain changes in synaptic (or neuronal) efficiency that are specific to paired, as opposed to randomly ordered stimuli?

Conditioning in *Aplysia*

Basic Behavioral Findings

A number of techniques have been used successfully to obtain conditioning in *Aplysia*. The procedure that has been most thoroughly examined physiologically concerns the gill- and siphon-withdrawal response. Carew, Hawkins, and Kandel (1983) explored discriminative conditioning using two types of CS, one being brief tactile stimulation of the siphon, the other brief (0.5 sec) weak electrical stimulation of the mantle. A strong 1-sec tail shock, which elicited a long-lasting siphon-withdrawal response, served as UCS, and the CR measured was siphon withdrawal. Each animal experienced both CSs. One (CS +) immediately preceded UCS onset (and terminated at UCS onset); the other (CS −) followed the UCS by 2.5 min, and preceded the next CS + by 2.5 min. For some animals, CS + was siphon stimulation, and CS −, mantle stimulation, and vice versa for other animals. Fifteen training trials were administered and, after an interval of 30 min, responding to CS + and CS − presented alone was measured. Figure 4.1 shows that CS + elicited a CR of significantly longer duration than that elicited by the CS −, and this constituted good evidence for differential conditioning to the two CSs.

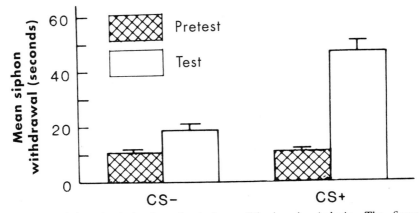

FIGURE 4.1. Discriminative classical conditioning in *Aplysia*. The figure shows mean siphon withdrawal (with standard error indicated) to CS + and CS − in a test carried out prior to training and in a test carried out 30 min after the end of training. Data are pooled over the two types of CS (mantle and siphon stimulation) used; for further details, see text. (*From* Carew, Hawkins, and Kandel 1983)

One important feature of this procedure is that both of the stimuli used as CSs in fact obtained siphon withdrawal prior to training. The major effect of the conditioning procedure was not to establish siphon withdrawal to CS +, but to prolong it. Another important feature is that the withdrawal response to CS − was also prolonged by the training, but to a lesser extent than that to CS +. The response to CS − was, then, sensitized by the training procedure, and the difference in the extent to which CS − was sensitized and the CS + response was increased may be presumed to reflect an associative process involving CS + and the UCS.

Carew, Hawkins, and Kandel (1983) further reported that both sensitization of CS − and the magnitude of the differential effect of training on CS − and CS + increased as the number of training trials increased from one to five to fifteen. Significant retention (up to three days later) of the discrimination was observed after one training trial. Perhaps more surprisingly, both sensitization and the degree of discrimination were larger 24 hours after training than one hour afterward. Exploration of CS-UCS intervals found optimal conditioning to CS + using the 0.5-sec interval referred to above: an interval of 1 sec produced weaker conditioning, and intervals of from 2 to 10 sec produced no conditioning. Finally, a backward-conditioning procedure, in which CS was delivered either immediately or .5 sec after UCS offset, produced no conditioning.

Using a similar paradigm, Carew, Hawkins, and Kandel (1983) found that differential conditioning could also be established to two stimuli delivered to different sites (one dorsal, one ventral) on the siphon. In this case, .5 sec weak electrical stimuli delivered through fine electrodes implanted in the siphon served as CSs. After five training trials, significant discrimination between CS + and CS − was demonstrated on testing 15 to 30 min later. Since all the cell bodies of the sensory neurons innervating the siphon lie in the LE cluster, this indicates that differential conditioning of the withdrawal response can be established using stimuli that activate neurons within the same cell cluster.

Physiological Correlates

Conditioning Involves a Change in Synaptic Efficacy

A number of studies agree in showing that conditioning obtains an increased effectiveness of monosynaptic connections between a sensory and a motor neuron. Hawkins et al. (1983) used a preparation consisting of the *Aplysia* central nervous system isolated from the rest of the body except for the posterior pedal nerve connectives to the tail region. Three cell bodies were impaled by microelectrodes. Two were of siphon mechanoreceptor neurons, the third was a siphon motoneuron from which monosynaptic EPSPs could be recorded when stimulating either mechanoreceptor neuron (see figure 4.2).

The experimental design used by Hawkins et al. (1983) was basically the same as that used by Carew, Hawkins, and Kandel (1983), except that the CS now consisted of stimulation of a mechanoreceptor neuron so that a train of five spikes was elicited, and the CR consisted of the resulting EPSPs in the motoneuron. UCS was a strong shock to either the tail or the posterior pedal nerve. Stimulation of one sensory neuron served as CS +, and preceded motoneuron stimulation by .5 sec; stimulation of the other neuron, CS −, followed the UCS by 2.5 min.

Figure 4.3 shows that over the course of five conditioning trials the magnitudes of the EPSPs (expressed as percentages of pretraining levels) to CS + and CS − rapidly diverged and, when tested 5 or 15 min after five trials, CS + showed a significant increase in EPSP, whereas CS − showed a decrease.

A similar rationale underlies an independent report by Walters and Byrne (1983). These workers measured monosynaptic EPSPs obtained by

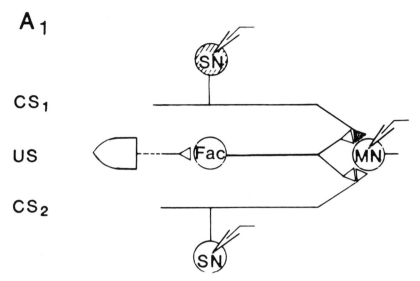

FIGURE 4.2. Schematic representation of the experimental arrangement used by Hawkins et al. (1983). Delivery of US (tail shock) activates facilitatory interneurons that obtain presynaptic facilitation of sensory neuron (SN) terminals onto motoneurons (MN). Shading indicates that stimulation of one sensory neuron is paired with US delivery. (*From* Hawkins et al. 1983)

intracellular stimulation of three individual tail mechanoreceptor neurons (in the left pleural ganglion) in a single tail motoneuron (in the left pedal ganglion). In the training phase, stimulation of one sensory neuron (CS+) was paired with the UCS, a strong tail shock, stimulation of a second neuron (CS−) was explicitly unpaired, and the third neuron, which served as a sensitization control, was not stimulated. Walters and Byrne (1983) reported that after five training trials EPSPs elicited by CS+ now were significantly larger than those elicited by stimulation of either CS− or the sensitization control neuron. EPSPs in fact increased over the course of training (and the CS− EPSPs tended to be larger than those of the sensitization controls). A subsequent report using similar procedures established that the enhanced EPSPs obtained following conditioning were maintained for 24 hours (Buonomano and Byrne 1990); it seems likely, therefore, that both short- and long-term retention of conditioning are mediated by enhanced synaptic efficacy.

The behavioral experiments of Carew, Hawkins, and Kandel (1983) assessed changes in the duration of siphon withdrawal, whereas the corresponding physiological studies (Hawkins et al. 1983) scored changes in

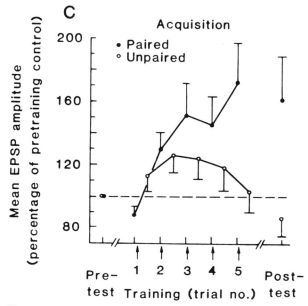

FIGURE 4.3. Development of differential facilitation of EPSPs elicited by stimulation of a sensory nerve when stimulation is paired with tail shock delivery. For further details, see text. (*From* Hawkins et al. 1983)

EPSP magnitude. There are, however, good reasons for supposing that increased EPSP magnitude could result in prolonged motoneuron activation (Hawkins et al. 1983), and it is reasonable to conclude that the physiological events discussed by Hawkins et al. (1983) do contribute to the behavioral changes of the sort reported by Carew, Hawkins, and Kandel (1983).

Conditioning Obtains Spike-Broadening in Sensory Neurons

The increase in efficacy of spikes in sensory neurons (as assessed by EPSP magnitude in motoneurons) recalls, of course, the physiological analysis of sensitization discussed in chapter 2. Hawkins et al. (1983) accordingly proceeded to ask whether the increased efficacy of the CS + mechanoreceptor neurons appeared due to the same processes that underlie sensitization.

Using similar general training procedures, Hawkins et al. (1983) went on to measure the duration of action potentials elicited in sensory neurons whose stimulation was either paired (CS +) or unpaired (CS −) with tail shock. When tested 5 to 15 min after a series of fifteen training trials, CS + neurons showed significantly prolonged action potentials, whereas those of CS − neurons were not significantly altered (see figure 4.4). Further experiments indicated that the increased duration of action potentials was associated with a decreased outward K^+ current. Since spike-broadening with a decreased K^+ current is the major mechanism of sensitization, these findings encourage the view that mechanisms of conditioning and sensitization in *Aplysia* have much in common.

Alternative Mechanisms for Pairing-Specificity

It is clear, from both the Hawkins et al. (1983) and the Walters and Byrne (1983) reports, that the differential effect of paired versus unpaired stimuli cannot simply be due to sensitization by UCS presentations: those reports agreed in finding that CSs that were presented against a background of UCSs but were not paired so that their onset reliably preceded UCS onset obtained significantly smaller CRs than did CSs that were explicitly paired. Temporal pairing of CS and UCS was, then, a critical factor and it is, of course, precisely that feature which implies that a genuine associative process is involved. A number of potential physiological interpre-

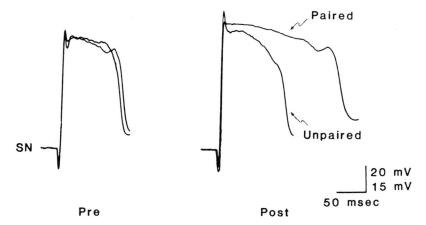

FIGURE 4.4. Superimposed action potentials of two sensory neurons before (Pre-) and three hours after (Post-) training in which stimulation of one neuron had been paired with tail shock and stimulation of the other neuron had been unpaired. The action potentials were recorded in the presence of tetraethylammonium, which decreases the K^+ current and thus broadens the action potential, making any changes in spike duration more apparent. (*From* Hawkins et al. 1983)

tations of the significance of temporal pairing have been made, of which two are currently of prime interest.

Hebb's Postulate. The first account to be considered here of the significance of pairing is due to Hebb, who proposed that: "When an axon of cell A is near enough to excite a cell B and repeatedly or persistently takes part in firing it, some growth process or metabolic change takes place in one or both cells such that A's efficiency, as one of the cells firing B, is increased" (Hebb 1949/1961:62). This postulate is sometimes known as the "successful use" postulate, since (see figure 4.5) the essential requirement for plasticity is that activity in the presynaptic cell is followed by activity in the postsynaptic cell.

Applied to *Aplysia,* Hebb's notion is that the synaptic connection between the paired sensory neuron and the motoneuron is strengthened because of the virtually simultaneous firing of the sensory and the motor neuron. Two implications of this proposal are, first, that direct stimulation of the motoneuron should serve as a successful UCS, and, second, that if firing of the motoneuron in response to the UCS is prevented, conditioning should not occur. Hawkins et al. (1983) report, however, that direct motoneuron stimulation does not serve as an effective UCS, and that conditioning *does* occur if the motoneuron is hyperpolarized and prevented from firing throughout the training period. Both of these findings suggest that the synapse is *not* modified according to Hebbian principles; and since CS activity is not sufficient in itself and UCS activity appears to be irrelevant, the implication is that interneurons are involved in modification of the relevant synapse.

Activity-Dependent Presynaptic Facilitation. A second interpretation (see figure 4.6), which does involve interneurons, is that presynaptic facilitation, the mechanism proposed for sensitization by Kandel and his colleagues, is amplified by recent preceding spike activity in a cell. This is the proposal, based on an early suggestion of Kandel and Tauc (1965), that is preferred by both Hawkins et al. (1983) and Walters and Byrne (1983). Two reports provide direct support for this notion of activity-dependent facilitation. Using preparations in which isolated clusters of sensory neuron cell bodies were exposed to a brief "puff" of serotonin-rich solution, both Abrams et al. (1984) and Ocorr, Walters, and Byrne (1985) have reported that the increase in cAMP content obtained by the serotonin puffs was enhanced if the puffs were immediately preceded by activation of the sensory neurons. Short-term sensitization is believed to be mediated by the increase in cAMP levels obtained by facilitatory stim-

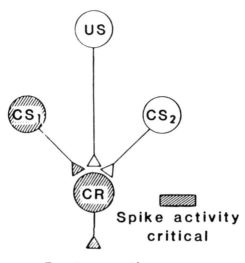

**Spike activity
critical**

**Postsynaptic
activity dependent
facilitation
(Hebb synapse)**

FIGURE 4.5. Schematic representation of Hebb's postulate. The synapse between a neuron activated by a CS paired with a US (CS_1) and a neuron involved in motor output (CR) is strengthened because activity in CS_1 coincides with activity (obtained by US activation) in CR. Neurons activated by unpaired stimuli (e.g., CS_2) show no facilitation of synaptic transmission because their activity does not coincide with CR activity. Cells whose activity is critical for synaptic facilitation are indicated by shading. (*From* Hawkins et al. 1983)

ulation; these results suggest that a similar mechanism could underlie short-term retention of conditioning.

If the degree of sensitization that is obtained by an intense stimulus is activity-dependent in the way suggested, one question that now arises is, how does the preceding spike interact with the processes of presynaptic facilitation? Kandel et al. (1983) suggest that it is the Ca^{2+} influx associated with the invasion of terminals by a spike which interacts with the

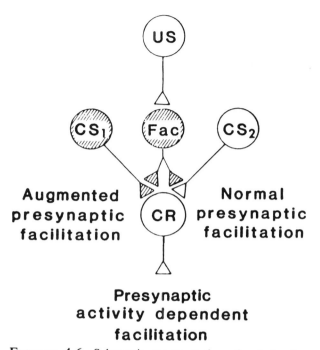

**Presynaptic
activity dependent
facilitation**

FIGURE 4.6. Schematic representation of activity dependent modulation of presynaptic facilitation. Activity in facilitatory interneurons (Fac) obtains presynaptic facilitation of all sensorimotor synapses, including those activated by unpaired stimuli (e.g., CS$_2$). But facilitation of the synapse between a neuron activated by a CS paired with a US (CS$_1$) and a neuron involved in the motor output obtained by the US (CR) is enhanced because activity in facilitatory interneurons (activated by the US) coincides with activity in CS$_1$. Cells whose activity is critical for enhanced presynaptic facilitation are indicated by shading. (*From* Hawkins et al. 1983)

facilitatory processes. Evidence for this view is provided by the finding that if spikes are elicited in sensory cells in a Ca^{2+}-free solution, then serotonin puffs do not obtain facilitation (spike-broadening) when subsequently tested in a standard solution. One final issue concerns the aspect of facilitation that Ca^{2+} influx might modulate. There is currently very little evidence on this issue, but Abrams and Kandel (1988) propose that the Ca^{2+} influx may "prime" the adenylate cyclase system which regulates the production of cAMP, and they cite evidence that Ca^{2+}, acting via the

Ca^{2+}-dependent regulatory protein calmodulin, does stimulate adenylate cyclase activity in *Aplysia*.

Although these proposals go a long way toward explaining the superior effectiveness of paired as opposed to unpaired stimuli in obtaining enhanced responding, they do not, as Abrams and Kandel (1988) acknowledge, fully account for the demanding temporal requirements of classical conditioning: in particular, they do not explain why CS onset should precede UCS onset. This is a problem that should be borne in mind when considering, at a later stage in this chapter, the difficulties encountered with temporal factors in conditioning in *Hermissenda*.

The account outlined above of the physiology of conditioning in *Aplysia* suggests that conditioning in those animals is a species of sensitization, so that by understanding the mechanisms of sensitization we would understand conditioning also. Currently, then, we may assume that short-term retention of conditioning may be mediated by elevated cAMP levels in sensory nerve terminals, and that long-term retention is mediated by some permanent structural change for which the building of new protein is required (figure 4.7 summarizes our current understanding of the mechanisms of activity-dependent presynaptic facilitation). Although we have seen support for both those propositions for short- and long-term retention of sensitization, comparable evidence specific to conditioning is not yet available.

Conditioning as a Form of Sensitization

The physiological analysis of association formation has progressed further in *Aplysia* than in any other species, vertebrate or invertebrate. The success of this work naturally leads to questions concerning the likelihood that conclusions reached using *Aplysia* may be generalized to other species, and to vertebrate species in particular. This is an issue that will be discussed more fully in a later section, in which the general relevance of molluscan conditioning to vertebrate conditioning is discussed. At this point it is appropriate, however, to note one difficulty facing acceptance of the mechanisms described for conditioning in *Aplysia* as models for mechanisms that may exist in other species. The major peculiarity in the account advanced for *Aplysia* is precisely the notion that conditioning might be a form of sensitization. This seems to imply that *Aplysia* could learn only associations in which excitatory connections between CS and CR exist prior to training (a type of conditioning known in the vertebrate literature as "alpha" conditioning). It is true that there have been reports of the development of CRs in *Aplysia* that differ in form from the UCR

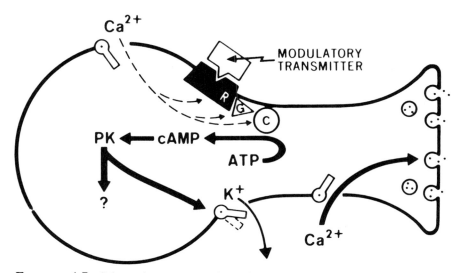

FIGURE 4.7. Schematic representation of activity-dependent enhancement of presynaptic facilitation. Initial influx of Ca^{2+}, caused by spike activity (obtained by CS delivery), affects one or more components of the adenylate cyclase complex: possible targets indicated here are the receptor (R) activated by the facilitatory transmitter, coupling proteins (G), and adenylate cyclase (C). Subsequent activation of cyclase through modulatory transmitter (a consequence of the activation by the UCS of facilitatory interneurons) results in amplification of cAMP production. This amplification obtains enhanced transmitter release to subsequent test stimuli relative to that produced by modulatory transmitter that has not been preceded by spike activity. For further details of mechanisms of sensitization, see fig. 2.10. (*From* Byrne 1987)

initially elicited by the CS, and resemble, instead, the UCR elicited by the UCS (e.g., Walters 1989; Hawkins et al. 1989). But these reports do not require rejection of the notion that classical conditioning involves the facilitation of preexisting excitatory connections. It will be recalled from chapter 2 that branch-specific heterosynaptic facilitation has been observed in *Aplysia,* and that different UCSs differentially sensitize different UCRs (the phenomenon of pseudoconditioning). Sensory neurons may be expected to be connected with a number of motor neurons, more strongly with some than with others. UCSs that selectively sensitize some of the initially less weak connections of a CS will result in changes in the form of the CR so that it now resembles the UCR to the UCS rather than the response initially elicited by the CS. This does not, however, violate the basic principle that we have extracted—namely, that classical conditioning in *Aplysia* is a form of sensitization that facilitates preexisting excitatory connections.

If that principle is valid, then conditioning in *Aplysia* may differ in important ways from conditioning in other species (vertebrate and invertebrate). It is important to emphasize at this point that such a conclusion does not invalidate (or, indeed, have any bearing on) the physiological interpretation of conditioning in *Aplysia*. The general question whether we should expect or require precise correspondence between behavioral processes of different species will be taken up again after introducing work on another mollusk that is of interest, not least because it focuses on an example of conditioning that does not seem to be a species of sensitization.

Conditioning in *Hermissenda*

Basic Behavioral Findings

A second invertebrate preparation that has attracted intensive investigation is another gastropod mollusk, belonging to the same (opisthobranch) order as *Aplysia*, the nudibranch *Hermissenda crassicornis*. *Hermissenda* is a strikingly colored carnivorous marine slug, which can grow up to about 8 cm in length. Alkon and his colleagues have studied changes in behavior to light which are obtained when light presentations are paired with whole-body rotation (with the animal's head oriented toward the center of rotation) (see figure 4.8). Two changes have been observed. First, when light has been paired with rotation the normal positive phototaxis of *Hermissenda* is reduced: after pairing, *Hermissenda* are slower to initiate locomotion toward a light source. Second, whereas prior to pairings *Hermissenda* react to light onset by lengthening the foot (possibly preparatory to initiating locomotion), *Hermissenda* after pairing react to light onset by shortening the foot.

These behavioral changes seen in *Hermissenda* may be retained for several weeks, and show extinction if trained animals are subjected to a series of light-alone presentations; these changes are also (subject to certain qualifications that will emerge in a later section) pairing-specific. The changes appear, then, to be instances of conditioning.

As was the case with *Aplysia*, the CS (light) used in the work on *Hermissenda* is not neutral, in the sense that it elicits a UCR (positive phototaxis and foot-lengthening). But, in this case, the effect of pairing is not to sensitize but rather to inhibit or, in the case of foot-lengthening, to reverse the UCR. It is therefore of interest to know what physiological processes underlie conditioning in *Hermissenda*.

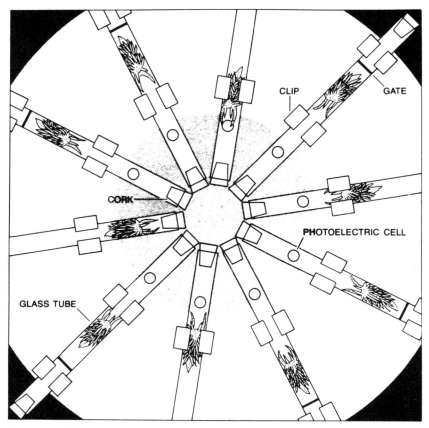

FIGURE 4.8. *Hermissenda* conditioning apparatus. The animals are placed in glass tubes on a turntable. The UCS consists in rotating the turntable while the *Hermissenda* are confined to the outer end of the tube and thus subjected to a centrifugal force that is sensed by the statocysts. CS consists of illumination of the whole apparatus. Strength of positive phototaxis response is assessed by directing a beam of light at the center of the apparatus and measuring the time taken by *Hermissenda* to interrupt the light detected by photoelectric cells at the central ends of the tubes. (*From* Alkon 1983)

Physiological Correlates

Increased Excitability of Type B Photoreceptors

Hermissenda possess two eyes, each of which contains five photoreceptors, two of which are labeled type A receptors, and three, type B. Type A and type B receptors are mutually inhibitory, and excitation of type A receptors obtains, via interneurons, excitation of motoneurons that drive the muscles involved in the locomotion of positive phototaxis (see figure 4.9). Alkon and his colleagues have traced the cause (at least in part) of the reduced phototaxis to an increased excitability of type B receptors: type B receptors following pairing react more strongly to light, which increases their inhibitory effect on type A receptors and so reduces the positive phototaxis elicited by type A activity. The increased excitability of type B cells can be shown to be localized to the cells themselves since they persist when the axons of the cells are severed, thus cutting off the soma from all synaptic input. The type B receptors also influence the activity of the motoneurons involved in foot contraction, but in this case their effect (mediated by interneurons) is excitatory (Lederhendler, Gart, and Alkon 1986; see figure 4.10). An increase in type B receptor excitability can therefore account for both reduced phototaxis and the foot-shortening response.

The increased excitability of type B receptors is associated with two consequences of pairings: first, the receptors show a cumulative long-lasting depolarization (LLD) following light offset and, second, they show an increased membrane input resistance. LLD contributes to increased excitability because a smaller potential change is required to obtain action potentials, and the increase in input resistance increases excitability because a given current across the membrane will induce a larger potential change. Since behavioral effects of conditioning may still be observed after the decay of LLD, it is the change in membrane resistance that is of central interest. The two effects are not, however, independent: in Alkon's scheme the cumulative LLD is responsible for the changes in input resistance.

Mechanisms of the Change in Excitability

The effects of rotation are detected by hair cells within two statocysts, the gravity organs of *Hermissenda*. When the animal's head points toward the center of rotation, rotation stimulates the caudal hair cells; when oriented away from the center, rotation stimulates the cephalad hair cells. The hair cells have direct reciprocal inhibitory connections with type B cells; hair cells also influence type B cell activity indirectly by inhibiting an interneuron cell pair in the optic ganglion (known as the S/E cell), which in turn excites type B cells. Those connections are summarized in figure 4.11.

In the absence of light, onset of rotation obtains a small hyperpolarization of type B cell activity, and offset is followed by a prolonged synaptic depolarization. The hyperpolarizing effect of rotation on type B cells is mediated by the direct and indirect inhibitory connections between the

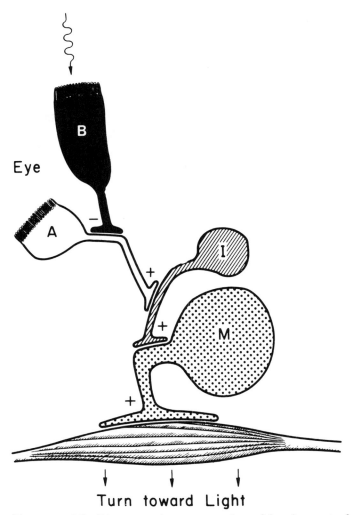

Eye

Turn toward Light

FIGURE 4.9. Diagrammatic representation of involvement of *Hermissenda* photoreceptors in positive phototaxis. Two types of photoreceptors (A and B) are activated by light. Type B receptors inhibit type A receptors, which activate excitatory interneurons (I) that in turn activate motoneurons (M) involved in positive phototaxis. (*Adapted from* West, Barnes, and Alkon 1982)

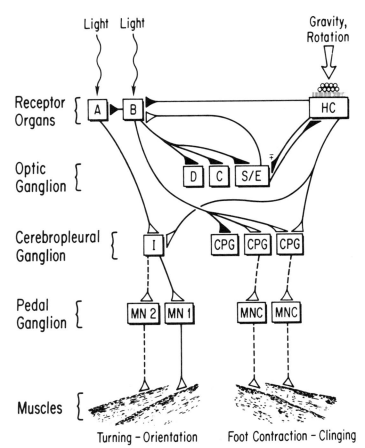

Light   Light

Gravity,
Rotation

Receptor
Organs

A   B   HC

Optic
Ganglion

D   C   S/E

Cerebropleural
Ganglion

I   CPG   CPG   CPG

Pedal
Ganglion

MN 2   MN 1   MNC   MNC

Muscles

Turning – Orientation   Foot Contraction – Clinging

FIGURE 4.10. Diagrammatic representation of established (solid lines) and hypothetical (broken lines) neuronal interconnections that underlie responses to light and rotation in *Hermissenda. Open endings:* excitatory synapses; *filled endings:* inhibitory synapses (with one exception, as indicated, from the hair cells to the S/E cell); A, B = photoreceptors, types A and B. HC = Hair cells; C, D, S/E = interneurons in the optic ganglion; I, CPG = interneurons in the cerebropleural ganglion; MN 1, MN 2 = motoneurons activating muscles involved in positive phototaxis; MNC = motoneurons activating muscles involved in foot-shortening. (*From* Lederhendler, Gart, and Alkon 1986)

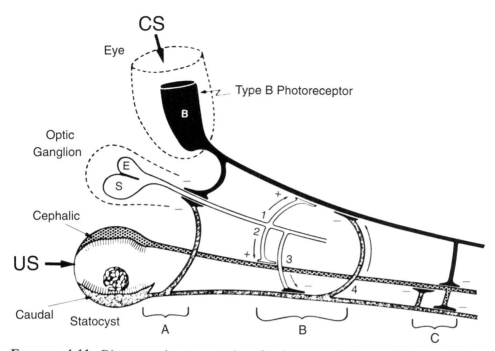

FIGURE 4.11. Diagrammatic representation of pathways mediating conditioning to light-rotation pairings in *Hermissenda*. A: Convergence of synaptic inhibition from type B photoreceptor and caudal hair cells on S/E cell. B: Positive feedback onto type B photoreceptor. 1, direct synaptic excitation. 2, indirect excitation (S/E cell excites cephalic hair cell that inhibits caudal hair cell and thus disinhibits type B cell). 3, indirect excitation (S/E cell inhibits caudal hair cell and thus disinhibits type B cell). C: Intra- and intersensory inhibition: cephalic and caudal hair cells are mutually inhibitory; type B cell inhibits mainly cephalic hair cell. Open endings: excitatory synapses (+); filled endings: inhibitory synapses (−). (*From* Byrne 1987)

hair cells and the type B cells. The depolarization following offset of rotation is believed to be due to the "rebound" activation of the S/E cell at the termination of inhibitory input from the hair cells; this rebound activation synaptically excites the type B cells.

In the absence of rotation, light onset obtains a depolarization of type B cells which is associated with a low input resistance; light offset is followed by an LLD of a few seconds or so, associated with a high input resistance. The major immediate effect (see figure 4.12) of simultaneous pairings of light and rotation is to enhance the LLD following light offset. This occurs partly because the LLD at light offset summates with the syn-

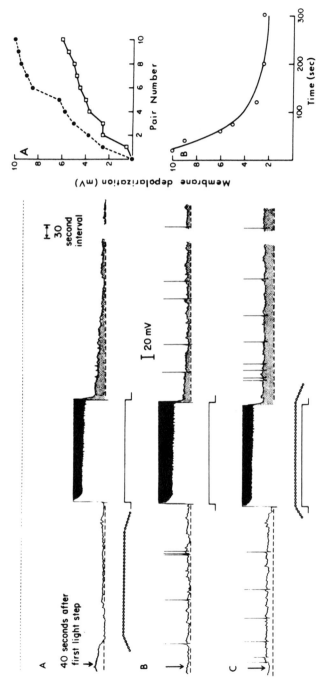

FIGURE 4.12. At left, intracellular recordings of *Hermissenda* neurons during and after light and rotation stimuli are shown; an isolated circumesophageal nervous system with intact eyes and statocysts was used in these experiments. (A) Responses of a type B photoreceptor to the second occurrence of rotation (beaded lower line) followed (after a 10-sec interval) by a 30-sec light step (solid lower line). The cell's initial resting potential, preceding the first of the two light steps in (A), (B), and (C), is indicated by the broken lines. Depolarization above the resting level after the second of the two light steps is indicated by shaded areas. (B) Responses of a type B receptor to the second of two light steps (no rotations were administered in this condition). (C) Responses of a type B photoreceptor to the second occurrence of a 30-sec light step accompanied simultaneously by rotation. The figure shows that 60 sec after offset of the second light step the greatest depolarization is seen in the condition in which light step and rotation occurred simultaneously, and the least in the condition in which rotation ceased 10 sec before onset of the light step.

At right is shown: (A) increases of type B cell depolarization with repetition of simultaneous pairings of rotation and light steps; membrane potential was measured either 20 sec (filled circles) or 60 sec (open squares) after each pairing; (B) decay of type B cell depolarization after ten simultaneous pairings of rotation and light steps. (*From* Alkon 1980)

aptic depolarization induced by the rebound S/E cell activity. But the effect is further enhanced because at offset the hair cells show reduced spontaneous activity (compared to prerotation levels), and so a tonic source of inhibitory synaptic input to the type B cells is also reduced. A series of pairings of light and rotation has a cumulative effect on LLD, which becomes progressively larger and more persistent. This cumulative enhancement of LLD is believed to mediate short-term retention and to be the first step in the establishment of long-term alterations in type B cell excitability.

Analysis of Membrane Currents

LLD is a light-dependent phenomenon: it cannot be produced simply by a depolarization of the type B cell. This in turn appears to reflect the fact that light onset initiates a (voltage-dependent) inward calcium current that persists after light onset and whose depolarizing effect is largely responsible for the LLD seen after light offset. LLD is abolished in a calcium-free solution, or if EGTA (a calcium chelator) is injected into a type B cell. Alkon's hypothesis is that this calcium current is responsible for the increased input resistance seen during LLD and, indirectly, for the long-term increase in input resistance seen following light-rotation pairings, an increase that may persist long after the decay of LLD.

An increase in membrane resistance reflects a change in the selective permeability of the membrane to ions. Alkon (e.g., 1984) has found that two (of at least four) voltage-dependent currents observed in the absence of light are reduced by the pairing procedure: both are outward potassium currents, one (IA) an early, rapidly inactivated current, the other (ICa^{2+}-K$^+$), an outward calcium-dependent current. There is evidence to show that each of these currents is reduced by high levels of intracellular calcium. The increased input resistance accompanying LLD is therefore plausibly accounted for by the proposition that the inflow of calcium during LLD directly reduces two outward potassium currents.

Physiological Basis of Long-Term Retention

Since the increase in calcium levels parallels the time course of the LLD, it cannot account for the more permanent change in resistance. In comparison with *Aplysia,* fewer details are currently available on the long-term correlates of conditioning in *Hermissenda;* some general similarities do, however, emerge. There is direct evidence for an increase in protein phosphorylation in eyes extracted from animals given paired training, when compared to those of animals subjected to control procedures

(Neary, Crow, and Alkon 1981); more recent work indicates that one of the proteins involved is a G protein (Nelson, Collin, and Alkon 1990).

There have been reports that suggest that the protein phosphorylation associated with conditioning in *Hermissenda* may be mediated by more than one type of protein kinase. Acosta-Urquidi, Alkon, and Neary (1984) found, for example, that injection of a Ca^{2+}/calmodulin-dependent kinase decreased the two outward potassium currents associated with conditioning; similarly, Alkon et al. (1986) found that activation of the Ca^{2+}/phospholipid-dependent kinase PKC obtained prolonged reduction of those same currents. Thus the persistent high levels of Ca^{2+} observed during cumulative LLD may trigger a protein phosphorylation that results in relatively permanent changes in membrane permeability. There is also evidence that those same currents may be prolonged by injection of a cAMP-dependent kinase (Alkon et al. 1983). A recent report, however, gave good support for a primary role of PKC, since current reductions elicited by an *in vitro* conditioning procedure were abolished by PKC inhibitors, but not by inhibitors of either Ca^{2+}/calmodulin-dependent or cAMP-dependent kinases (Farley and Schuman 1991). A further interesting finding of this report concerned the effect of PKC inhibitors on the electrophysiological activity of B photoreceptors from animals that had been trained behaviorally two days previously. Reductions in K^+ currents were, as anticipated, seen in control cells but were not seen in cells subjected to the inhibition of PKC activity. PKC inhibition, in other words, blocked the (cellular) expression of a long-term memory. It appears, then, that in *Hermissenda,* as in *Aplysia,* protein phosphorylation plays an important role in the mediation of long-term retention of conditioning and that in *Hermissenda* a pathway involving PKC may be of particular importance in both the establishment and the maintenance of that phosphorylation. Figure 4.13 summarizes the sequence of events involved in obtaining increased excitability of type B cells.

We saw that in *Aplysia* inhibition of protein synthesis disrupted long-term retention; by way of contrast, protein synthesis inhibition in *Hermissenda* appears to prolong calcium-induced decrements in potassium channels (Alkon et al. 1987). This somewhat unexpected finding may be associated with the equally unexpected finding (Alkon et al. 1990) that one long-term consequence of conditioning in *Hermissenda* is a reduction in the arborizations of the terminal branches of type B photoreceptors. The total number of those branches was not influenced by training, and there were significant correlations between the boundary volumes of the arborizations of cells taken from individual animals and both their behavioral

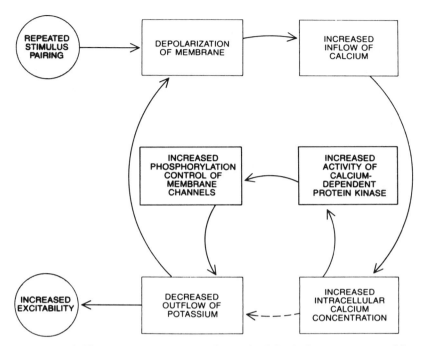

FIGURE 4.13. Summary diagram of the physiological events proposed by Alkon to account for increased excitability of type B photoreceptor cells (see text for further details). (*From* Alkon 1983)

CR performance (a negative correlation) and their B cell soma input resistances (a positive correlation).

Optimal Temporal Relationships of CS and UCS

The explanation outlined above for the importance of pairing light and rotation suggests that one critical factor is the coincidence of the offset of the UCS and the CS, and that their relative times of onset may be less important. A number of reports provide experimental support for this conclusion. One relevant study was reported by Farley et al. (1983), who impaled single type B photoreceptors in relatively intact *Hermissenda* with microelectrodes. Farley and his colleagues found that when positive (depolarizing) current injections were presented to coincide with offset of light presentation, increases in membrane resistance and reductions in behavioral phototaxis were obtained. The current injections were analogues of the synaptically mediated depolarizations believed to follow light- and rotation-pairings, and were not effective unless paired with light offset. One major virtue of this experiment is that it provides direct evidence for a causal role in reduced phototaxis of increases in B cell excitability.

A second relevant report (Grover and Farley 1987) involved physiological experiments carried out *in vitro* and behavioral experiments on intact *Hermissenda*. The *in vitro* experiments involved dissecting out the circummesophageal nervous system (including the eyes, the statocysts, and the optic ganglia). Grover and Farley compared the effects on cumulative LLD of forward, backward, and simultaneous pairings of light and direct caudal hair cell stimulation (via an implanted electrode, simulating the effects of rotation). The light and hair cell stimuli were 30 sec in duration, and in the case of forward and backward pairings, the offset of one stimulus coincided with the onset of the other. Simultaneous pairings obtained greater LLD than either forward or backward pairings. Other conditions, using stimuli of varying durations, were run to see whether the simultaneous condition was more effective because of the simultaneous onset of the stimuli, or because of their simultaneous offset. The findings were clear-cut: relative time of onset had no significant influence (when offsets were simultaneous), whereas simultaneity of offset had a major influence on LLD (when onsets were simultaneous). A comparable series of conditions using light and rotation stimuli was then run in intact *Hermissenda*, and behavioral phototaxis was measured. The results paralleled those of the physiological experiments, finding maximal reduction in phototaxis when stimulus offsets were simultaneous.

A more recent report (Matzel et al. 1990) used CSs and UCSs of relatively short duration (CS durations ranged from 2 to 12 sec, and UCSs were 2-sec duration). These authors found optimal conditioning using a 4-sec CS that coterminated with the UCS; simultaneous presentation of a 2-sec CS and the 2-sec UCS obtained a somewhat lower level of conditioning, a level comparable to that found in a condition in which a 2-sec CS terminated at UCS onset. A condition in which onset of a 12-sec CS preceded UCS onset by 10 sec did not sustain conditioning, nor did explicitly unpaired presentations of the stimuli. Taken altogether, the Matzel et al. (1990) results provide further support for the importance of the simultaneous offset of CS and UCS; they also, however, provide evidence that, at least when short-duration stimuli are used, conditioning may be enhanced when CS onset precedes UCS onset by a relatively brief interval.

But other reports raise doubts concerning the optimal temporal relationship between CS and UCS in *Hermissenda*, particularly when relatively long-duration CSs and UCSs are used. One problem is that it is difficult to decide precisely when UCS onset is effective: rotation begins from a stationary position and accelerates to an asymptote from which it, again gradually, reduces at offset. Although in most of Alkon's recent work light and rotation onset and offset are simultaneous, the onset and offset of the effective rotating stimulus clearly are not coincidental with light onset and offset. Moreover, in certain conditions (Alkon 1974; Crow 1983) no difference is found between the effects of paired versus unpaired periods of light and rotation. Other studies have found that CS onset must precede UCS onset by a rather precise interval (Lederhendler and Alkon 1986). And Farley (1987) has reported that inhibition of phototaxis may even be potentiated in animals in which onset of a 60-sec UCS precedes CS onset by 30 sec, compared to animals in which CS and UCS onsets and offsets are simultaneous (each stimulus lasting 30 sec). It seems, to say the least, odd that simultaneous offset of two stimuli should be an important factor in their association, and that their relative times of onset should be so unimportant that associations are formed efficiently even where UCS onset precedes CS onset.

Contrasts Between *Hermissenda* and *Aplysia*

One feature of conditioning in *Hermissenda* that originally encouraged interest was that whereas in *Aplysia* the conditioning explored was a type of alpha conditioning, in *Hermissenda* the CR was either a reduction (in the case of phototaxis) or a reversal (in the case of foot shortening) of the original UCR to the CS. The physiological analysis of conditioning in *Hermissenda* does not, however, suggest that this difference is of real theoretical significance: no new connections are activated, nor is the nature (excitatory versus inhibitory) of any synaptic connection changed. In effect, we see in *Hermissenda,* as in *Aplysia,* facilitation of an excitatory response (depolarization of the B cell) to a stimulus (light) that originally elicited that same response.

Despite the uncertainties of interpretation that have emerged from consideration of temporal factors, it is clear that experience-induced changes in B cell excitability do occur in *Hermissenda,* and there is good support for the notion that their basis lies in the reduction of specific membrane currents, and that the relatively permanent changes are due to calcium-dependent closure of potassium channels by a process of protein phosphorylation, and to morphological changes. These conclusions indicate at least some congruence with conclusions reached from work on *Aplysia.*

One major difference in conclusions lies in the fact that changes in *Aplysia* have been attributed to restricted presynaptic sites, whereas the changes in *Hermissenda* appear to affect the excitability of the entire cell and are in effect postsynaptic since the effect of pairing is mediated by an interaction between UCS-induced synaptic excitation and ongoing CS-induced activity of B cells. Alkon (e.g., 1984) therefore suggests that we should look in vertebrates for conditioning-induced changes in excitability of postsynaptic membranes. Alkon does not, however, suggest that we should expect to find changes in whole-cell excitability; in agreement with the general consensus of current work, Alkon expects to see changes in excitability specific to particular synapses. More specifically, he points to similarities between the ionic currents detected in B cells and currents observed in mammalian hippocampal cells, and suggests that calcium-dependent changes in postsynaptic potassium currents may be found in them also (and that is an issue to which we shall return in chapter 6).

Although the final result of plasticity in both *Hermissenda* and *Aplysia* may be reflected in similar biophysical modifications, it can be seen that the mechanism proposed for *Hermissenda* might, in contrast to that proposed for *Aplysia*, lead one to expect to find "Hebbian" synapses in vertebrates. The analogy is indirect since the effect of conditioning in *Hermissenda* is to render more effective not a synapse but a generator potential (induced by the light CS). But since this effect depends upon synaptically mediated UCS-evoked activity—activity that must coincide with CS-induced activity—analogous modification of a synapse would imply plasticity of the kind envisaged by Hebb.

Behavioral Aspects of Learning in Mollusks

In chapter 2 and in this chapter, we have discussed physiological analyses of learning in mollusks. In the course of these discussions, it has become evident that the mollusks concerned, *Aplysia* and *Hermissenda*, are capable of at least some forms of learning. The correspondence between vertebrates and mollusks in the parametric characteristics of habituation and sensitization drawn up by Thompson and Spencer (1966) gave good grounds for the conclusion that the processes involved in those forms of learning are comparable in the two groups. But there is no similar catalog of associative (and other) processes of learning and of their characteristics. It is therefore no simple matter to find a way of deciding whether the processes involved in association formation in mollusks are comparable to those used by vertebrates; we have, moreover, seen certain aspects of molluscan conditioning (the notion that conditioning in *Aplysia* is a species of sensitization; the role of simultaneous offset of CS and UCS in *Hermissenda*) that highlight the possibility that association formation in mollusks involves processes somewhat different from those involved in vertebrates. It is appropriate now, therefore, to consider two questions: first, to what extent are molluscan processes of associative learning comparable to vertebrate processes; second, what would be the implications of demonstrations of substantive qualitative differences in learning processes between mollusks and vertebrates? I shall begin by tackling this latter question, in a somewhat indirect way, by considering first the potential implications of similarities in behavioral processes.

Although the properties of the basic unit of the nervous system—the neuron—are similar in mollusks and in vertebrates, there are, as we have seen, large differences, both quantitative and qualitative, between the systems considered as a whole. The molluscan nervous system contains many fewer neurons and shows so different a basic organization that no part of the molluscan central nervous system can reasonably be taken to be homologous to any part of a vertebrate central nervous system. In one sense, then, it is clear that no event that takes place in the molluscan central nervous system could have a direct parallel in a vertebrate nervous system; the physiological events that accompany learning in mollusks necessarily differ from those that accompany learning in vertebrates.

The clear disparity in physiological events does not, however, rule out comparability of behavioral processes. The parallels between molluscan and vertebrate habituation encourage a similar behavioral analysis (in terms, for example, of opposing processes of habituation and sensitization). And when a similar behavioral analysis seems appropriate, it is sensible to ask whether any of the principles detected in the physiological implementation of those behavioral processes in one group might not be involved in the other group also. Thus the demonstration that habituation in *Aplysia* is mediated by homosynaptic depression in a monosynaptic pathway encourages the search for a comparable phenomenon at some (or all) of the multiple synapses within an S-R pathway in a vertebrate. And should homosynaptic depression be demonstrated in vertebrates, it would be natural then to ask whether that depression was in turn mediated by reduced transmitter release.

A similar argument would apply if it was concluded that associative learning processes were comparable in mollusks and vertebrates. If, for example, it did emerge that no substantive qualitative difference could be drawn between the two groups in the characteristics of the behavioral processes involved in association formation, then it would make good sense to look in vertebrates for, say, activity-dependent modulation of presynaptic facilitation as a specific mechanism used in the detection of CS-UCS contingency.

One possible objection to the above argument is that, given the long history of independent evolution of mollusks and vertebrates, it is likely that similar behavioral processes developed independently and show parallels through convergence, rather than that those processes were inherited from a common ancestor. If the similarity is the result of convergence rather than common ancestry, then, it might be argued, there is no reason to suppose any parallel in neurophysiological implementation. Persuasive as this argument is, it omits the fact that the invertebrate and vertebrate nervous systems employ the same basic unit. Given this fact it is likely—but not, of course, inevitable—that if there is some optimally efficient way of solving a particular problem using those units, different nervous systems will converge upon the same solution. There does not seem to be any way of resolving this issue other than finding out precisely how tasks are solved behaviorally in different species, and how behavioral solutions are in fact implemented at the cellular level in those species. It is, however, reasonable to suggest that a useful strategy would be to seek in one species a mechanism that has been shown to operate in another, however distant phylogenetically the species might be.

What, however, would be the consequence of demonstrations of substantive differences in behavioral processes? Should it then be concluded that the physiological analysis of molluscan learning is not relevant to vertebrate neurophysiological analysis? There are good reasons for arguing that this is not so. The analyses achieved using mollusks provide the only reasonably detailed accounts at the cellular level of learning in any species. If it turns out that molluscan associative learning differs importantly from vertebrate learning, what that will mean is that the molluscan nervous system is performing different complex tasks from those performed by the vertebrate nervous system; the molluscan nervous system is, nevertheless, solving problems and, when the behavioral processes involved are well understood, it will be possible to show how at least one nervous system solves a particular set of problems. It is clear that an overview of how different nervous systems—all using the same basic units—solve a range of complex problems is likely to give rise to a more general understanding of the relationship between neurophysiological activity at the cellular level and behavioral processes. That understanding could in turn generate insights into ways in which the vertebrate nervous system might implement behavioral processes that are specific to vertebrates.

The general conclusion to be drawn here is that there are advantages to be gained from comparative research whether behavioral analyses in different groups of animals reveal diversity or relative uniformity of processes involved in associative learning. Diversity of processes would allow the determination of general principles concerning ways in which different problems may be solved at the cellular level; uniformity of process would allow the possibility of a relatively direct generalization to other animal groups of physiological mechanisms used by one group.

A major implication of the foregoing discussion is that a full interpretation of physiological work on learning in any species requires a detailed behavioral analysis of the processes of learning in that species. Since the behavioral analysis of learning in vertebrates (and particularly in mammals) is currently much more advanced than in mollusks, one sensible strategy is to use vertebrate learning as a framework, and to see whether phenomena well established in vertebrates are seen in mollusks also. Parallels between phenomena will support the view that comparable processes are involved; contrasts will invite further investigation aimed at comprehending the contrast and identifying more precisely the properties of a behavioral process that may exist in vertebrates but not in mollusks (or vice versa). That strategy is adopted in the following sections, which review briefly performance of mollusks in learning tasks other than the basic Pavlovian conditioning procedure, in which pairings of a discrete CS and UCS obtain a specific CR. We shall in fact find in these sections what may appear to be a surprising degree of correspondence between molluscan and vertebrate associative learning.

Instrumental Conditioning

Aplysia have been shown to be efficient performers in paradigms other than those discussed previously. Susswein, Schwartz, and Feldman (1986), for example, showed that two European species of *Aplysia* (*A. fasciata* and *A. oculifera*) rapidly learned to inhibit feeding responses to food made inedible by being wrapped in netting. Susswein and colleagues argue that because occurrence of the negative reinforcer is contingent upon the animal's response, this constitutes an instance of instrumental learning. A more convincing case for instrumental learning is provided by a report by Cook and Carew (1986), who showed that head waving in *Aplysia* (held suspended by their parapodia) could be modified by punishing waving to one side with presentation of a bright light. *Aplysia* are, then, capable of learning in tasks that may involve instrumental conditioning and that do not involve strengthening of a withdrawal response.

Fear Conditioning

There is evidence that aversive conditioning in *Aplysia* may show motivational parallels with aversive conditioning in vertebrates. Walters, Carew, and Kandel (1981) paired a presentation of a chemosensory stimulus (shrimp extract) to *Aplysia* with delivery of a strong head shock. Figure 4.14 shows that, compared to unpaired controls, shrimp extract now elicited a stronger head withdrawal response. More interestingly, however, it also facilitated other defensive responses that were not originally elicited by shrimp extract. These responses (escape locomotion, inking, and siphon withdrawal) were elicited at a low level by a test stimulus (a weak shock to the tail), and were strengthened when elicited in the presence of the shrimp extract; this strengthening was seen in paired but not in unpaired animals.

Recordings (Carew, Walters, and Kandel 1981) from individual motoneurons involved in each of the three defensive responses indicated that more spikes were elicited by weak tail shock in the presence of shrimp extract (in paired animals) but that neither the resting potential nor the input resistance of the motoneurons had changed as a result of pairing. These results indicate that the facilitation was not due to a subthreshold activation of the motoneurons and imply that as a result of the pairing procedure the shrimp extract now activated facilitatory interneurons common to a wide variety of defensive responses.

Walters, Carew, and Kandel (1981) went on to show that presentation of shrimp extract which had been paired with tail shock inhibited an appetitive response—biting. For this experiment, food-deprived *Aplysia* were presented with a strip of seaweed, which elicited orientatory head lifting and biting: in the presence of shrimp extract, the latency of both head lifting and biting (see figure 4.14) was lengthened in paired animals (although the subsequent rate of biting was not affected).

The behavioral results of pairing a CS with an aversive UCS suggest that central motivational states may modulate responding in *Aplysia*, that a state like fear may potentiate defensive responses and inhibit appetitive responses (see figure 4.15). Apart from the evidence that fear-inducing stimuli do not directly excite defensive motoneurons, little is known of the physiology of these phenomena. It may be that the same interneurons both facilitate defensive and inhibit appetitive responses, or that different interneurons mediate opposing actions. It is worth noting that one general implication is that CSs paired with aversive UCSs not only become more likely to elicit responses in motoneurons: they also come to elicit responses in interneurons. And if association formation proceeds in *Aplysia*

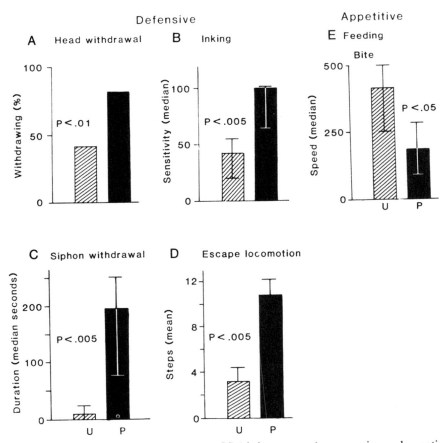

FIGURE 4.14. Effects of an aversive CS (shrimp extract) on aversive and appetitive responding in *Aplysia*. In each graph, P refers to animals that had previously experienced nine CS-shock pairings, U to animals that had experienced unpaired presentations of CS and shock. Test stimuli were applied after delivery of the CS. (A) The percentage of animals showing strong withdrawals to CS delivery in the first test. (B) Median duration of siphon withdrawal to weak tail stimulation. (C) Median sensitivity of ink release in response to a series of progressively stronger shocks to the tail (sensitivity expressed as the reciprocal of the threshold, in mA, x 10⁴). (D) Median number of steps in response to weak tail stimulation. (E) Median speed to take the first bite after stimulation of the head with seaweed (speed expressed as the reciprocal of the latency to bite, in sec, x 10⁴). Graphs showing medians indicate interquartile ranges; graph D shows the standard error of the mean. (*From* Walters, Carew, and Kandel 1981)

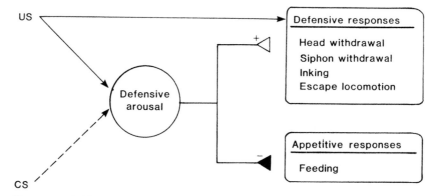

FIGURE 4.15. Proposed model of conditioned fear in *Aplysia*. According to the model, aversive UCSs produce not only motor responses but defensive arousal, a central state that selectively facilitates (open triangle) defensive responses and inhibits (filled triangle) appetitive responses. An initially neutral CS, when paired with an aversive UCS, becomes capable of eliciting this same defensive central state. (*From* Walters, Carew, and Kandel 1981)

by a process of activity-dependent enhancement of presynaptic facilitation, then the synapses between stimuli and interneurons are strengthened by feedback from interneurons on to the synapses between sensory neurons and interneurons.

The Role of Contingency

Recent analyses of classical conditioning in vertebrates have focused attention on the fact that pairing per se does not guarantee efficient association formation. Investigations of the conditions that are necessary for the effectiveness of pairings have led to the development of new theories of association formation (e.g., Rescorla and Wagner 1972; Mackintosh 1975; Pearce and Hall 1980).

Effects of Extra UCSs

Rescorla (1968) demonstrated that if "extra" shock UCSs were presented amongst a series of CS-UCS pairings, the ability of the CS to elicit fear was reduced. This result suggests that animals detect the contingency between a CS and a UCS in the sense that they somehow assess the probability of a UCS in the presence of the CS relative to its probability in the absence of the CS. The more likely a UCS is when no CS is presented, the less effective will a CS paired with the UCS become.

Hawkins, Carew, and Kandel (1986) have reported that "extra" UCS presentations detract from the effectiveness of CS-UCS pairings in *Aplysia*, and Farley (1987) has reported a similar result in *Hermissenda*. Hawkins, Carew, and Kandel (1986) used the basic procedures that were employed by Carew, Hawkins, and Kandel (1983) and have been described previously. CSs were, then, either tactile siphon stimulation or weak mantle shocks, and UCS was strong tail shock. Inter-trial interval was 5 min, CS+ preceded UCS by .5 sec, and CS− occurred 2.5 min after UCS presentation. When "extra" UCSs were added 1 min before the CS+ presentation on each trial, no conditioning to CS+ occurred. Both CS+ and CS− showed sensitization (to a level somewhat greater than that seen to CS− in a group that did not receive extra UCSs), but there was no difference in response to CS+ and CS−. This report, then, provides prima facie evidence of a role for contingency in association formation in *Aplysia*. The report is, however, limited since no exploration was made of the effects of varying temporal parameters. This is potentially of importance, since Farley (1987) did vary the temporal location of the UCS relative to CS-UCS pairings, and obtained results from *Hermissenda* that did not encourage the view that the phenomenon is properly to be compared with the effects of contingency in vertebrates.

In Farley's (1987) experiment, UCS and CS durations were 30 sec, and subjects received 50 pairings with simultaneous CS (light) and UCS (rotation) onset and offset. Interstimulus interval was 2 min, and extra UCSs were delivered which began 30, 45, or 60 sec before each pairing. In the two conditions in which the extra UCSs terminated (either 15 or 30 sec) before each pairing, poorer conditioning was obtained; but where the extra UCS onset preceded the pairing onset by 30 sec (so that in effect a 60-sec continuous UCS was presented), conditioning was actually enhanced by the extra UCS. Physiological analysis suggested that the deleterious effect of extra UCSs was retroactive, since the effect of the interpairing rotation was to reduce the LLD of the type B cell, which followed the preceding pairing trial. As noted above, hair cell activation tends to hyperpolarize type B cells.

The fact that an extra UCS whose termination coincides with pairing onset actually enhances conditioning detracts from the parallel with experiments on mammals. And the physiological mechanism proposed implies a substantially different process from any currently proposed to underlie the effect obtained in mammals. The influential Rescorla-Wagner model (1972), for example, can account for the detrimental effects of extra UCSs by supposing (Randich and LoLordo 1979) that an association is formed between these UCSs and the context, an association that reduces the subsequent effect of pairings of CS and UCS (an example of blocking, a phenomenon that will be discussed in the following section). This account finds no role for any analogue of a reduction by UCSs of type B cell depolarization, such as, say, weakening by the UCS of some trace of the CS which might persist throughout the interpairing intervals.

No physiological analysis of the mode of action of extra UCSs in *Aplysia* is yet available, so that we do not know whether problems similar to those seen in the analysis of *Hermissenda* will emerge also in *Aplysia*. We shall, however, see evidence that *Aplysia* do show conditioning to contextual cues, and that at least some mollusks (including, perhaps, *Aplysia*) show blocking: it is therefore plausible that the Rescorla and Wagner account (1972) of the disruptive effect of extra UCSs may apply to *Aplysia*.

Effects of Extra CSs

Rescorla (1968) also demonstrated the less surprising fact that extra CS presentations diminish the effectiveness of CS-UCS pairings. Farley (1987) reports a similar effect in *Hermissenda*, but once again the mechanism proposed suggests a very different process from that in effect in mammals. The effects of extra CS (light) presentations depended, as with extra UCS presentations, upon the position of the extra CS within the interpairing interval. Extra CSs (each 30 sec in duration) were without effect when their onset preceded pairing onsets by either 30 or 60 sec. They did impair conditioning when they preceded pairings by 45 sec. Physiological analysis indicated that this effect was proactive, since it appeared that extra light presentations reduced the type B cell depolarization seen during a subsequent pairing—the consequence, perhaps, of a transient light-adaptation process. No suggestion of a similar temporal dependency of extra CSs is found in the vertebrate literature, and accounts of the effects of extra CSs do not suppose that these effects are mediated by a reduction in the sensory impact of CSs within pairings.

Blocking

We shall consider now the phenomenon of blocking, a phenomenon that has not yet been demonstrated unequivocally in *Aplysia* or *Hermissenda*, but has been shown in another gastropod, *Limax maximus*, a common garden slug. It is not unreasonable to suppose that there may be much in common between the learning mechanisms of gastropods in general, and there is (from experiments on contextual conditioning, to be described in the following section) evidence that suggests that blocking does occur in *Aplysia*.

Sahley, Rudy, and Gelperin (1981) reported a striking series of experiments that demonstrated the occurrence in *Limax* of three phenomena known in vertebrates, phenomena strongly suggestive of parallels between the processes of conditioning in mollusks and vertebrates. The phenomena concerned were higher-order conditioning, blocking, and the UCS preexposure effect. We shall consider here only their demonstration of blocking (for an account and theoretical analysis of the other two phenomena in vertebrates, see Mackintosh 1983).

Blocking provides another example of the fact that the strength of conditioning is not simply a function of number of CS-UCS pairings. Originally demonstrated by Kamin (1969), blocking is observed in a procedure that involves two stages. In Stage 1, an originally neutral CS, CS1, is paired with a UCS; in Stage 2, CS1 is presented simultaneously in compound with a second CS, CS2, and that compound stimulus is paired with the UCS used in Stage 1. In such a procedure, vertebrates show less conditioning to CS2 than does a control group for which Stage 1 is omitted. The presence of the previously trained stimulus CS1 is said to block learning about CS2.

The Sahley, Rudy, and Gelperin (1981) demonstration of blocking proceeded as follows: in Stage 1, animals in a Blocking Group received three pairings, separated by two hours, of a carrot odor and a bitter taste. Such pairings consisted of a slug being placed for two minutes in a plastic dish with a carrot odor followed by two minutes in a petri dish lined with filter paper soaked in quinidine sulphate. In Stage 2 the slugs experienced three pairings of a carrot and potato compound odor with the same bitter taste. In a test phase (see figure 4.16), the slugs' preference for the (normally preferred) potato odor relative to rat-chow odor was assessed: the Blocking Group showed significantly stronger preference for the potato odor than did a control group for which Stage 1 had been omitted; in other words, the Blocking Group had apparently not associated the potato odor with the aversive taste stimulus. Two other control groups showed that blocking did not occur if the order of presentation of the bitter taste and the carrot odor was reversed in Stage 1 (in other words, that forward pairing was required), and did not occur if the potato odor alone was paired with quinidine in Stage 2.

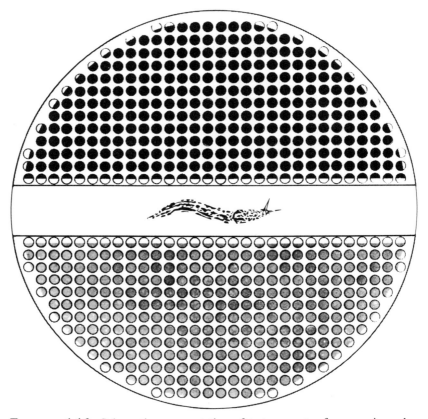

FIGURE 4.16. Schematic representation of test apparatus for assessing odor preferences in *Limax*. The animal is placed in a neutral zone bordered on each side by two different odor-generating food sources directly under the perforated floor of the chamber. Choice is assessed by measuring the time for which the slug's head leaves the neutral zone to rest on the side over one odor source relative to the total time spent with the head outside the neutral zone. (*From* Sahley, Rudy, and Gelperin 1981)

Contextual Conditioning

For a final specific example of learning in *Aplysia* we shall consider a report by Colwill, Absher, and Roberts (1988) of contextual conditioning. Contextual conditioning is of interest because it differs from more conventional conditioning procedures in that there is no discrete CS, with a specific time of onset and offset. In one experiment, Colwill, Absher, and Roberts exposed *Aplysia* to each of two contexts for 20 min a day for eight days. One context was a smooth round bowl containing lemon-flavored seawater; the other was a rectangular tank with a ridged surface that contained unscented seawater and was gently vibrated. Each *Aplysia* was given four UCSs (moderate shocks to the mantle surface) daily in one of the two contexts (the lemon-flavored context for some animals, the unscented context for others). Two days following the final contextual training session, *Aplysia* experienced two sessions of conditioning in each of which there were four pairings of an explicit CS (mild tactile stimulation of the siphon) with the mantle shock UCS. For some animals, pairings took place in the context in which shocks had previously been experienced; for others, the pairings were carried out in the context in which no shocks had been experienced. Following those pairings, CRs to the siphon CS were assessed in a third, neutral, context (the home tank). The results are summarized in figure 4.17, which shows that stronger CRs were elicited in those animals that had received paired training in the context in which UCSs had *not* previously been delivered.

An obvious implication of the Colwill, Absher, and Roberts result is that the *Aplysia* had learned in the first stage of the experiment that one of the two contexts was associated with shock delivery. It is difficult to conceive any other interpretation of the differential performance observed following CS-UCS pairings in the two contexts. A further implication is that *Aplysia*, like *Limax*, may be capable of blocking. We have seen that UCS preexposures in a given context can lead, in mammals, also to impaired subsequent acquisition of a CS-UCS association in that environment, and that a prominent account of that phenomenon supposes that the prior association of the context with the UCS blocks the subsequent learning about the CS-UCS relationship (Randich and LoLordo 1979). Although, as Colwill, Absher, and Roberts point out (1988), further controls are necessary before an unequivocal demonstration of blocking can be claimed, their report clearly provides good prima facie evidence of the occurrence of the phenomenon in *Aplysia*.

Conclusions

Parallels Between Molluscan and Vertebrate Learning

The behavioral data surveyed here have provided overall an impressive series of parallels between learning phenomena observed in gastropod

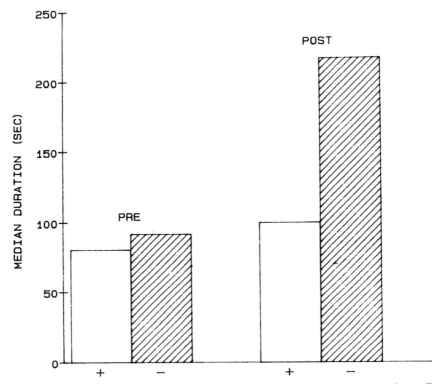

FIGURE 4.17. Evidence for contextual conditioning and blocking in *Aplysia.* The figure shows median duration of siphon withdrawal in response to mild tactile siphon stimulation delivered in the home tank. Scores are shown separately for the group conditioned in the reinforced context (open bars) and the group conditioned in the nonreinforced context (striped bars). The pretest scores obtained prior to conditioning are displayed on the left, and the posttest scores obtained after conditioning, on the right. (*From* Colwill, Absher, and Roberts 1988)

mollusks and those observed in vertebrates, parallels that encourage the view that there may be much in common between gastropod and vertebrate mechanisms of learning. If, moreover, we extend the hunt to other mollusks, and to other invertebrate groups, we find more demonstrations of phenomena originally demonstrated in vertebrates. The cephalopod mollusk *Octopus vulgaris,* for example, shows such effects as transfer along a continuum, the overtraining reversal effect, and serial reversal improvement (for a review, see Sutherland and Mackintosh 1971). And the range of phenomena exhibited by an insect, the honey bee (*Apis mel-*

lifera), in a series of experiments by Bitterman and his colleagues, is even more impressive (for a list see Macphail 1985a).

The phenomena actually demonstrated to date in *Aplysia* are not, perhaps, all that remarkable. But other gastropods, other mollusks, and other invertebrates have demonstrated abilities that encourage the conclusion that *Aplysia* may indeed be capable of greater feats. A similar argument applies of course to *Hermissenda,* although there is here the difference that only one basic procedure, involving one type of CS and one type of UCS, has so far been explored physiologically, and there do appear to be some important differences between the features of conditioning obtained using that procedure in *Hermissenda* and those typically seen in vertebrates. As noted above, the experiments on contingency (Farley 1987) serve to emphasize differences rather than similarities between conditioning in vertebrates and in *Hermissenda.* Moreover, Farley (1987) has reported that preexposure of either CS (light) or UCS (rotation) has no effect on subsequent conditioning: numerous studies have found that CS preexposures retard learning in mammals (the phenomenon of latent inhibition: Lubow 1973), and UCS preexposures, as we have seen, retard conditioning in both *Limax* and mammals. It therefore becomes necessary to raise the possibility that the behavioral changes induced by light-rotation pairings are not typical of conditioning in gastropods and not even, perhaps, typical of conditioning in *Hermissenda.*

Problems in Interpretation of the Hermissenda *Findings*

A conditioning-induced increase in the excitability of a primary sensory receptor in response to any input does not seem intuitively likely to provide a satisfactory general mechanism of learning: it is hard to see, for example, that such a mechanism could allow discrimination between two light stimuli, one associated with rotation, the other not. Nor is it clear why light-alone presentations should obtain extinction of both behavioral CRs and pairing-induced increases in input resistance (Richards, Farley, and Alkon 1984): a series of light-induced depolarizations and their subsequent LLDs might be expected, on the contrary, to potentiate preexisting increased input resistances.

There remain also questions about the behavioral status of the changes seen. Pairing of light with rotation elicits a foot-shortening response, an index of "clinging" to the substrate, and it is supposed that this response is due to the increased activity of B cells. But if *Hermissenda* are subjected to a rotation in which the head of the animal is oriented away from the center of rotation, then decreases in B cell excitability are observed (Alkon 1980), and animals show enhanced positive phototaxis (Farley and Alkon 1980). Alkon explains this finding (which of course does provide further support for the causal role of B cells in phototaxis) in terms of differential connections of cephalad and caudal hair cells. But if B cell activity declines, the clinging response in this paradigm should decline. Evidence on the clinging-response to rotation with a cephalic orientation is not yet available. But if clinging declines in response to rotation with a cephalic orientation and increases with a caudal orientation, its adaptive significance will be far from clear. And if clinging does not decline following pairings of light with rotation having a caudal orientation, then the role of changes in B cell excitability in the control of the foot-shortening response will be placed in doubt.

Finally, although Grover and Farley (1987) make out a case for an adaptive utility of a system that detects cotermination of light and perturbation of water (for which rotation is taken to be an analogue), it seems very much a post hoc account. Alkon (1983), for example, writing of the adaptive significance of conditioning, suggests that following "experience of encountering turbulence in association with light at the surface . . . the light would [for *Hermissenda*] come to presage the onset of turbulence" (Alkon 1983:64). It is difficult to see the advantage of a system that is designed to detect that one stimulus presages another but which in fact detects only that stimuli coterminate. The Grover and Farley account, moreover, fails to make sense of the fact that *Hermissenda* will apparently learn to swim away from lights that coterminate with perturbations which activate the caudal hair cells of the statocysts, but toward lights that coterminate with perturbations which stimulate the cephalad receptors.

It is not currently possible to decide whether similar problems will apply to other instances of conditioning in *Hermissenda,* or whether these problems are peculiar to the light-rotation pairing procedure. The differences between the phenomena associated with the light-rotation pairing procedure and those associated with conditioning in vertebrates do not alter the fact that the *Hermissenda* preparation has provided a detailed cellular analysis of a complex behavioral change. It constitutes, at the least, an example of a way in which the nervous system may solve a complex problem. The general import of this section is, however, that extrapolation from procedures used with *Aplysia* to vertebrates seems more plausible than would extrapolation from the light-rotation procedure in *Hermissenda.*

A Reductionist Analysis of Complex Learning Phenomena

The most striking evidence of parallels between invertebrate and vertebrate learning has been obtained in animals other than *Aplysia* and *Hermissenda*. But in none of those animals has so detailed an analysis of the processes involved yet been achieved. It might then be thought that although the learning processes of gastropods were comparable with those of vertebrates, the physiological analyses available concerned only the simplest of those processes and were of restricted relevance to more complex and more interesting phenomena. This concern is the subject of an important theoretical paper by Hawkins and Kandel (1984) in which it is claimed that a number of superficially complex phenomena may be understood in terms of phenomena already demonstrated in *Aplysia*. I shall attempt to convey at least the flavor of their approach by considering their account of blocking.

Application to Blocking

As we have already noted, the account proposed by Kandel and his colleagues for conditioning in *Aplysia* supposes that stimuli paired with the firing of facilitator interneurons will become conditioned so that their presentation alone now elicits facilitator firing (and this forms the basis of "fear" conditioning). Hawkins and Kandel (1984) argue that firing of facilitator interneurons declines rapidly owing to the influence of accommodation and recurrent inhibition (and they cite independent evidence for these processes in facilitators). Thus in Stage 1 of a blocking paradigm, CS1 will come to elicit a burst of firing of the facilitator interneuron (see figure 4.18), which will cease owing to the effects of accommodation and recurrent inhibition. Those same inhibitory effects will affect the firing of the facilitators that would normally be elicited by the UCS. Thus, in Stage 2, there will be a burst of facilitator firing at the onset of the compound CS1 and CS2, but no facilitator firing at the offset of the compound, when the UCS is delivered.

This account of blocking has much in common conceptually with that advanced by Kamin (e.g., 1969) and by Rescorla and Wagner (e.g., 1972). Kamin proposed that learning does not occur unless there is a surprising event: because CS1 predicts a UCS after Stage 1 training, there is no surprise in Stage 2, and hence no learning about CS2. Rescorla and Wagner formalized the notion of surprise in a model that supposed that UCSs lose capacity to support new learning to the extent to which they

STAGE 1

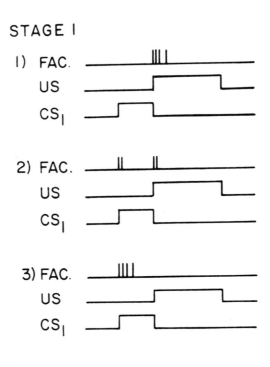

STAGE 2

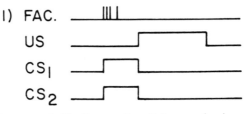

FIGURE 4.18. Proposed cellular mechanism of blocking. As conditioning of CS1 proceeds (Stage 1: trials 1, 2, and 3), the facilitator neurons (FAC) fire more during the CS period. This firing produces accommodation and recurrent inhibition, which reduce firing during the US period. When compound conditioning starts (Stage 2), CS2 is not followed by firing of the facilitator neurons and therefore does not become conditioned. (*From* Hawkins and Kandel 1984)

are already predicted. The Hawkins and Kandel (1984) suggestion also attributes blocking to a loss of effectiveness of the UCS following Stage 1 training.

Difficulties for the Reductionist Analysis

Sensory Preconditioning

Hawkins and Kandel (1984) have succeeded in showing that it is possible to interpret a surprisingly wide range of phenomena observed in *Aplysia* or in other gastropods in terms of rather simple processes, the most fundamental of which are homosynaptic depression and heterosynaptic facilitation. They suggest also that a range of other phenomena (such as, for example, overshadowing and latent inhibition) may also be explained in similar terms. But, as they also point out, there are phenomena that are readily observed in vertebrates for which their mechanisms do not provide a ready account. Sensory preconditioning provides one example (for a discussion of this phenomenon in mammals see Mackintosh 1974): if (in an experiment using rats) two neutral stimuli, CS1 and CS2, are paired in Stage 1 and CS2 is paired with shock in Stage 2, a subsequent test of CS1 will reveal that it now elicits fear. This observation indicates that in Stage 1 an association was formed between two neutral stimuli. Since there is no presentation of intense stimuli in Stage 1, there is no reason to suppose that facilitators were activated and so no mechanism for the association of CS1 and CS2.

Although no experiments on sensory preconditioning in *Aplysia* have yet been reported, the problem for the Hawkins and Kandel (1984) scheme is clear. If *Aplysia* are capable of sensory preconditioning, then the current account of conditioning in *Aplysia* is seriously incomplete; if sensory preconditioning cannot be obtained from *Aplysia,* then conditioning in *Aplysia* may employ mechanisms very different from those employed by, say, rats.

Inhibitory Conditioning

A further example of learning that cannot yet be explained in terms of mechanisms known in *Aplysia* is inhibitory conditioning (see Mackintosh 1974 for a discussion of this phenomenon in mammals). When a UCS is less likely in the presence of a CS than in its absence, then in vertebrates that CS tends to become a conditioned inhibitor, endowed with the capacity to weaken the CR normally elicited by a conditioned excitor: a conditioned inhibitor established with a shock UCS—a safety signal—will reduce the fear elicited by a CS paired with shock (Rescorla 1969). We do not yet know whether conditioned inhibition can be obtained in mollusks, nor do we know whether latent inhibition (which would be expected by Hawkins and Kandel) can be found in them (we have seen that latent inhibition is not obtained in the *Hermissenda* light-rotation pairing procedure: Farley 1987)

The absence of evidence on learned inhibitory processes in *Aplysia* focuses attention on one major barrier in the way of accepting the aversive conditioning explored by Kandel and his colleagues as being an example of the sort of conditioning that is obtained in vertebrates. In Kandel's work, as has been noted, the CRs that are obtained are strengthenings of preexisting responses to CSs rather than de novo responses; they are, then, instances of alpha conditioning. Since the stimuli typically used as CSs in vertebrate classical conditioning experiments may equally well become conditioned inhibitors as conditioned excitors, it is clear that at least in vertebrates strengthening of excitatory connections is not the only way in which conditioning proceeds. But in some sense the pathways involved in association formation must exist prior to the conditioning procedure, and there may be little significance in the question whether conditioning consists in the strengthening of excitatory (or inhibitory) connections or of the activation of previously inactive connections.

Contextual Learning

We have seen that *Aplysia* can learn about contexts (Colwill, Absher, and Roberts 1988). The demonstration of contextual conditioning poses problems for the reductionist account, problems that stem from the Hawkins and Kandel (1984) proposal that extinction is mediated simply by habituation. Contextual cues are continuously present and (assuming that sensory adaptation to them is incomplete) would obtain a steady train of impulses in a subset of sensory neurons. Those impulses should then amplify the facilitation engendered in their terminals by UCSs, so that contextual cues should indeed come to elicit CRs. The problem is, however, that those CRs should extinguish (habituate) in the relatively long periods of exposure to the context in the absence of UCSs. Habituation is the mechanism of extinction proposed by Hawkins and Kandel (1984), and there would be, in the inter-UCS intervals of exposure to the context, long trains of impulses in the sensory neurons activated by the context (it cannot, of course, be argued that those neurons would adapt since in that case conditioning could not take place in the first place). It is, then, difficult to see how, in terms of the reductionist model, conditioning could be obtained and extinction *not* obtained by the presentation of intermittent brief UCSs against a background of continuously present CSs. One intriguing possibility is raised by Colwill, Absher, and Roberts, who suggest "that different cellular mechanisms may be involved in different associative learning paradigms" (1988:4438). This is the first hint of a notion that will form the focus of interest in chapter 7—namely, that learning about contexts may proceed in a way different from learning about discrete stimuli.

S-S Versus S-R Associations

Perhaps the most serious problem facing the Hawkins and Kandel reductionist analysis—at least insofar as it aims to draw parallels between molluscan and mammalian learning—is the nature of the elements in the association formed by a conditioning procedure. The physiological analyses of the events accompanying conditioning in *Aplysia* (and in *Hermissenda*) concern a direct connection between the sensory stimulus and the motor response—an S-R connection. But there is general agreement now (see Mackintosh 1983) that classical conditioning in vertebrates results in an association between (representations of) CS and UCS, not between CS and UCR. Some of the most compelling evidence for this conclusion comes from experiments on the effects of altering the "value" of a UCS after conditioning has taken place. If the aversive properties of, for example, a shock are reduced after conditioning by, say, habituation training with the shock, then the fear-inducing properties of the CS previously associated with it are reduced; similarly, if the value of a UCS is inflated postconditioning, then a stronger CR is elicited (e.g., Rescorla 1973, 1974). Since manipulations involving the UCS affect the CR, the implication is that the critical association is between the CS and the UCS, an S-S association: presentation of the CS elicits a representation of the UCS, which in turn elicits the response. Given that we accept the physiological analysis offered of them, it is clear that no such analysis is to be applied to the *Aplysia* conditioning data currently available (nor, of course, to the *Hermissenda* data).

Conclusions

We have seen that there are a number of difficult questions which await answers before a confident assessment may be made of the relevance of neurophysiological work on gastropods to vertebrate investigators. The types of learning that have been subjected to detailed physiological analysis are indeed simple and may not be comparable to the learning observed under similar conditions in vertebrates. And although Hawkins and Kandel (1984) have been able to demonstrate the possibility that more complex learning phenomena could reflect the operation of the processes that have been analyzed, there is as yet no direct support, either physiological or behavioral, for their reductionist analysis. We do not, for example, know whether facilitator activity in response to a UCS *is* reduced in a blocking procedure. We should therefore be cautious about accepting the suggestion that "there may be a cellular alphabet of learning and that surprisingly complex forms of learning might be generated from combinations of this alphabet of simple cellular mechanisms" (Hawkins and Kandel 1984:389).

The problems of interpretation should not, however, obscure what is the central achievement of the invertebrate work, which has provided for the first time detailed analyses of cellular and subcellular changes that are associated with experience-induced behavioral changes. These achievements will be further emphasized by a consideration of studies on the physiology of learning in spinal vertebrates, and we shall return to mollusks at the end of this chapter in a discussion of the extent to which the questions initially set out have been answered by studies on simple systems.

Conditioning in Spinal Animals

Attempts to demonstrate associative learning in spinal animals remained controversial for several decades. Successful reports were subjected to the criticism that controls were inadequate, particularly to rule out the possibility that behavior changes were due to a nonassociative sensitization effect (for a review see Patterson 1976). But recent work on cats has made it clear that conditioning may indeed be obtained in spinal animals.

Classical Conditioning in Spinal Cats

Patterson and his colleagues have reported a series of experiments on cats whose spinal cord was sectioned at the junction of the thoracic and lumbar regions (T12–L1). The animals were paralyzed and respirated, and the superficial peroneal sensory nerve and the deep peroneal motor nerve were dissected out from one hind limb. CSs were shock trains to the sensory nerve, and CS intensity was adjusted to produce a small electrophysiological response in the motor nerve. The UCS was a strong shock to the ankle skin of the leg, which obtained a large electrophysiological response in the motor nerve (actual flexion being prevented by the paralysis). Patterson, Cegavske, and Thompson (1973) showed that a series of CS-UCS pairings obtained a substantial increase in the motor nerve response elicited by CS-alone presentations, and that unpaired presentations of CS and UCS found no such increase; the results of their experiment are summarized in figure 4.19. A subsequent study (Patterson 1975) found that "backward" pairings, in which UCS onset preceded CS onset (by 100 or 250 msec) did not obtain an increase in motor nerve response to CS presentation. This finding confirms that the effects should not be attributed to sensitization, not even to a modified account that suggests that sensitization is more effective when it occurs in conjunction with a CS: it is the relative time of onset of the stimuli that is critical, a result that strongly supports an interpretation of the findings in terms of genuine conditioning.

Subsequent work with this preparation (Beggs et al. 1983) has shown: that the CR is established very rapidly, reaching asymptote after approximately ten trials; that the CR may be retained for at least four hours; and that the response extinguishes as a consequence of CS-alone presentations (but not as a result of the passage of time). Beggs, Steinmetz, and Patterson (1985) have shown that differential conditioning may be established. When stimulation of the peroneal nerve was paired with UCS and stimulation of the tibial nerve was not paired, CRs were obtained to peroneal nerve stimulation and not to tibial nerve stimulation (and both CSs obtained small motor nerve responses prior to training).

There is, then, good evidence that classical conditioning may proceed efficiently in the isolated spinal cord, and a good general agreement between its properties and those of conditioning in intact animals. But there are at least some differences. Intact animals generally show a decrease in response latency to CS as training proceeds (e.g., Gormezano et al. 1962); but Patterson and his colleagues have found no change in latency in their conditioning studies (Beggs et al. 1983). And although good differential conditioning was obtained when peroneal nerve stimulation served as CS + and tibial nerve stimulation as CS − , no such discrimination occurred in the reverse condition: when tibial nerve stimulation served as CS + and peroneal stimulation as CS − , a marked increase in response to *both* stimuli was obtained. We may, then, agree with Patterson that the data "suggest that the machinery for the basic pairing or associative effects of classical conditioning is present [in the spinal cord]," but that "the spinal cord may lack the elegant machinery for response selection and adaptation of the cortex or upper brain stem" (Patterson 1980:270).

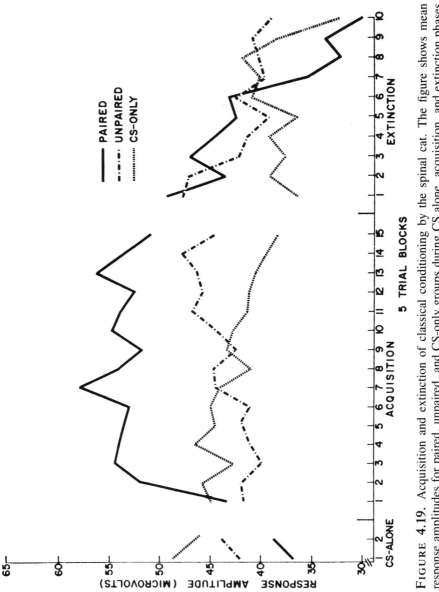
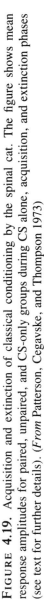

FIGURE 4.19. Acquisition and extinction of classical conditioning by the spinal cat. The figure shows mean response amplitudes for paired, unpaired, and CS-only groups during CS alone, acquisition, and extinction phases (see text for further details). (*From* Patterson, Cegavske, and Thompson 1973)

Physiological Basis

Although the reality of spinal conditioning is now firmly established, little progress has been made on identifying the physiological basis of this learning. Since the studies described above used direct nerve stimulation and recordings as CSs and CRs, changes in either receptors or muscles need not be considered. Patterson (1980) reports that preliminary data indicate no changes following conditioning in excitability of either afferent terminals or motoneurons, and these results point to the interneuron pool as the source of alterations, an unsurprising and not very helpful conclusion.

Efforts to throw light on physiological mechanisms have been made by Durkovic and his colleagues, who have worked with an unparalyzed spinal cat preparation, in which the cord was sectioned at T10 of the thoracic region. They have found that the intensity of both CS (stimulation of the cutaneous saphenous nerve) and UCS (stimulation of the cutaneous portion of the superficial peroneal nerve) must be sufficiently strong that both large-diameter (Aα) and small-diameter (Aδ) fibers are stimulated; stimulation that recruited only large-diameter fibers was not adequate either as a CS (Misulis and Durkovic 1984) or as a UCS (Durkovic and Light 1975).

The investigations reported by Misulis and Durkovic (1984) and by Durkovic and Light (1975) used conventional forward-conditioning procedures, and unpaired presentations of CS and UCS as controls. Subsequent work (Durkovic and Damianopoulos 1986) with this preparation has found that backward conditioning (in which UCS onset precedes CS onset) can be obtained (the optimal UCS-CS onset interval being 0.25 sec). Onifer and Durkovic (1988) have gone on to show that although CS intensities that are set below the threshold required for Aδ fiber activation do not obtain reliable forward conditioning, they do obtain reliable backward conditioning. Durkovic and his colleagues (e.g., Onifer and Durkovic 1988; Hoover and Durkovic 1989) suggest that activation of Aα fibers mediates the acquisition of backward conditioning, whereas activation of Aδ fibers mediates forward conditioning. Since Aα and Aδ fibers are largely segregated in the spinal cord, where they terminate in different laminae, this conclusion suggests a difference in the physiological mechanisms that underlie backward as opposed to forward conditioning. The existence of backward (excitatory) conditioning in vertebrates has long been a contentious issue, although there are by now a number of reports of its successful demonstration (Spetch, Wilkie, and Pinel 1981; Hall 1984). What Durkovic's work suggests, then, is that it may be advantageous to seek a qualitatively different account of backward as opposed to forward conditioning rather than to attempt to explain both varieties through the operation of a single process. At this stage, however, the physiological analysis of backward conditioning in spinal animals does not give any clue to the properties that a backward-conditioning mechanism might possess.

Activity-Dependent Presynaptic Facilitation in Spinal Cord?

One important feature of the preparations discussed thus far is that prior to any training the CS alone elicits the target CR at a low level. We are, then, seeing, as in *Aplysia,* an example of alpha conditioning, the strengthening of preexisting excitatory connections. It therefore makes sense to ask (e.g., Durkovic 1986) whether the mechanism believed to be responsible for conditioning in *Aplysia*—activity-dependent presynaptic facilitation—might be involved in vertebrate spinal cord conditioning. There appears to be little positive experimental support for this possibility.

The mechanism proposed for *Aplysia* assumes a nonspecific sensitization by the UCS of the excitatory connections, which is selectively amplified in the case of terminals that have recently been active. But most studies of spinal cats find no increase in CS-alone effectiveness (and frequently a decrease) when UCSs are presented in an explicitly unpaired condition (e.g., Patterson, Cegavske, and Thompson 1973; Durkovic 1983; see figure 4.19).

A further difficulty for an activity-dependent presynaptic-facilitation account of spinal conditioning emerges from a report of Durkovic (1983). In this study, responses (contractions) were recorded in three muscles (semitendinosus—ST; tibialis anterior—TA; and extensor digitorum longus—EDL). Prior to training, CSs elicited small contractions in all three muscles. The UCS, a strong shock to the cutaneous superficial peroneal nerve, elicited contractions from ST and TA, but tended to inhibit activity in the EDL muscle. CS-UCS pairings in this preparation obtained CRs in ST and TA but had no effect on EDL responses. In other words, the UCS did not facilitate *all* excitatory connections activated by the CS prior to UCS delivery: it strengthened only those connections involving muscles that were also excited by the UCS. These findings may not conclusively rule out a conditioning mechanism based on selective amplification of a sensitizing effect of UCSs, but they offer no support for such a mechanism and indicate that its application to the spinal cord preparation will require considerable modification of the processes proposed for *Aplysia.*

Implications for Behavior Theory

This review of conditioning in spinal cats has concluded that genuine classical conditioning is obtained in this preparation, and this is a conclusion that has implications for contemporary theories of classical conditioning.

Whereas the dominant view of classical conditioning over the first half of this century was that it reflected an association between the CS and the UCR, most current theorists now believe that the effective association is between CS and UCS, or, somewhat more specifically, between internal representations of the CS and the UCS (e.g., Dickinson and Mackintosh 1978). We have already noted some differences between spinal conditioning and conditioning in intact animals, and these may well be attributable to the less refined representations available at the spinal level. But successful spinal conditioning may be problematical for one proposal, which derives from a widely held view of UCS representations that supposes that effective UCSs have multiple attributes which may be distinguished into two broad classes—those related to "preparatory" responses, and those related to "consummatory" responses (e.g., Mackintosh 1983).

Preparatory responses in general constitute the animal's emotional reaction to the affective properties of the UCS, and include relatively nonspecific alterations in activity, and in autonomic indices such as heart rate; consummatory responses are precise skeletal actions specific to the sensory attributes of the UCS—responses such as an eyeblink, leg flexion, and so on. Many authors argue that conditioning to different attributes of the UCS may involve distinct processes, and some (e.g., Konorski 1967; Thompson, Clark, Donegan, Lavond, Lincoln et al. 1984) that establishment of consummatory CRs is dependent upon the prior establishment of a preparatory CR. This proposal is supported by evidence that unless a UCS produces an emotional impact, CRs are not obtained even when a UCR reliably occurs. Colavita (1965), for example, showed that although acid injected directly into a dog's mouth produced a reliable salivary UCR, conditioned salivation with acid injections as the UCS was not obtained unless the acid was also injected into the stomach (this latter injection had no effect on the UCR). This finding may be taken to reflect the fact that acid injected into the mouth had little aversive effect, whereas acid in the stomach produced a strong aversive consequence. In other words, motivation is held to be essential for successful conditioning. While this may seem intuitively perfectly reasonable, it would seem to imply that successful leg flexion CRs in spinal cats indicates the existence of motivation—fear, in this instance—in that preparation. And that may not seem at all reasonable, particularly as it is well known (see chapter 8) that damage to the amygdala (a telencephalic structure) appears virtually to eliminate fear in otherwise intact animals, animals whose spinal cords are, of course, undamaged.

Conditioning in Spinal Rats

This section will describe two phenomena observed in spinal rats that are of general psychological interest because (like aversive conditioning in spinal cats) they suggest that if current behavioral analyses (applied to intact animals) are valid, then surprisingly high-level information-processing devices are available to spinal animals.

Conditioned Antinociception

A particularly interesting example of an apparently high-level behavioral process in a spinal animal emerges from the second of two experiments reported by Grau et al. (1990) in a study of the phenomenon of antinociception. When a CS is paired with an aversive UCS, that CS gains (in intact mammals) antinociceptive properties, in the sense that its presentation subsequently may reduce the aversiveness of some (novel) noxious stimulus. The mechanisms of this antinociceptive response are currently a subject of intense research activity but are not relevant here: our concern is to use conditioned antinociception as a behavioral index of association formation in a classical paradigm.

The first experiment of the Grau et al. (1990) report demonstrated antinociception in spinal rats, and demonstrated also that discriminative conditioning was possible in this preparation. The cord was cut at level T2, and a strong tail-shock was used as UCS. Mild shocks to either the left or the right hind limb served as CSs; shocks to one hind limb (CS +) were consistently paired with the UCS, shocks to the other hind limb (CS −) were unpaired. Following 30 CS(+)-UCS pairings and 30 CS − presentations, the rats were placed in a restraining tube with their tails on a plate that was heated until there was a tail-flick response (a measure of sensitivity to the heat stimulus). The latency to tail-flick was longer when heat was administered accompanied by CS + than when accompanied by CS − (or when administered with no CS). CS + had, then, acquired antinociceptive properties, and the spinal rats had discriminated between the two CSs.

The second experiment of the Grau et al. report has some striking implications. The procedure was simple: spinal rats were placed in the restraining tube and given three strong tail shocks at 20-sec intervals. Tail-flick latencies on the hot plate were then tested five times, at 2-min intervals. Four groups of rats were run: one group received UCSs alone; a second group received no UCSs; a third group received UCSs each of which was immediately followed by a "distractor" (a weak tail shock); the fourth group received presentations of the distractor alone. Figure 4.20 summarizes the results and shows that an antinociceptive CR developed in both the groups given UCSs and, to a lesser extent, in the group given only distractors. The figure also shows, however, that extinction proceeded more rapidly in the animals given distractors following UCSs than in the animals given UCSs alone. This result suggests that the presentation of distractors had resulted in a weaker antinociceptive CR. Since presentations of the distractor alone obtained a significant increase in tail-flick latencies (compared to no-shock controls), this is a surprising result: how is it to be explained?

The explanation favored by Grau et al. (1990) is foreshadowed in their description of the mild tail-shocks as "distractors." We have already seen

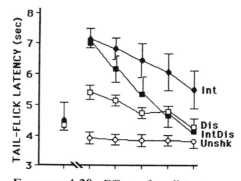

FIGURE 4.20. Effect of a distractor on the magnitude of intense shock-induced antinociception in the spinal rat. After baseline testing, subjects received either three intense shocks alone (Int: filled circles), a distracting stimulus after each intense shock (IntDis: filled squares), the distractor stimulus alone (Dis: open squares), or remained unshocked (Unshk: open circles). Tail-flick latencies were measured five times at 2-min intervals; error bars show the standard error of the mean. (*From* Grau et al. 1990)

(in chapter 3) Wagner's (e.g., 1976) proposal that there exist discrete short- and long-term memory stores. One property of the short-term store is that it has a limited capacity, so that access of an item to the short-term store is likely to displace some other item currently represented in it. The longer an event is represented in short-term memory (the longer it is rehearsed), the stronger will be the memory of it. Support for this theoretical stance has been provided by experiments (on intact mammals) that show that the occurrence shortly after the presentation of some target event of a distractor (a stimulus that is likely to gain access to short-term memory) results in poorer memory for the target event (e.g., Wagner, Rudy and Whitlow 1973; Grau 1987). The effectiveness of distractors in the spinal rat therefore argue the presence in that preparation of a short-term memory store. To the extent that this seems an implausible suggestion, behavioral psychologists may be encouraged to seek alternative explanations for the disruptive effects of distractors on memory in intact animals.

Instrumental Conditioning

Before leaving the spinal cord, mention should be made of one preparation that, although less well explored than the spinal cat preparation, has two intriguing features. Work has been carried out using spinal rats in a modification of a procedure originally introduced by Horridge (1962) for the study of leg-position learning in headless insects. A spinal rat is suspended over a water-filled container, and entries of a hind limb into the water are recorded. When leg entries are followed by a strong shock, the rats come to hold the leg out of the water much more than control rats who receive the same series of shocks, independent of their leg position (Chopin and Buerger 1975). A later report finds that the rats may also successfully be trained to hold the leg in the water when shocks are delivered for lifting it out of the water (Sherman, Hoehler, and Buerger 1982).

The points of interest in this preparation are, first, that it appears to demonstrate instrumental as opposed to classical conditioning (a demonstration of instrumental learning in a spinal preparation would pose difficulties for those—e.g., Dickinson 1980—who suppose that instrumental conditioning involves "imperative logic"). And second, bidirectional response changes as a consequence of learning suggest that a form of conditioning other than alpha conditioning is being shown in the spinal cord. Unfortunately, however, there are difficulties in interpretation of the data. First, it is not clear that appropriate control procedures have been established (e.g., Church and Lerner 1976); second, as Sherman, Hoehler, and Buerger (1982) acknowledge, since the delivery of shocks is consistently preceded by a particular complex of proprioceptive stimuli, an interpretation in terms of classical conditioning cannot be ruled out. Because of these problems, along with the fact that there are no physiological data on the nature of the changes underlying performance, we shall not consider further this potentially important preparation.

Pointers for Work on Intact Vertebrates

I shall conclude this chapter by referring back to the questions raised in chapter 3 and at the beginning of this chapter, and by asking to what extent those questions have been answered by work on simple systems; to the extent that answers have been obtained, they may provide pointers for the approach to the physiology of learning in intact vertebrates. It may be noted first that work on spinal preparations has contributed little if anything to the answers of any of those questions. That work has, however, raised issues of considerable interest to behavioral psychologists, all of which center on the fact that the spinal preparation shows behavioral phenomena (e.g., classical aversive conditioning; instrumental conditioning; distractor effects) whose current interpretations suppose a role for relatively high-level motivational and cognitive capacities (e.g., fear, imperative logic, short-term memory). Given that it seems unlikely that such capacities are represented in the spinal cord, these results suggest that somewhat less sophisticated interpretations of those phenomena in intact animals should be sought.

One problem raised in the discussion of habituation was—given that transmission in S-R pathways becomes progressively less efficient with repeated stimulation—how could learned responses be elicited consistently to many repetitions of a stimulus? The work on *Aplysia* suggests a clear answer—namely, that habituation does indeed continue to play a role in conditioning tasks and does reduce the effectiveness of a CS, but that the process of habituation is successfully opposed and counteracted by sensitization, a process that is engaged by UCSs of motivational significance.

Questions raised in the introduction to this chapter concerned the location and the nature of changes induced by conditioning. The changes observed in *Aplysia* and *Hermissenda* clearly occur in the S-R pathway, in the direct route from sensory stimulus to motor response. In *Aplysia* the changes concern specific synapses, and are presynaptic; in *Hermissenda* the excitability of an entire cell is altered through a postsynaptic mechanism. Investigators of both preparations agree, however, that in vertebrates we should look for synapse-specific changes, while differing over the question whether pre- or postsynaptic mechanisms are likely to be primarily involved.

A further issue concerned the distinction between short- and long-term retention of associations. Conditioning in *Aplysia* is in effect a special case of sensitization, and we saw in chapter 2 that there was evidence for important differences between the mechanisms of short- and long-term sensitization. In particular, long-term sensitization, unlike short-term sensitization, requires the synthesis of new proteins and involves major morphological changes. We have seen that those same two features apply also to long-term retention of conditioning in *Hermissenda*. In general, then, we should be alert to the possibility that different mechanisms may serve short- as opposed to long-term retention of conditioning in (intact) vertebrates.

Finally, the question was raised of what mechanism might account for the pairing-specificity of conditioning at a neuronal level. Two postulated mechanisms—the Hebbian synapse and activity-dependent presynaptic facilitation—have been considered. Work on *Hermissenda* favored the former, and work on *Aplysia* the latter mechanism. We should, then, approach work on mammals with an open mind on this issue.

5. Association Formation in Vertebrates: The Role of the Cerebellum

Brain Structures and Conditioning in Vertebrates

Chapter 4 documented the considerable achievements of work on the physiological basis of classical conditioning in invertebrates. The success of that work encourages the search for comparable synaptic changes in the much less amenable nervous systems of vertebrates. We saw in chapter 4 that although the isolated spinal cord was capable of conditioning, little progress had been made in identifying the physiological basis of that learning, and this was largely because it has proved so difficult to establish precisely *where* the critical changes are occurring. Our review of conditioning in spinal animals also concluded that although genuine conditioning, at least of the alpha variety, could be found in spinal preparations, supraspinal centers might nevertheless play some modulating role. In this and the following chapter I shall discuss the potential role in conditioning of two vertebrate brain regions (the cerebellum, in this chapter, and the hippocampus in chapter 6). We shall see, for both structures, evidence that allows us to pinpoint, in a way that was not possible for the spinal cord, specific synapses that may exhibit the plasticity that underlies learning.

A Role in Conditioning for the Cerebellum

The cerebellum is, perhaps surprisingly, one of very few structures in the vertebrate nervous system for which there is now convincing evidence of a general role in conditioning; it will be recalled from chapter 3 that it has also been shown that the cerebellar vermis is essential for acquisition of long-term habituation of the startle reflex. These recent findings have focused the attention of physiological psychologists on the cerebellum as a site of prime interest, an attitude that stands in sharp contrast to the traditional stance, which supposed that the cerebellum played a relatively uninteresting role, as part of the extrapyramidal motor system, in control of movement (Watson 1978).

The first ground for supposing a role for the cerebellum in conditioning is that electrophysiological recordings have found cells in regions of the cerebellum whose activity is clearly tied to the development and occurrence of CRs. The second ground is that lesions of some of those same regions prevent the acquisition and retention of CRs. Subsequent work, much of which has employed brain stimulation techniques, has concentrated on the route through the cerebellum of information critical for CR formation. That work has pointed to a pathway that carries information about the CS, and a pathway that carries information about the UCS. The cerebellar site at which those pathways interact promises to be a region of synaptic plasticity critically involved in conditioning. Before discussing the findings in detail, preliminary introductions will be given to cerebellar anatomy and to rabbit eyelid conditioning, a paradigm that has played a central role in almost all the work to be discussed here as well as in much of the work to be discussed in chapter 6.

FIGURE 5.1. Architecture of the cerebellar cortex shown diagrammatically for a section of tissue from cat brain. The location of the tissue section is indicated in the drawing at top right; the same array of cells is repeated throughout the cortex. The cortex is organized around Purkinje cells, whose cell bodies form a layer between the superficial molecular layer and the deeper granule-cell layer. A single axon can be seen leaving each Purkinje cell body and passing through the granule-cell layer. In the molecular layer can be seen Purkinje cell dendrites, which are arrayed in flattened networks like pressed leaves, and parallel fibers, which pass through the dendrites perpendicularly. This layer also contains stellate cells and basket cells, which have similarly flattened arrays of dendrites. A stellate cell can be seen drawn in the right-hand part of the figure, near the molecular-layer surface; beneath and to the right of the stellate cell can be seen a basket cell, lying deep in the molecular layer, near the Purkinje cell layer. In the deep layer are granule cells and Golgi cells. The dendrites of the small granule cells receive inputs from mossy fibers, and their axons rise into the molecular layer, where they split (assuming the shape of a capital T) to form the parallel fibers. A Golgi cell, characterized by a cylindrical dendritic array and an axon showing multiple arborizations, can be seen drawn toward the left of the figure, just below the Purkinje cell layer. (*From* Llinás 1975)

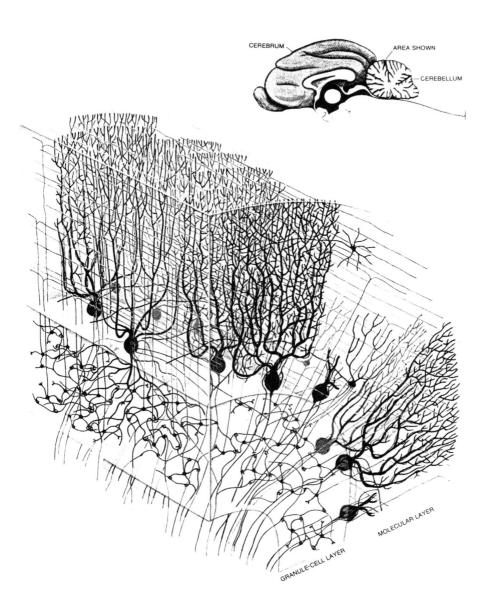

CEREBRUM

AREA SHOWN

CEREBELLUM

MOLECULAR LAYER

GRANULE-CELL LAYER

Cerebellar Neuroanatomy

The dorsally located cerebellum constitutes the major structure of the vertebrate hindbrain and consists of a cortical mantle that is separated by white matter from the underlying cerebellar deep nuclei. Figure 5.1 shows the location and general appearance of the cerebellum in the cat, and shows also a diagrammatic representation of the architectonic appearance of a cross-section through the cerebellar cortex. The cerebellar surface is marked by a series of transverse sulci and fissures that serve to increase the available area of thin cortical tissue. The fissures divide the cerebellum into folia that are conventionally assigned to groups that form an anterior-posterior series of lobes and lobules, the nomenclature for which varies according to the species and the neuroanatomist concerned. For our purposes, however, the major important division of the cerebellum is into the medial zone, the vermis (with its associated deep nucleus, the fastigial nucleus) and the lateral cerebellar hemispheres (with their associated deep nuclei—the dentate and the interpositus nuclei).

The organization of the cerebellum appears strikingly simple and is summarized schematically in Figure 5.2A. The cerebellar cortex consists of three layers: a superficial molecular layer, a deep granular layer, and, lying between them, a layer of Purkinje cells. The cortex contains only five types of neuron: small granule cells, Golgi cells, Purkinje cells, basket cells, and stellate cells. Golgi cells and granular cells are found in the granular layer, and basket cells and stellate cells in the molecular layer. Each cell type possesses ordered connections with the others. The pattern of connectivity is invariant throughout the cortex, and the architectonic appearance of the cortex correspondingly varies little within or between folia.

Inputs

Input to the cortex is derived exclusively from two types of fiber. Climbing fibers (whose cells of origin lie in the inferior olive) synapse onto dendrites of the large Purkinje cells, which constitute the middle layer of the cortex; and mossy fibers (that originate from pontine and other brainstem nuclei) synapse onto the small granule cells of the deep cortical layer. The mossy fibers derive their name from their enlarged terminals (shown on figure 5.2B) in the glomeruli of the granular layer. Axons of the granule cells project up to the superficial layer of the cortex where they bifurcate and run parallel to the cortical surface, constituting the major part of the superficial molecular layer. These parallel fibers synapse onto dendrites of the underlying Purkinje cells (whose dendritic tree is oriented

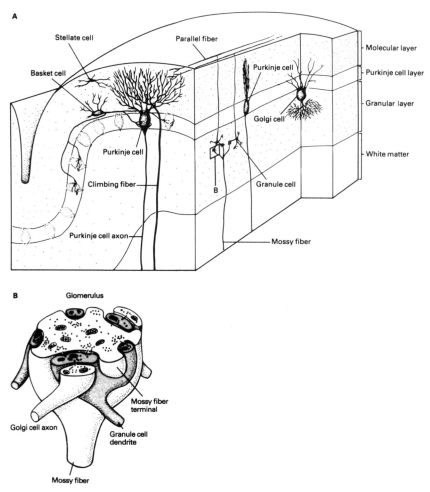

FIGURE 5.2. At the top, fig. 5.2A shows a single cerebellar folium sectioned vertically in both longitudinal and transverse planes, and illustrates the general organization of the cerebellar cortex. Fig. 5.2B shows the structure of a cerebellar glomerulus (a blowup of region B in fig. 5.2A). (*From* Kandel and Schwartz 1985)

orthogonally to the plane in which the parallel fibers run), and also onto basket cells and stellate cells, whose somata lie in the molecular layer. The cell bodies of the fifth class of cortical cell, the Golgi cell, lie in the deep granular layer, where their axons synapse onto granule-cell dendrites (see figure 5.2B); Golgi cell dendrites receive input from synapses made in the molecular layer with parallel fibers.

One further feature of cerebellar anatomy is of considerable importance here. The mossy/parallel fiber input is widely distributed across a region of the cortex; each mossy fiber contributes to the activation of several hundred granule cells, and each Purkinje cell receives many tens of thousands of parallel fiber synapses. But each climbing fiber projects to only one Purkinje cell, and each Purkinje cell receives input from only one climbing fiber; that single fiber does, however, make a large number of dendritic synapses onto the Purkinje cell and has a powerful excitatory effect upon it. We see, then, one precise and one diverse type of input to the cerebellar cortex.

Outputs

The sole output of the cerebellar cortex is provided by the axons of the Purkinje cells, which terminate in the deep cerebellar nuclei; intermediate and lateral regions of the cerebellar cortex project upon the dentate and interpositus nuclei, and the medial (vermal) cerebellar cortex, upon the fastigial nucleus. Since the dentate and interpositus nuclei merge into one another in the rabbit, they will generally be referred to henceforth jointly as the dentate/interpositus nucleus. The Purkinje cells exert an inhibitory influence on the cells of the cerebellar nuclei, and in fact all the cerebellar cortical neurons except the granule cells are inhibitory in their effect. The mossy fibers provide excitatory input to the granule cells, and the parallel fibers excite the other cerebellar cortex neurons (with all types of which, as we have seen, they make synaptic contact). Similarly, the climbing fibers excite Purkinje cells (the only cortical cell type that they contact). But apart from those inputs, the other actions of the cortex are entirely inhibitory. The Golgi cells inhibit granule cells; basket cells and stellate cells inhibit Purkinje cells, and Purkinje cells inhibit the cells of the cerebellar nuclei. The net result of the interactions between all cell types in the cortex is, then, to modulate the inhibition exerted by Purkinje cells upon the cerebellar nuclei.

A Vertebrate "Model System"

Most of the experiments discussed in this chapter will, as was the case in chapter 4, concern classical conditioning: this is probably for the same reason—the control given to the experimenters by that technique—and there are no very good grounds for supposing that the conclusions established may not equally be applicable to instrumental learning. One procedure that will receive particular attention is eyelid conditioning in the rabbit. This is a classical conditioning preparation that has been well characterized behaviorally, and that promises to be particularly suitable for physiological analysis. These features have contributed to its wide adoption as a vertebrate "model system" for the study of learning, so that results from its use will be discussed not only in the discussion of cerebellar function in this chapter but also in the discussion of the role of the hippocampus in chapter 6.

The rabbit eyelid-conditioning paradigm owes much of its current popularity as a vertebrate model system to the pioneering early work of Gormezano and his colleagues, who established its reliability as a technique for establishing classical conditioning and provided the controls necessary to show that results were not contaminated by nonassociative factors (see, for example, Gormezano 1972). The procedure itself is simple. A restrained rabbit receives pairings of a CS (which is, in most studies, a tone) and a UCS which may be either an airpuff delivered to the eyeball or a mild electrical shock to the periorbital region. The UCR (and CR) recorded is usually either closure of the eyelid or the nictitating membrane response; the nictitating membrane is a third eyelid, which lies between the external eyelids and the eye in some mammals, and which sweeps laterally across the eye. The nictitating membrane response is in fact a passive consequence of eyeball retraction, a response that has itself been used as a response measure. All three response measures correlate very highly with one another (e.g., McCormick et al. 1982), and we shall describe the responses measured from this preparation as eyelid responses, whether the original data collected were eyelid responses, nictitating membrane responses, or eyeball retractions.

Although the target CR for most of the studies to be discussed is the eyelid CR, other response systems are affected by the conditioning procedure. The airpuffs and periorbital shocks used are aversive UCSs, and autonomic changes indicative of fear are obtained during conditioning: CSs, for example, come to elicit conditioned decelerations of heart rate. It is important to note that these conditioned emotional responses do not show the same time course of acquisition as the skeletal eyelid response: in general, the emotional changes emerge more rapidly (within a very few trials) and tend to decline with further training (e.g., Schneiderman 1972).

Unconditioned eyelid-response latency is approximately 20 msec, and the UCR pathway appears to be disynaptic: UCS input is carried by the trigeminal nerve, which synapses in the trigeminal nucleus onto interneurons which in turn synapse in the cranial motor nuclei concerned with eyelid and eyeball-retraction responses—the facial nucleus, and the abducens and accessory abducens nuclei. Efferents from these nuclei directly innervate the muscles responsible for eyelid and eyeball-retraction responses (Cegavske, Harrison, and Torigoe 1987).

Basic Evidence for Cerebellar Involvement in Conditioning

A Neuronal Model of the CR in the Cerebellum

McCormick et al. (1982) used chronically implanted extracellular electrodes that could be used to record the activity of clusters of units in a variety of mesencephalic and metencephalic regions in rabbits during acquisition of a classically conditioned eyelid response, in which CS was a tone and UCS a corneal airpuff. Recordings from sites in the lateral and intermediate (but not the vermal) cerebellar cortex and in the dentate/interpositus nucleus found neuronal responses that mirrored the growth and final form of the learned eyelid CR. Figure 5.3 shows a series of recordings from a site in the dentate/interpositus nucleus. Initially, responses were obtained to onset of both UCS and CS. As training proceeded, those evoked responses diminished, and activity was seen that preceded CR initiation by some 50 msec or so. At this site, activity was also seen during UCRs. Figure 5.4 shows activity at another site in the dentate/interpositus nucleus. In this case, CS and UCS onset evoked no activity, and a "model" of the CR but not of the UCR developed as training proceeded. It should be noted here that these cells model only one aspect

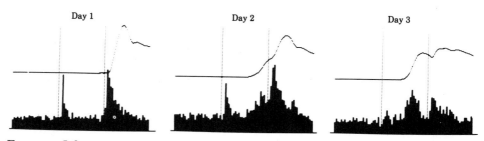

FIGURE 5.3. Development of a neuronal model of the CR in the cerebellum. The figure shows unit histograms obtained from the medial dentate nucleus during classical conditioning of the eyelid response. Each histogram bar is 15 msec wide, and each histogram is summed over an entire day (120 trials) of training. The first vertical line represents the onset of the tone and the second vertical line represents the onset of the airpuff. The trace above each histogram represents the averaged movement of the animal's nictitating membrane for an entire day (with up being extension of the nictitating membrane across the cornea). The total duration of each histogram and trace is 750 msec. (*From* McCormick et al. 1982)

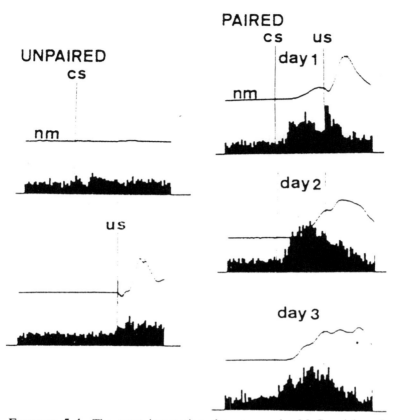

FIGURE 5.4. The most impressive change seen by McCormick and Thompson (1984) in neuronal unit activity within the medial dentate–lateral interpositus nuclei during unpaired and paired presentations of training stimuli. The animal was first given pseudorandomly unpaired presentations of the tone and corneal airpuff, in which neurons responded very little to either stimulus. However, when the stimuli were paired together in time, the cells began responding within the CS period as the animal learned the eyelid response. The onset of this unit activity preceded the behavioral CR within a trial by 36 to 58 msec. Each histogram bar is 9 msec in duration. The upper trace of each histogram represents the movements of the nictitating membrane (with up being extension across the cornea). (*From* McCormick and Thompson 1984)

of conditioning, namely, the eyelid CR; the activity of the cells that exhibit models of the eyelid CR does not parallel the course of all the CRs that result form CS-UCS pairings and, in particular, does not model conditioned autonomic responses. Similar development of "models" of the CR was also seen in many extracerebellar sites in the brainstem, and the most striking evidence for a critical role of the cerebellum in conditioning comes from lesion studies.

Effects of Dentate/Interpositus Lesions

McCormick et al. (1981) were the first to report that large unilateral cerebellar lesions abolished a learned CR when the UCS was delivered to the ipsilateral eye; that finding was confirmed in a more detailed report by McCormick et al. (1982), whose principal results are summarized on figure 5.5. Clark et al. (1984) went on to show that smaller cerebellar lesions confined to the dentate/interpositus nucleus had a similar effect, and subsequent work indicates that the critical site for disruption of conditioning

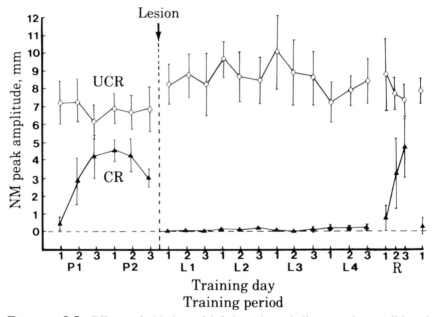

FIGURE 5.5. Effects of ablation of left lateral cerebellum on the conditioned eyelid response. *Filled triangles:* amplitude of CR; *open diamonds:* amplitude of UCR. All training was to the left eye (ipsilateral to lesion), except where labeled R (right eye). The lesion abolished the CR of the ipsilateral eye but had no effect on the UCR. P1 and P2, initial learning on the two days prior to the lesion; L1–4, four days of postoperative training to the left eye; R, right eye training (showing rapid acquisition). After training to the right eye, the left eye was again trained and showed no learning. Left eye, 40-trial training periods; right eye, 24-trial training periods. (*From* McCormick et al. 1982)

is a dorsolateral region in the anterior interpositus nucleus (Lavond, Hembree, and Thompson 1985; Welsh and Harvey 1989).

McCormick et al. (1982) found that following cerebellar damage reacquisition using the ipsilateral eye was not possible, but that acquisition using the contralateral eye was rapid and efficient. And, perhaps the most significant finding of all, although ipsilateral cerebellar lesions abolished CRs, they "had no effect at all on the unconditioned reflex response" (McCormick et al. 1982:2731). Subsequent lesion studies have shown: that cerebellar lesions also abolish eyelid CRs in rats (Skelton 1988); that cerebellar lesions in rabbits may abolish leg-flexion CRs established to tone CSs (Thompson et al. 1987); and that such lesions abolish instrumentally conditioned (avoidance) eyelid CRs in rabbits (Polenchar et al. 1985). In none of these cases is the relevant UCR affected. There is also one report (Solomon, Stowe, and Pendlbeury 1989) of a human patient having damage to cerebellar afferents who (unlike appropriate controls) failed to acquire a conditioned eyelid response (using a tone CS and an airpuff UCS); in her case also, the unconditioned eyelid response to airpuffs was normal.

The absence of effect on the UCR indicates that the deficit is not motor in origin. Nor is there any reason to suppose that it reflects a primary sensory deficit. Cerebellar lesions that disrupt CRs established using auditory CSs do not disrupt the primary auditory pathway (from the cochlear nuclei to the inferior colliculus, medial geniculate body, and auditory cortex). There is evidence, moreover, that the deficit is independent of sensory modality. Lewis, LoTurco, and Solomon (1987) found that lesions of the middle cerebellar peduncle, the major source of afferents to the cerebellar hemispheres, disrupted retention of conditioned eyelid responses in rabbits to both light and tone stimuli, and prevented acquisition of CRs to light, tone, or tactile (vibration of a plate on the animal's back) stimuli. Finally, although dentate/interpositus lesions abolish the conditioned eyelid response, they do not disrupt fear conditioning. Lavond et al. (1984) found that (bilateral) dentate/interpositus lesions had no effect on acquisition of a conditioned deceleration of heart rate to a tone CS paired with a face shock; the lesions did totally prevent acquisition of a conditioned eyelid response in the same rabbits.

Exploration of CS, UCS, and CR Pathways

The findings from lesion studies encourage exploration of the cerebellum as a potential site of formation of new links, or of the strengthening of existing links, as a consequence of CS-UCS pairings that establish skeletal CRs. We turn now to a consideration of the routes by which information about the CS and the UCS might reach the cerebellum, and of the route by which information essential to the occurrence of skeletal CRs might leave the cerebellum. Establishment of these routes should allow the pinpointing of sites at which changes in synaptic strengths as a consequence of stimulus pairings should be sought.

CS Pathway

Mossy fibers project to the cerebellum from their origin in pontine nuclei via the middle cerebellar peduncle; climbing fibers project from their cells of origin in the inferior olive via the inferior cerebellar peduncle. Thompson and his colleagues suggest that CS information is carried by the mossy fibers, and we shall review the support for that proposition here.

As noted above, lesions of the middle cerebellar peduncle prevent acquisition and abolish retention of conditioned eyelid responses in rabbits (Lewis, LoTurco, and Solomon 1987). Retention is immediately abolished by lesions; it does not seem, therefore, that the deficit can be attributed to a postlesion failure of the UCS information to be processed, since in that case one might expect not a sudden loss, but a gradual extinction of the previously acquired response. Electrical stimulation of the middle cerebellar peduncle, or of pontine nuclei which give rise to mossy fibers running in the peduncle, serves as an effective CS when paired with a corneal airpuff (Steinmetz et al. 1986). The pontine nuclei concerned (the dorsolateral, lateral, and medial pontine nuclei) do receive afferents from both neocortical and subcortical regions concerned with various sensory modalities.

Steinmetz et al. (1987) explored the role of the pontine regions in the projection of specifically auditory information to the cerebellum. They found both electrophysiological and anatomical evidence that auditory information reaches the lateral pontine nuclear region by a variety of routes, including direct projections from the cochlear nuclei. Moreover, lesions of this same region abolished CRs to auditory, but not to light, CSs. Detailed information on the routes taken by other sensory modalities is not yet available, but the current assumption (supported by the abolition by middle cerebellar peduncle lesions of CRs to CSs of at least three modalities) is that information from the visual and tactile senses is relayed via other pontine regions in a manner comparable to that established for audition.

UCS Pathway

Thompson proposes that UCS information is carried by the climbing fibers, and the primary supporting evidence comes from lesion and stimulation studies.

The inferior olive, from which most if not all climbing fibers originate, receives sensory input from the face region, and lesions of part of the olive (the dorsal accessory nucleus, DAO) prevent the acquisition of an eyelid CR but have no effect upon the UCR (McCormick, Steinmetz, and Thompson 1985; Yeo, Hardiman, and Glickstein 1986). Two contrasting effects of DAO lesions on retention of prelesion CRs have been reported. McCormick and his colleagues and Yeo and his colleagues agree that DAO lesions abolish CRs, but whereas Yeo and colleagues find immediate abolition, McCormick and colleagues report a gradual loss of CRs, comparable to the behavioral extinction seen when UCSs are no longer delivered. This latter effect is, of course, what should be expected if UCS information was transmitted via the inferior olive.

Stimulation of DAO may produce a variety of behavioral responses (including leg flexion, eyelid closure, and head turns), and stimulation of DAO serves as an adequate UCS when paired with a tone CS, the CR produced matching the response obtained by DAO stimulation (Mauk, Steinmetz, and Thompson 1986). Stimulation of brain-stem regions adjacent to the inferior olive, but which do not give rise to climbing fibers, may obtain movements; stimulation at these sites does not, however, serve as an effective UCS (Thompson 1988).

These observations do, then, give good support to the notion that UCS information is carried by climbing fibers from the inferior olive, although it should be borne in mind that McCormick and his colleagues (1985) and Yeo and his colleagues (1986) hold opposing views on the consequences of DAO lesions on retention.

CR Pathway

Thompson proposes (see figure 5.6) a somewhat circuitous route for the efferent limb of the cerebellar associative system: the pathway originates in the dentate/interpositus nucleus and runs in the superior cerebellar peduncle to the contralateral red nucleus, from which fibers again cross the midline to act directly upon the motor neurons controlling the eyelid movements. Both lesion and stimulation data support this proposal. Lesions of either the superior cerebellar peduncle (McCormick, Guyer, and Thompson 1982) or the red nucleus (Rosenfield and Moore 1983) abolish

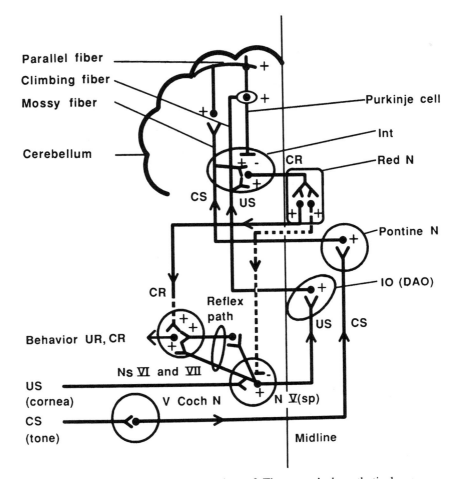

FIGURE 5.6. Schematic representation of Thompson's hypothetical memory-trace circuit for discrete behavioral responses learned as adaptations to aversive events. The US (corneal airpuff) pathway consists of somatosensory projections to DAO and its climbing fiber projections to the cerebellum. The tone CS pathway consists of auditory projections to pontine nuclei (Pontine N) and their mossy fiber projections to the cerebellum. The efferent (eyelid closure) CR pathway projects from the interpositus nucleus (Int) of the cerebellum to the red nucleus (Red N) and via the descending rubral pathway to act ultimately on motor neurons. The red nucleus may also exert inhibitory control of the transmission of somatic sensory information about the US to the inferior olive (IO). NV (sp): spinal fifth cranial nucleus; N VI: sixth cranial nucleus; N VII: seventh cranial nucleus; V Coch N: ventral cochlear nucleus. + indicates excitatory synaptic action; − indicates inhibitory synaptic action. (*From* Thompson 1986)

established eyelid CRs and prevent their acquisition; the lesions are without effect on the UCR. As would be expected if this pathway transmitted information generated subsequent to the "link" between the CS and UCS paths, stimulation of the red nucleus, which may elicit eyelid responses, does not serve as an effective UCS (Chapman, Steinmetz, and Thompson 1988). Figure 5.6 shows in diagrammatic form the CS, UCS, and CR pathways proposed by Thompson.

Site of Conditioning-Induced Changes

One preliminary observation to be made here is that although there is currently debate on precisely which regions of the cerebellum are necessary for eyelid conditioning, it is generally agreed that neither the vermis nor the fastigial nucleus (the deep nucleus to which the vermal cerebellar cortex projects) is involved. We have seen above that neuronal "models" of the CR have not been observed at vermal sites; and neither lesions of the vermis nor lesions of the fastigial nucleus disrupt eyelid conditioning (McCormick and Thompson 1984; Yeo, Hardiman, and Glickstein 1985a, 1985b). The vermal mechanism necessary for acquisition of long-term habituation of the startle reflex (see chapter 3) is not, then, involved in classical eyelid conditioning. It is worth remarking also that although vermal lesions do not affect short-term habituation, dentate/interpositus lesions totally prevent acquisition of eyelid conditioning.

A Site in Cerebellar Cortex?

When McCormick et al. (1981) originally reported the involvement of the cerebellum in eyelid conditioning, they suggested that the cerebellar cortex was the most likely site of the plasticity involved in conditioning. The proposal was not entirely original; that the cerebellum might play a critical role in learning of motor skills was suggested by, amongst others, Marr (1969) and Eccles (1977b). The McCormick et al. proposal was, however, the first to be based on a clear and specific learning deficit, and it has in fact proved extremely difficult to specify any of the "motor skills" proposals sufficiently well to allow convincing proof or disproof (e.g., Watson 1978). Early proponents of a role in learning for the cerebellum were stimulated not so much by direct behavioral evidence as by cerebellar anatomical organization. As we have seen, Purkinje cells see the coming together of a diffuse and a specific input system (the former mediated by mossy/parallel fibers, the latter by climbing fibers). Applied to the conditioning paradigm, the diffuse system may be seen as "learning" input, the specific system as "teaching" input. (e.g., Thompson and Donegan 1986). Learning would be affected by a modulation of the effectiveness of those parallel fiber–Purkinje cell synapses that were active at the time of arrival of input from a climbing fiber. The activity dependence of the modulation would ensure specificity of conditioning to the appropriate CS (the "learning input"); and the previously wired connection between the specific climbing fiber, the Purkinje cell, and the cerebellar nuclear cells would ensure the appropriate CR.

Effects of Cortical Lesions on Acquisition and Retention

Evidence for a potential role of cerebellar cortex in conditioning comes from the electrophysiological observation that some cortical cells do exhibit "models" of the CR which occur prior to the emission of the CR (McCormick et al. 1982). But it is doubtful whether cerebellar cortex is necessary for conditioning to occur. Yeo, Hardiman, and Glickstein (1984, 1985b) have reported that restricted unilateral lesions of cerebellar cortex abolish, and prevent reacquisition of, a conditioned eyelid response (using either white noise or a light as CS, and periorbital shock as UCS). The critical cortical region—hemispheric lobule HVI in Larsell's (1952, 1953) nomenclature—receives afferents from DAO and projects to the dentate/interpositus nucleus (parts, respectively, of the UCS and the CS pathways). Thompson and his colleagues, however, have repeatedly failed to find a comparable effect of lesions restricted to cortical tissue, even when using the same procedures as Yeo and his colleagues (Thompson 1986). But there are reports by Thompson and his colleagues to indicate that cerebellar cortex may indeed play a role in eyelid conditioning.

Lavond and Steinmetz (1989) established that extensive unilateral cerebellar cortical lesions slowed but did not prevent the original acquisition of conditioned nictitating membrane responses: thus cerebellar cortex may play an important (but not critical) role in acquisition, as opposed to retention, of conditioned eyelid CRs. There is, however, evidence also that retention may in certain circumstances be disrupted by cortical lesions.

Woodruff-Pak, Lavond, and Thompson (1985) investigated the effects of removal of lobule HVI on retention in a more difficult conditioning paradigm—trace conditioning—in which the CS (tone) offset preceded UCS (corneal airpuff) onset by .5 sec. Cortical lesions did impair retention of trace-conditioned CRs, but the effect was temporary and responding returned to preoperative levels by the third postoperative session, showing considerable savings when compared to the original rate of acquisition. By contrast, just as in the standard delay-conditioning paradigm, lesions of the dentate/interpositus nucleus permanently abolished trace-conditioned CRs.

Cerebellar cortical lesions may also disrupt retention of the conditioned eyelid response when the CS used is direct stimulation of a brain-stem source of mossy fiber afferents. Knowlton, Lavond, and Thompson (1988), for example, reported that restricted cerebellar cortex lesions abolished retention of eyelid CRs when stimulation of the lateral reticular nucleus (a source of mossy fibers) served as CS. Knowlton and his colleagues suggest that whereas a conventional CS, such as a tone, probably activates widely distributed areas of cerebellar cortex, direct brain-stem stimulation may obtain a more localized cortical response. This work throws open once again the question of cerebellar cortical involvement in conditioning: perhaps if *all* cerebellar cortex was removed, retention of eyelid conditioning with a tone CS *would* be disrupted.

The electrophysiological and lesion findings argue, then, that the cerebellar cortex does play a role in conditioning, but it is not yet clear that it is an essential part of the conditioning circuit in the way that the dentate/interpositus nucleus clearly is. Perhaps, then, the site of plasticity should be sought in the deep nuclei.

A Site in the Deep Nuclei?

The principal features of the afferent and efferent cerebellar pathways have been outlined in preceding sections. But it will be noticed that although the deep nuclei formed part of the CR pathway, they were not part of either the CS or the UCS pathways, which converged on the cortical Purkinje cells. If the cortical site of convergence of those pathways is not necessary for conditioning, where does the critical modulation occur?

Thompson's proposal (e.g., 1986) is that modulation of synaptic activity occurs in parallel in the cortex and at the dentate/interpositus nucleus, and that convergence occurs at the latter site of collaterals given off by both climbing fibers (the UCS pathway) and mossy fibers (the CS pathway) en route, respectively, to Purkinje cells and to granule cells in the cortex. There is anatomical evidence for such collaterals of both climbing fibers (Courville, Augustine, and Martel 1977) and mossy fibers (McCrea, Bishop, and Kitai 1977), although Yeo, Hardiman, and Glickstein (1985b) point out that anatomists disagree on whether mossy fibers originating from pontine nuclei (that is, those fibers presumed to form part of the CS pathway) do in fact give off collaterals to the cerebellar nuclei (see, for example, Dietrichs, Bjaalie, and Brodal 1983).

Nature of the Modulation

Eyelid Conditioning as Alpha Conditioning

If there remain doubts about the precise site of the conditioning-related modulation in the cerebellum, even less is known of the nature of that modulation. A preliminary question is whether eyelid conditioning using a tone CS is an example of "alpha" conditioning. We have spoken so far only of excitatory connections between mossy (CS) fibers and the dentate/interpositus nucleus, and in figure 5.6 these are shown as excitatory. But prior to training, any such excitatory influence on the eyelid response appears to be minimal: Thompson, Clark, Donegan, Lavond, Madden et al. (1984) point out that although intense auditory stimuli may elicit reflex eyelid (alpha) responses, these are of much shorter latency than the CRs obtained to trained tone CSs. Moreover, a tone may readily be established as a conditioned inhibitor of the conditioned eyelid response (e.g., Mis 1977). It seems safe to assume therefore that the change brought about by conditioning to a tone CS activates a previously inactive synapse (or synapses) and that that activation could result not only in excitatory but also in inhibitory influences on the postsynaptic cell (although we shall encounter a quite different account of the potential basis of conditioned inhibition when we discuss SOP—"sometimes opponent process"—theory in a later section).

Although tone CSs do not elicit unconditioned eyelid responses of a similar topography to conditioned eyelid responses, light CSs do. If a light is used as a CS in the eyelid-response paradigm, the resultant CR is, then, an example of alpha conditioning. It is therefore of interest that cerebellar lesions (in the dentate/interpositus nucleus) also disrupt alpha conditioning to dim-light CSs without having any detectable effect on the UCRs elicited by dim (or bright) lights (Skelton, Mauk, and Thompson 1988). One implication of this result is that the mechanisms concerned in the establishment of conventional (non-alpha) conditioning are concerned also in alpha conditioning: although conventional conditioning involves the strengthening of a response without prior excitatory connections to the CS, and alpha conditioning involves strengthening previously existing connections, the physiological processes involved may well be the same.

Mechanism of Activity-Dependent Modulation

The data reviewed above led to the proposal that the effectiveness of the synapses between collaterals from the CS pathway (the mossy fibers) and cells in the dentate/interpositus nucleus is modified as a consequence of the excitatory influence upon dentate/interpositus of activity in the UCS pathway, carried by collaterals of the climbing fibers. As noted above, the modulation is clearly activity dependent, since it is specific to pairings of CSs and UCSs. Two candidates for a mechanism of activity-dependent modulation were introduced in chapter 4—Hebb's postulate (the "successful use" postulate), and activity-dependent presynaptic facilitation (the mechanism that appears to mediate classical conditioning in *Aplysia*).

Applied to the cerebellar data, Hebb's postulate would assume that the increased effectiveness of mossy fiber–deep nuclei synapses was due to the pairing of mossy-fiber activity with deep-nuclei activity (the latter being activated via the climbing-fiber activity induced by UCS presentation). But direct stimulation of the deep nuclei, despite eliciting discrete skeletal responses, does not serve as an effective UCS (Chapman, Steinmetz, and Thompson 1988): if, therefore, the effective synaptic modulation is at the level of the deep nuclei (and not, for example, in the cerebellar cortex), then it appears that the synapse is not modified according to Hebbian principles.

If Hebb's postulate is rejected, activity-dependent presynaptic facilitation may be the preferred mechanism, but by default only, since there is no direct evidence in its support. There is no anatomical evidence of terminals of climbing-fiber collaterals on presynaptic terminals of mossy-fiber collaterals, nor any physiological evidence of presynaptic facilitation of mossy-fiber collaterals as a consequence of conditioning. Nor indeed is there evidence that UCS presentations sensitize unpaired CS presentations.

There is evidence (Mamounas, Thompson, and Madden 1987) that GABA-ergic synapses may be involved, since injection of bicuculline (a GABA receptor antagonist) into the dentate/interpositus nucleus of trained animals abolishes both CRs and the recorded "models" of CRs. GABA is a prominent inhibitory transmitter in the cerebellum, so that this is not, perhaps, a surprising result, and it tells us little about the precise nature of the modulation.

There is good evidence for both anatomical and physiological plasticity of the cerebellum following various environmental manipulations (e.g., Floeter and Greenough 1979; Ito 1984). But that evidence does not relate directly to standard conditioning procedures, and in fact the best evidence we have on the nature of a plasticity involved in vertebrates as a correlate of learning will be found when we consider hippocampal involvement in conditioning.

The foregoing discussion has assumed that eyelid conditioning does not require the formation of new connections: the proposals outlined could be satisfied by altering the strengths of preexisting synapses. But it should be borne in mind that there is currently no *direct* evidence either for or against the proposition that no new cerebellar synapses are formed as a result of conditioning.

The use of the conditioned eyelid response in the investigation of the role of the cerebellum in learning is an important example of the development of a "model system" in vertebrates. One of the major payoffs of this model system, the precise specification of the anatomical and physiological nature of the plasticity involved, lies in the future. At present, we can consider issues already raised for behavior theorists by the results described above.

Implications for Behavioral Theory

The effects of dentate/interpositus lesions on conditioning have a considerable bearing on three issues in behavior theory. The first concerns the notion that there is an important difference between the learning of preparatory as opposed to consummatory CRs: this is an issue that was raised previously, in the discussion of learning in the spinal cord (in chapter 4). The second issue concerns theorizing by Wagner, whose work has also been referred to previously (in chapter 3, in which his notions of priming and of the distinction between short- and long-term memory were introduced). We shall see in this chapter a formalization of some of his notions and discuss his view that CRs invariably differ in at least some respect from UCRs. The third issue concerns the nature of the association formed in classical conditioning, and in particular, the question whether an S-S association is formed so that the CS comes to substitute for the UCS.

Preparatory Versus Consummatory Responses

The pertinent facts may be rapidly summarized: dentate/interpositus lesions disrupt conditioning of skeletal CRs (eyelid closure; leg flexion) but have no effect on the corresponding UCRs and no effect on fear conditioning.

The differential sensitivity to lesions of skeletal and autonomic CRs supports the view (Konorski 1967; Dickinson 1980) that consummatory and preparatory CRs are indeed mediated by different systems. But this conclusion may not be as strong as at first appears, since those systems may have much in common. This possibility merits serious consideration because lesions of another cerebellar region—the vermis—do disrupt heart-rate conditioning. Supple and Leaton (1990) have reported that although vermal lesions did not disrupt the unconditioned heart-rate response of rats to either a tone CS or a shock UCS, vermal-lesioned rats given a series of tone-shock pairings did not (unlike controls) develop a conditioned bradycardia response. Thus just as interpositus lesions disrupt skeletal CRs without affecting UCRs, vermal lesions disrupt at least one autonomic CR without affecting the UCR. The parallel may, however, be incomplete since it is not clear that the vermal-induced deficit is specific to learning. Other work has shown that vermal lesions have a general taming effect: Supple, Cranney, and Leaton (1988) found that vermal lesions (but not lesions of the cerebellar hemispheres) much reduced fear (assessed, for example, by freezing) in the presence of a cat. The fear induced by cats is presumably unlearned, and such a result suggests that vermal lesions may disrupt motivation so that fear may no longer be experienced. If conditioned bradycardia is a consequence of fear, the disruptive effects of vermal lesions can be accommodated without supposing an effect on learning. Thus the interpretation of the effects of vermal lesions on fear-related CRs is complicated, and so, in consequence, is the relevance of those findings to the proposal that consummatory and preparatory CRs employ very different neuronal systems. Further complications may be introduced by recalling that vermal lesions disrupt the acquisition (but not the retention) of long- (but not of short-) term habituation of the acoustic startle response (see chapter 3). One clear implication of all these findings—perhaps the only clear implication—is that the functions of the cerebellum extend far beyond those of motor control.

The Nature of the Association Formed

A cerebellar pathway involving the dentate/interpositus nucleus is, then, involved selectively in the formation of consummatory CRs, responses that are specific to the specific sensory qualities of the particular UCS used. The data reviewed above suggest that the cerebellar system influences the most direct "reflex" UCR pathway at its terminal region of synapse formation, onto the brain-stem motoneurons directly responsible for the eyelid response. The modulation of synaptic strengths responsible for conditioning appears to occur some synapses away from that motor region, and is between pathways that carry CS information and UCS information. The nature of this link suggests that eyelid-response conditioning does involve an S-S association, a physiological finding congruent with the dominant current view of the nature of classical conditioning. But there is a difficulty with this conclusion.

The problem arises when we ask why, given that an animal detects the contingency between, say, bell and food, the animal salivates to the bell in the absence of the food. The standard response of those who hold an S-S interpretation of classical conditioning is that the bell activates a representation of the food, which in turn elicits food-related responses (e.g., Mackintosh 1974; Dickinson 1980). Implicit in this stimulus-substitution account of response generation is the notion that the UCS itself activates its own representation, and that that activation is in turn responsible for the UCR. But the rabbit's eyelid response appears to be elicited by corneal airpuff UCSs through a pathway that is clearly independent of the cerebellar UCS pathway described by Thompson and his colleagues, since cerebellar damage does not affect the unconditioned eyelid response. It would appear, therefore, that although UCS presentation would be expected to activate the cerebellar UCS pathway, activation of that pathway does not contribute to the UCR. But it is now difficult to see why modulation of synaptic strengths so that CS activity potentiates activity at any point in the cerebellar pathways activated by the UCS should engender a CR. We know that electrical stimulation of the dentate/interpositus nucleus may elicit discrete skeletal responses (McCormick and Thompson 1984); but if damage to those regions has no effect on UCRs, the implication would seem to be that endogenous synaptic activation does not obtain a behavioral response.

In view of the wealth of evidence that converges on the conclusion that the final result of the conditioning procedure is to enhance dentate/interpositus activity, it seems most economical to conclude that these pathways are indeed normally activated by UCSs and that such activation does obtain behavioral output but that *either* the effects of activation of the cerebellar pathways are normally lost in the much more substantial response obtained through the "reflex" pathway, *or* a more detailed examination of UCRs following cerebellar ablations may yet yield evidence of lesion-induced changes.

Support for the notion that cerebellar damage may obtain subtle changes in UCRs is provided by Welsh and Harvey (1989) in a report on rabbits with interpositus lesions. Welsh and Harvey found that their lesions had, as anticipated, a disruptive effect on conditioned eyelid-response acquisition and no perceptible effect on UCRs to the UCS used (a corneal airpuff). However, when the intensity of the airpuff was reduced to levels below those normally used to support conditioning, the interpositus-lesioned animals showed both substantial reductions in the probability of occurrence of a UCR and increases in the latency to peak amplitude of UCRs. The general point to be made here is that in the absence of some account of the anomalous lack of effect of cerebellar lesions on UCRs, it will not be possible to accommodate the physiological findings within a stimulus-substitution account of response generation in classical conditioning.

"Sometimes Opponent Process" Theory

We may turn now to consideration of an interpretation of the physiological data derived from a behavioral theory that offers an alternative to the traditional stimulus-substitution theory of classical conditioning; the theory has the advantage that it can accommodate the fact, troublesome for stimulus-substitution theory, that CRs do not always resemble UCRs.

"Sometimes opponent process" (SOP) theory (e.g., Wagner 1981) has at its base the notion that UCRs to all UCSs (indeed to all stimuli) consist of two components—a primary followed by a (longer-lasting) secondary response. An important feature of the theory is that CRs reflect only the secondary component of the UCR, so that when the secondary component differs in form from the primary component, the CR does not resemble the (immediate) UCR. Thus the immediate UCR of rats to electric shock is violent activity: but this is succeeded by behavioral inhibition (freezing). And when a stimulus is paired with shock, the CR to that stimulus is not activity, but freezing. The theory derives its name from the fact that not all secondary components do contrast in nature from the primary components. Thus some CRs do resemble (immediate) UCRs, others do not.

In formalizing SOP theory, Wagner (e.g., Wagner and Donegan 1989) speaks of the internal representations of stimuli as nodes, elements of which may be either inactive or in one of two active states, A1 and A2. A1 states obtain the primary response process, and A2 states the secondary response process. Presentation of any stimulus (UCS, CS, or neutral) moves elements in the node representing that stimulus from an inactive state into the A1 state (from which decay into the A2 state occurs rapidly).

When an excitatory connection exists between nodes representing a CS and a UCS, presentation of the CS obtains, in the UCS node, movement of the elements in the UCS node from the inactive state to the A2 state; thus only the physical occurrence of a stimulus can obtain (brief) activation of the A1 state. The A2 state corresponds to the short-term memory store referred to in the discussion (in chapter 3) of Wagner's account of habituation in terms of priming. Stimuli are primed when they are in the A2 state, and this may occur either as a result of the recent occurrence of that stimulus (self-generated priming, the occurrence of the A2 state as a result of rapid decay from the A1 state) or as a result of the occurrence of some other stimulus whose node has an excitatory connection with the stimulus (retrieval-generated priming). The notion (encountered in chapter 3) that primed stimuli are less effective than unprimed stimuli in gaining access to short-term memory is captured by the SOP model in the following way: the more elements of a node that are currently in the A2 state, the fewer elements will be promoted from the inactive to the A1 state by presentation of the appropriate stimulus; and, of course, the fewer elements that are promoted to the A1 state, the fewer will in turn decay from that state to the A2 (short-term memory) state. The entire collection of nodes and their interconnections constitutes long-term memory.

Excitatory connections between nodes are formed when both nodes are simultaneously in the A1 state; inhibitory connections between nodes are formed where one node (CS) is in the A1 state while the other (UCS) is in the A2 state. Figure 5.7 summarizes some of the principal features of SOP theory.

The preceding thumbnail sketch of SOP theory will, it is hoped, be sufficient to allow an understanding of its application to the cerebellar work, and of how its novel predictions are generated.

Wagner and Donegan contend that the A1 state obtained by airpuff presentation is reflected by activity in the primary eyelid-response pathway (from the trigeminal nucleus via one or two brain-stem relays to the motoneurons), *plus* activity in the cerebellar UCS pathway (from the DAO via the climbing fibers to the cerebellar cortex and deep nuclei). The transition from the A1 to the A2 state (see figure 5.8) occurs either at the cerebellar cortex or the deep nuclei, so that the secondary process engendered by UCS presentation involves activation of the deep nuclei and of the other stations of the CR pathway including the red nucleus. The conditioning procedure results in the activation by the CS of those systems involved in the A2 state—of, that is, the CR pathway. Wagner and Donegan also assume that these same systems mediate the secondary component of the UCR, and so the UCR must be altered by lesions that disrupt them. In other words, Thompson's CR pathway "can be regarded as an obligatory branch of the UCR pathway" (Wagner and Donegan 1989:178).

Since the conditioned eyelid response resembles the unconditioned eyelid response, the secondary component of this UCR must resemble the primary component, but it will represent the later components of the eyelid response. The first prediction made by Wagner and Donegan is, therefore, that a close examination of the *late* components of the UCR following cerebellar lesions will reveal their disruption. Although Welsh and Harvey (1989) have reported deficits in UCRs (to weak UCSs) in cerebel-

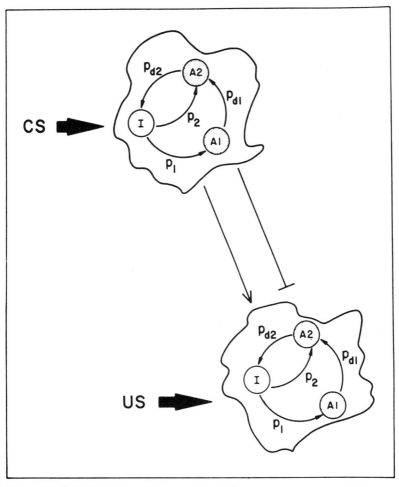

FIGURE 5.7. Depiction of two nodes in the memory system of SOP, one presumed to be directly activated by a CS and the other by a US in a Pavlovian conditioning procedure. The connected circles within each node represent the three activity states (inactive, I; primary active state, A1; secondary active state, A2) in which nodal elements may momentarily reside, and the connecting paths represent the allowable state transitions. When a node is acted upon by the stimulus it represents, some proportion (p1) of the elements in the I state will be promoted to the A1 state, from which they decay first to the A2 state, and then back to the inactive state. But when a node is acted upon by excitation propagated over an associative connection, some proportion (p2) of the elements in the inactive state will be promoted to the A2 state, from which they will decay to the inactive state. Momentary decay probabilities are represented by pd1 and pd2, and pd1 is assumed to be greater than pd2. The two nodes are joined to suggest the manner of directional excitatory (pointing arrows) and inhibitory (stopped line) linkages that are commonly assumed to be formed. (*From* Wagner and Donegan 1989)

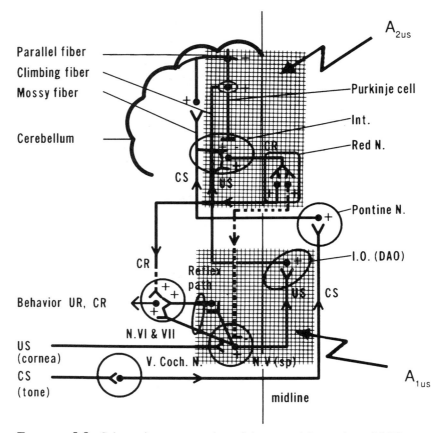

FIGURE 5.8. Schematic representation of the potential mapping of SOP upon the hypothetical circuit (fig. 5.6) underlying the rabbit conditioned eyelid response. Segments of the US pathway that are taken to correspond to the A1 activation state are shown in the lower shaded area, and segments of the US pathway that are taken to correspond to the A2 activation state are shown in the upper shaded area. (*From* Wagner and Donovan 1989)

lar-lesioned rabbits, those deficits were not confined to late UCR components, and this is therefore a prediction that has yet to receive support.

Striking support for a second prediction of this theory comes from a recent report (Sears and Steinmetz 1991) on multiple-unit recordings from DAO cells during UCS (airpuff) presentations in rabbits. It will be recalled that DAO is believed to form a station in the UCS pathway, and as figure 5.8 shows, activity in DAO constitutes, according to Wagner and Donegan (1989), promotion of elements of the UCS node to the A1 state.

Sears and Steinmetz (1991) found that UCS-elicited DAO activity showed a dramatic decrease following a series of CS (tone)-UCS pairings; the DAO response to UCS-alone presentations did not decline. According to the Wagner and Donegan account, CS-UCS pairings would result in the capacity of the CS to promote elements of the UCS node from the inactive to the A2 (short-term memory) state (retrieval-generated priming); this is, of course, the mechanism of CR production. But stimuli appropriate to nodes whose elements are currently in the A2 state are, according to this account, less likely to gain access to the A1 state. What the Sears and Steinmetz (1991) report shows, then, is that, in accordance with predictions derived from the Wagner and Donegan (1989) account, a primed UCS is indeed less effective in obtaining access to the A1 state, represented here by DAO activity.

A third prediction concerns the role of the red nucleus, part of the system underlying the A2 state. We have seen that inhibitory links between nodes are formed, in SOP theory, when a CS node is in the A1 state and a UCS node is in the A2 state. It should therefore be the case that pairing of a CS with stimulation of part of the CR pathway, the red nucleus for example, should lead to an inhibitory association between CS and UCS, to the CS being a signal for a reduced probability of UCS delivery. As noted above, there is evidence that although stimulation of either the deep nuclei or the red nucleus may obtain eyelid responses, in neither case does that stimulation serve as an effective UCS. Wagner and Donegan (1989) make the striking prediction that in fact pairing of a CS with red nucleus stimulation should lead to an *inhibitory* connection being formed between the CS and the node representing the UCS whose presentation normally elicits the response obtained by red nucleus stimulation. Conversely, damage to the A2 system should disrupt the growth of conditioned inhibition.

We know that, in agreement with Wagner and Donegan's predictions, red nucleus stimulation does not serve as an effective UCS for excitatory conditioning; but we do not yet know whether it serves to set up inhibitory connections. As yet there is very little evidence from any source on the physiological basis of conditioned inhibition, but it is encouraging for Wagner and Donegan's view to note that there is some evidence from both lesion and stimulation experiments for a role of an anterior region of the red nucleus in conditioned inhibition (Mis 1977, although Mis's report concluded that the critical locus for inhibition of conditioned eyelid responses lay in the accessory oculomotor nuclei). It is clear that if it turns out that stimulation of the red nucleus elicits an eyelid response, but, when paired with a CS, endows that CS with the power to inhibit conditioned eyelid responses, such physiological findings will provide convincing support for SOP, a behavioral theory.

Cerebellum and Learning: Two Reservations

The preceding sections have documented an important role for the cerebellum in conditioning of discrete skeletal responses. An assessment of the overall significance of the cerebellum in learned behavior should, however, take into account two sets of observations, one of which refers back to the spinal cord review.

Spinal animals, which possess, of course, no cerebellum, are capable of acquiring conditioned leg-flexion responses; but, at least when tone CSs are used, rabbits with cerebellar damage cannot acquire leg-flexion CRs. Similar UCSs are involved, and although the most convincing demonstrations of spinal conditioning have involved alpha conditioning, we have seen evidence that cerebellar damage disrupts alpha conditioning as well as conventional conditioning. A similar point is made in a recent report by Kelly, Zuo, and Bloedel (1990), who investigated eyelid conditioning using a tone CS in decerebrate rabbits with extensive unilateral cerebellar damage. Kelly and his colleagues found that a substantial level of CR acquisition was possible in these rabbits (so that up to about 50 percent of CS presentations obtained CRs). Most of their animals were trained following decerebration and then subjected to cerebellar damage: these animals generally showed no retention of CRs but nevertheless did show successful acquisition, attaining levels of performance considerably in excess of those reported for animals having lesions limited to the cerebellum.

Nordholm, Lavond, and Thompson (1991) have pointed out that Kelly and his colleagues used an unconventional procedure that involved a very short (9 sec) intertrial interval and an idiosyncratic measure of CR (any response occurring in the CS-UCS interval that was at least 10 percent of the average UCR magnitude). In a carefully controlled study using intact rabbits, Nordholm and his colleagues failed to detect CRs when a 9-sec intertrial interval was used (CRs were obtained when a 30-sec interval was used). Nordholm and his colleagues argue that the Kelly, Zuo, and Bloedel (1990) report did not control adequately for pseudoconditioning, and that the CRs they reported were not genuine CRs—CRs that reflected the detection by the rabbits of the CS-UCS contingency. Given, however, the fact that spinal animals do show genuine CRs, the Kelly, Zuo, and Bloedel

(1990) report carries at least a prima facie plausibility, and further work may be expected shortly to resolve this issue.

Successful skeletal conditioning in spinal animals and in animals that are both decerebrate and decerebellate raises the uncomfortable possibility (Kelly, Zuo, and Bloedel 1990) that animals having cerebellar damage are capable of forming associations but that the level of excitability of the pathway involved in the expression of the CR is depressed by some rostrally located brain structure or structures. Some support for the possibility that cerebellar lesions may not disrupt association formation is provided by two studies reported by Welsh and Harvey.

The first study (Welsh and Harvey 1989) found that rabbits having anterior dorsolateral interpositus lesions showed, as anticipated, virtually no CRs (on less than 2 percent of CS presentations) in the period between CS onset and UCS onset (285 msec, in their study). This is the period within which CRs typically occur in normal animals, and is the time-window that is conventionally adopted. Welsh and Harvey did, however, occasionally present CS-alone trials, and on those trials scored as CRs any responses that occurred within 800 msec of CS onset. The same animals that had shown a virtually total lack of CRs using the 285-msec window now showed a mean of approximately 14 percent CRs.

The second study (Welsh and Harvey 1991) explored the effects of continuous microinfusion of an anesthetic (lidocaine) into the right interpositus nucleus of rabbits during right eyelid conditioning. Lidocaine infusion prevented both the expression of CRs to a previously trained (light) CS and the development of CRs to a novel (tone) CS. As would be anticipated, the infusion had no effect on UCRs. However, when the rabbits were tested two days later, after the effects of the anesthetic had dissipated, normal CRs were seen to both the light and the tone CS, despite the fact that tone-UCS pairings had occurred only when the interpositus nucleus had been inactivated by lidocaine. In other words, although inactivation of the interpositus nucleus prevented the expression of CRs, it did not prevent the detection by the rabbits of the CS-UCS contingency, nor the formation of CRs that could not be expressed in the absence of normal functioning of the interpositus nucleus. We should, then, be alert to the possibility that cerebellar damage does not disrupt association formation but instead depresses a pathway necessary for the expression of CRs, a pathway that is also subject to tonic depression from rostral brain structures.

A second observation concerns the restriction of the effects of cerebellar damage to specific skeletal responses. Cerebellar damage does not consistently impair human intelligence, although it does impair equilibrium and motor control. And Lashley and McCarthy (1926) found that a rat with its entire cerebellum destroyed was, despite grave abnormalities of movement, quite capable of learning to choose accurately in locomoting through a maze. Lashley's rat could, then, learn the significance of the different alleys of a maze and could adjust its movements so as to approach those alleys leading to the goal-box and avoid the blind alleys. Similarly, rabbits with cerebellar damage clearly appreciate the "emotional" significance of tones that signal airpuffs. In the light of recent work on the cerebellum, we would now surely wish to qualify Lashley's conclusion that "the associative connexions of simple conditioned reflexes are not formed in the subcortical structures of the brain" (Lashley 1950:490), while nevertheless agreeing with another of Lashley's conclusions, namely that "the cerebellum of the rat plays no significant part in the habit systems involved in maze running" (Lashley and McCarthy 1926:431).

The cerebellum plays a major role in the expression of specific conditioned skeletal responses. But the potential for learning and memory in the absence of the cerebellum may seem so considerable that the cerebellum should be regarded as at best a minor member of the set of mechanisms that taken as a whole constitute intelligence. Chapter 6 looks at the role of telencephalic structures in conditioning and is largely concerned with the hippocampus, a structure that, when damaged, leads in humans to dramatic changes in cognitive function.

6. Association Formation in Vertebrates: The Role of the Hippocampus

The Hippocampus: A Structure of Special Interest to Neuroscience

The word "hippocampus" was the Latin for seahorse, and was in turn derived from the Greek words for "horse" and "caterpillar." It appears that the brain structure now known as the hippocampus was first so named in the sixteenth century by Julius Caesar Arantius, a "rather dull" pupil of Andreas Vesalius. It is, however, not entirely clear why he used the term (for an entertaining and fascinating account of this topic, see Lewis 1923). According to Lewis, "The flight of fancy which led Arantius, in 1587, to introduce the term *hippocampus* is recorded in what is perhaps the worst anatomical description extant. It has left its readers in doubt whether the elevations of cerebral substance were being compared with fish or beast, and no one could be sure which end was the head" (ibid.:213). However dubious its origin, the term has stuck, and recent explorations suggest that the function of the hippocampus may be sufficiently exotic to justify the fancifulness of its name.

The hippocampus now attracts more attention from neuroscientists than any other brain structure, and more than one thousand papers on the hippocampus appeared in research journals in 1991 alone. This chapter will introduce two of the major reasons for the recent dramatic growth of interest. The first is the demonstration of the development in the hippocampus of neuronal models as a consequence of conditioning procedures.

These models suggest a potentially important role for the hippocampus in conditioning; a similar argument was made out for the cerebellum, but we shall find that the models seen in hippocampal activity differ in important ways from those seen in the cerebellum. A second major reason for interest in the hippocampus is the discovery there of the phenomenon of long-term potentiation (LTP), a long-lasting physiological change in synaptic efficacy brought about by a relatively short-lasting initiating event. We shall see that there are good grounds for supposing that LTP represents a mechanism that could well provide a physiological substrate for conditioning.

The data to be reviewed here will be derived from experiments on non-humans and so will exclude reference to a third major cause of interest in the hippocampus—namely, the fact that hippocampal damage has a profound effect on memory in humans. The effects of hippocampal damage on memory in nonhumans will be discussed in chapter 8, with explicit reference to the question whether memory deficits comparable to those reported in humans with hippocampal damage are found in nonhumans also. But it will be useful here to set the background for the discussion of the potential role of the hippocampus in association formation by anticipating some of the work to be introduced more fully in chapter 8. It will be recalled from chapter 3 that hippocampal damage in nonhumans does not disrupt habituation but does slow the rate of decline of active exploratory responses. It was argued there that this might reflect a critical involvement of the hippocampus in recognition, and that the hippocampus might play a similar role, in "conscious" recognition, in humans also. We shall find in chapter 8 rather compelling evidence that recognition memory is impaired in nonhumans by hippocampal damage. But we shall see in this chapter that hippocampal damage does not prevent successful acquisition of at least some types of learning, and this seems to imply that a hippocampectomized animal may acquire, through learning, an appropriate response to a stimulus that it does not recognize. This somewhat paradoxical conclusion points to what will emerge as one of the most forceful implications of work on hippocampal function—namely that learning is mediated by a number of processes or systems that can operate relatively independently of one another. Spinal animals are, after all, capable of classical conditioning, although we might find it hard to accept that they are capable of recognition. Intact animals do, presumably, normally recognize the stimuli to which they show learned responses; but it may be that the process or processes involved in recognition are independent of those involved in acquiring conditioned responses. The general notion that learning may involve a multitude of processes operating in parallel and with a degree of independence is one that should, then, be borne in mind throughout this and the following two chapters.

Chapters 6, 7, and 8 will concentrate on the hippocampus but will not exclude consideration of other areas. A major aim of these chapters is to consider light thrown by physiological work on psychological issues: it is because analyses of hippocampal function carry so many implications for the behavioral analysis of learning and memory that the hippocampus warrants the degree of attention devoted to it here. Investigations of other brain areas are, as we shall see, also relevant to the topics—classical conditioning, contextual learning, differences between memory stores—on which attention will be focused in these chapters, and we shall, accordingly, also consider at various points functional analyses of such regions as the neocortex and the amygdala.

The case for a role of the cerebellum in conditioning was based on both electrophysiological and lesion data, but the lesion data carried the most conviction. This chapter will concentrate on electrophysiological phenomena—neuronal models and LTP—which imply for the hippocampus also a role in association formation. However, before discussing electrophysiological work on the hippocampus, early notice should be given that hippocampal damage (in contrast to cerebellar damage) does not prevent either acquisition or retention of eyelid conditioning (e.g., Solomon and Moore 1975). In fact, Mauk and Thompson (1987) have shown virtually perfect retention of preoperatively established eyelid CRs following acute decerebration (involving removal of the entire telencephalon and the diencephalon). It appears, therefore, that *no* forebrain structure is necessary for classical conditioning of the eyelid response.

It may be useful in attempting to provide a context in which to view the work on hippocampal electrophysiology to note also that although the hippocampus is not necessary for all types of association formation, hippocampal damage does disrupt conditioning in some circumstances: hippocampectomy does not prevent acquisition of the eyelid CR using the standard delay procedure (in which CS onset precedes UCS onset and in which the CS either overlaps the UCS or terminates at UCS onset); but hippocampectomized rabbits do show impairments in certain other classical-conditioning procedures—when, for example, a trace procedure (in which there is an interval between CS termination and UCS onset) is used (Solomon et al. 1986; Moyer, Deyo, and Disterhoft 1990). The effects of hippocampal damage on classical conditioning will be taken up in more detail when electrophysiological evidence has been presented; that evidence will be further placed in context by an introduction to the anatomy and physiology of the hippocampus.

Hippocampal Anatomy

The hippocampus develops, phylogenetically and ontogenetically, from the medial region of the pallial zone of the telencephalon. In mammals, the expansion of the central dorsal zone of the pallium—the neocortex—results in a ventral and lateral displacement of the medial pallium so that in primates the hippocampus is found in the temporal lobe; Figure 6.1(a) shows the location, size, and general shape of the hippocampus in the rabbit. The hippocampus is sometimes (unhelpfully) known as archicortex, while the lateral pallial zone, represented in primates by the prepiriform cortex, is known as the paleocortex. The mammalian hippocampus does not immediately adjoin true neocortex, but is divided from it by zones of "transitional" cortex—the subicular complex and the entorhinal cortex.

The absolute size of the hippocampus in mammals increases with brain size, which in turn increases with body size. But just as brain size does not keep pace with body size—so that smaller mammals tend to have larger brain-to-body-weight ratios than larger mammals—hippocampal size does not keep pace with brain size. Although the hippocampus does show an orderly increase in size as brain size increases, the percentage of total brain volume taken up by the hippocampus becomes progressively smaller as absolute brain size increases. The human hippocampus, for example, constitutes less than 1 percent of the total brain volume whereas the hippocampus of the shrew *Sorex araneus* constitutes some 12 percent of its total brain. The human hippocampus is nevertheless a very large structure (some 10,000 mm^3), and that of the shrew very small (some 22 mm^3; Stephan and Manolescu 1980). A further anatomical indication of the potential importance of the hippocampus is provided by the fact that the human fornix (which consists of fibers, both afferent and efferent, that connect the hippocampus with subcortical regions) contains some one million fibers; it is, then, approximately the same size as the human optic tract (Nauta and Feirtag 1986).

Intrinsic Hippocampal Connections

Figure 6.2 illustrates diagrammatically the basic features of intrahippocampal organization. The hippocampus consists of two interlocking parts,

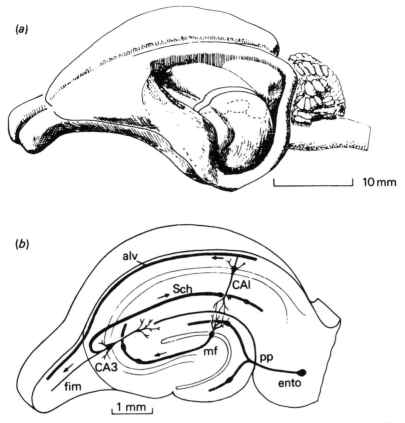

FIGURE 6.1. Location and lamellar organization of the hippocampus. Fig. 6.1(a): Lateral view of the rabbit brain with the parietal and temporal neocortex removed to expose the hippocampal formation. Fig. 6.1(b): Lamellar organization of the hippocampus. The lamellar slice indicated in fig. 6.1(a) has been presented separately to show the trisynaptic pathway. Alv = alveus (fiber bundle consisting primarily of axons of pyramidal cells); ento = entorhinal cortex; fim = fimbria fornicis (region formed by the fibers of the fornix, fanning out as they enter the hippocampus or collecting together as they leave the hippocampus); pp = perforant path; Sch = Schaffer collateral. (*From* Andersen, Bliss, and Skrede 1971)

the hippocampus proper (cornu ammonis, or Ammon's horn) and the dentate gyrus, or fascia dentata. The principal cells of the hippocampus proper are pyramidal cells, possessing both apical and basal dendritic trees; the principal cells of the dentate gyrus are granule cells. The hippocampus proper consists of two major regions—an inferior region, con-

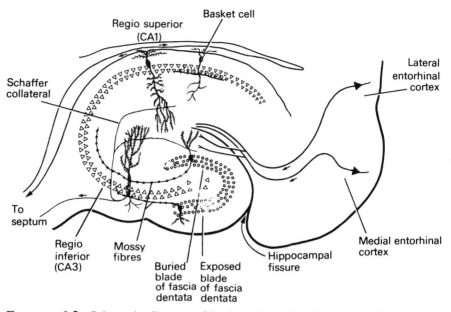

FIGURE 6.2. Schematic diagram of horizontal section through the right hippo-campus of a mouse, showing intrahippocampal connections. Caudal is to the right. (*From* O'Keefe and Nadel 1978)

ventionally labeled CA3, and a superior region, CA1. The pyramidal cells in the CA3 region are giant cells, whereas the CA1 cells are medium sized. A relatively small number of other types of cell are found in the hippocampus, of which the most prominent are the basket cells, which function as inhibitory local interneurons.

One striking feature of hippocampal organization is that different sources of synaptic input to the granule and pyramidal cells are segregated so that they make contact with dendritic zones that lie at different distances from the cell body. This may be illustrated by considering synaptic input to the dentate gyrus in a little detail. The entorhinal cortex, source of the major input to the hippocampus, projects extensively via the perforant path onto the dendritic trees of the dentate gyrus granule cells (as well as, to a lesser extent, onto the dendrites of both CA3 and CA1 pyramidal cells). Perforant path axons make contact with dendritic spines on the outer two-thirds of the dendritic trees of the dentate gyrus granule cells—with, that is, the two-thirds of the dendritic tree located distal from the granule cell bodies. The proximal third of the dendritic tree is invaded by commissural fibers from the contralateral dentate gyrus, and by longitudinal associational fibers from neighboring granule cells. There is also, between the associative-commissural layer of synaptic contact and the cell body, a thin zone in which axons from the medial septal nucleus make contact. Finally, there are on the cell bodies themselves synaptic terminals of basket cells.

The output from the dentate gyrus is carried by mossy fibers, which are axons of the granule cells, and which make contact both with the proximal zone of the apical dendrites of the CA3 pyramidal cells and with the basal dendrites of those cells. Mossy fibers show a unique pattern of synaptic swellings along the axon, and contact is made with a complex dendritic spine, which is totally enveloped by the swelling.

Axons of CA3 pyramidal cells divide and provide a number of collateral outputs. Some CA3 axon collaterals run outside the hippocampus, to the lateral septal nucleus; others cross the midline to provide commissural input to the proximal zone of the apical dendrites, and to the basal dendrites of contralateral CA1 and CA3 pyramidal cells; others give rise to associational fibers which make contact with ipsilateral CA3 pyramidal cells (terminating in the same zone as the commissural fibers); still others, known as Schaffer collaterals, project to both the basal dendrites and the inner zone of the apical dendrites of the CA1 pyramidal cells, whose axons in turn project heavily out of the hippocampus onto the subicular complex.

Two important features of hippocampal organization emerge from the data summarized above. First, extrahippocampal output derives exclusively from pyramidal cells: CA3 cells project to the lateral septal nucleus, CA1 cells to the subicular complex. Second, hippocampal circuitry shows an intrahippocampal trisynaptic pathway beginning with the perforant path, which synapses onto dentate gyrus granule cells; granule-cell axons (mossy fibers) synapse onto CA3 pyramidal cells, and CA3 cells, via Schaffer collaterals, project onto CA1 pyramidal cells. These connections are all excitatory, and so form a feed-forward circuit. Since the CA1 cells project onto the subicular complex, one of whose many projections is onto the entorhinal cortex (source of the perforant path), the anatomical foundation for a closed loop exists in the hippocampus and its associated structures.

Andersen (e.g., 1975) has drawn attention to a further feature of hippocampal organization, which is that the hippocampus consists of a series of strips or "lamellae" lying in a plane orthogonal to the long (septotemporal) axis of the hippocampus. Stimulation of a discrete locus in the entorhinal cortex obtains excitation in a relatively narrow zone of the dentate gyrus; stimulation of the dentate gyrus (and of subsequent stations of the trisynaptic circuit) in turn obtains excitation that is maximal within the same lamella. The functional independence of these lamellae should not be exaggerated since there are numerous longitudinal associational fibers (and commissural fibers) so that activity within a given lamella does affect activity in other lamellae. This point has been made forcibly by Amaral and Witter, who have emphasized that "the major hippocampal projections are as extensive and highly organized in the long or septotemporal axis of the hippocampus as in the transverse axis" (Amaral and Witter 1989:571). But the existence of the complete trisynaptic circuit within a thin lamella has the important consequence that hippocampal slices may be excised which, when investigated *in vitro,* show a functional trisynaptic pathway; figure 6.1(b) illustrates schematically a lamellar slice and the basic trisynaptic lamellar pathway.

Extrinsic Hippocampal Connections

Some insight into the potential functional role of the hippocampus may be gained by considering its major extrinsic connections with cortical regions, connections that are channeled through adjoining transitional cortex. The account that follows is based largely on work with primates, although there is evidence for similarities in basic organization in nonprimate mammals (Rosene and Van Hoesen 1987).

Inputs

The major input to the hippocampus derives from the entorhinal cortex, so that to understand the nature of hippocampal input we need to consider what are the major projections to the entorhinal cortex. All the sensory systems project to the entorhinal cortex, but only one of them, olfaction, does so relatively directly: there are projections from primary olfactory cortex (the destination of fibers from the olfactory epithelium) to the entorhinal cortex. Projections from the other sensory modalities are much less direct and require a brief consideration of the cortical organization of those modalities.

The primary cortical areas for vision, hearing, and the somatic senses receive unimodal input from their respective thalamic relays (the lateral geniculate nucleus, the medial geniculate nucleus, and the ventrobasal complex). Those primary cortical areas project to adjoining unimodal association cortex and these first-order parasensory association cortices in turn project to second-order unimodal parasensory association areas that do not receive direct input from the primary sensory cortex. The great majority of neocortex (excluding frontal cortex) is occupied by primary sensory cortex and unimodal (first- and second-order) parasensory association cortices. There are, however, a number of multimodal association areas that show convergence of inputs from more than one sensory modality. Multimodal regions are found in parietal cortex, at the junction of unimodal parasensory association areas serving different modalities, and in (at least) four other areas: in temporal polar cortex, in the cingulate gyrus, in the parahippocampal gyrus, and in orbitofrontal cortex. Figure 6.3 shows the location of the major areas of association cortex in the rhesus monkey.

The entorhinal cortex does not receive direct projections from either first- or second-order unimodal association cortices: its input derives from multimodal areas and, in particular, from all of the multimodal regions mentioned above. And in the words of O'Keefe and Nadel: "This pattern of inputs to the entorhinal area strongly suggests that the hippocampus is concerned not with information about any particular modality, but rather with highly analyzed, abstracted information from all modalities" (1978:126).

Although the major synaptic input to the hippocampus derives from entorhinal cortex, there are important projections from subcortical regions that appear to have general modulating effects on hippocampal activity. Serotonergic fibers from the raphe nucleus of the caudal midbrain project via the fornix and are distributed widely through the hippocampus. Noradrenergic fibers from the locus coeruleus, which straddles the midbrain/hindbrain boundary, are also widely distributed and reach the hippocampal formation caudally, after coursing through retrosplenial cortex. Finally, there are cholinergic fibers that originate in the forebrain, in the nucleus of the diagonal band of Broca and in the medial septal nucleus, which project via the fornix; the significance of the projection from the medial septal nucleus will be considered further in chapter 7.

Outputs

When we turn to consider hippocampal efferents to cortical sites, we find that the subicular complex (which receives direct hippocampal projections) shows connections with parasensory association cortices—with both the multimodal areas that project to the entorhinal cortex and with unimodal parasensory association cortices. The subicular complex pro-

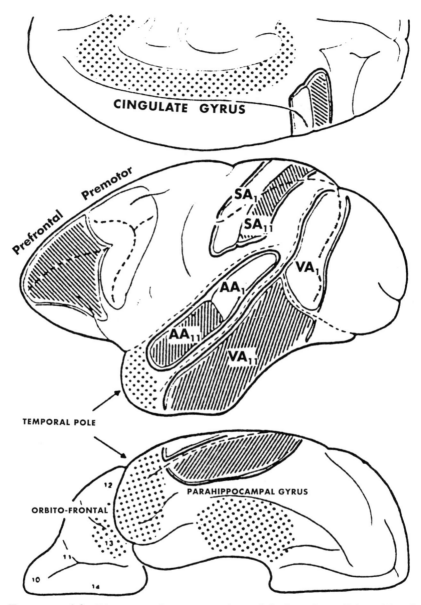

FIGURE 6.3. Diagrammatic representations of the lateral, medial, and basal surfaces of the cerebral hemispheres of the rhesus monkey, showing locations of regions of association cortex. The regions shown may be classified into three major divisions: (1) parasensory cortex (auditory association areas AAI and AAII; somatic sensory association areas SAI and SAII; visual association areas VAI and VAII); (2) frontal association cortex (premotor and prefrontal areas); (3) paralimbic association cortex (cingulate gyrus, parahippocampal gyrus, temporal pole, and orbitofrontal cortex). (*From* Pandya and Seltzer 1982)

jects also to the entorhinal cortex, and it appears therefore that the hippocampus is well placed not only to monitor highly processed perceptual input but also to modulate its own intake of that information.

The bulk of the fornix consists of efferent fibers from the hippocampal formation to a number of subcortical zones, including the anterior thalamic nucleus, the lateral septal nucleus, and the mammillary bodies of the hypothalamus. The projection to the mammillary bodies (which derives from the subiculum rather than from the hippocampus proper) forms part of a series of connections which form the circuit first described by Papez (1937) and since then known as the Papez circuit. The mammillary bodies project via the mammillothalamic tract to the anterior nucleus of the thalamus; the anterior nucleus projects to the cingulate gyrus of the medial telencephalon, which in turn projects to the entorhinal cortex. The projection from the entorhinal cortex to the hippocampus completes the circuit. Subsequent work has confirmed the projections of the Papez circuit but has shown also that the flow of information is not necessarily unidirectional: there are projections, for example, from the hippocampal formation to the anterior thalamic nuclei and to cingulate cortex.

The hippocampal formation also shows reciprocal connections with the amygdala, a structure that forms part of the so-called limbic system. The term "limbic" was originally introduced by Broca to refer to a ringlike set of structures bounding the cerebral hemispheres and visible on the medial surface of the hemispheres. The major components of the limbic system are the hippocampal formation, the cingulate gyrus, and the amygdala. There is no universally accepted list of structures that belong to the limbic system, but Nauta and Feirtag (1986) point out that the major components of the limbic system have strong connections with the hypothalamus, and on those grounds the septal area is usually regarded as forming part of the limbic system.

Summary

In summary, the hippocampal formation shows extensive and largely reciprocal connections with sensory association areas and with limbic structures that in turn show connections with the hypothalamus. The involvement with processed sensory information might suggest a cognitive role for the hippocampus, and striking effects of damage on certain types of learning and memory are found: these will be the focus of most of the following two chapters, which will discuss (in chapter 7) the notion that the hippocampus plays a central role in the processing of contextual (and particularly spatial) information, and (in chapter 8) proposals that the hippocampus is the site of one of a number of memory stores. The association of the hippocampus and other limbic structures with the hypothalamus suggests a potential role for the limbic system in establishing the motivational significance of stimuli: this possibility will be explored, with particular reference to the amygdala, in chapter 8. Notions about the functions of the limbic system and the Papez circuit have enjoyed a checkered history, and the more general question whether either the limbic system or the Papez circuit functions as a coordinated system concerned with learning will be taken up in chapters 7 and 8.

A Neuronal Model in the Hippocampus

Characteristics of Hippocampal Neuronal Models

Thompson and his colleagues have carried out an extensive series of investigations of the electrical activity of rabbit hippocampal cells during acquisition of the eyelid CR. Early results using multiple-unit recording techniques indicated that hippocampal cell activity increased as a consequence of CS-UCS pairings, those increases being seen in both CS and UCS periods (Berger, Alger, and Thompson 1976). Subsequent work (Berger and Thompson 1978) has shown that when data are pooled over a block of trials, the probability of response of hippocampal cells in trained animals closely matches the amplitude and time course of the behavioral eyelid response—both the CR and the UCR (see figure 6.4 for examples). Data from control animals showed that the discharge rate of hippocampal cells was not affected by unpaired presentations of CS and UCS; the parallel between hippocampal activity and the eyelid response does not, therefore, reflect any simple motor involvement of the hippocampus in eyelid-response production: the increased activity is related to learning.

Further evidence against the possibility of a motor account of hippocampal involvement derives from two important temporal dissociations between the electrical activity and the behavioral response. First, increases in hippocampal activity may be detected early in training, and substantially earlier than the first overt behavioral CR: Berger and Thompson (1978), for example, obtained hippocampal activity increases within the first eight conditioning trials in an experiment in which eyelid CRs were not obtained until some 50 to 70 pairings had occurred; the earliest increases in hippocampal activity were seen during UCS presentations, being followed some trials later (but before eyelid CRs were seen) by increases during CS presentations. Thus although hippocampal activity at asymptote models the behavioral response, the earliest increases in hip-

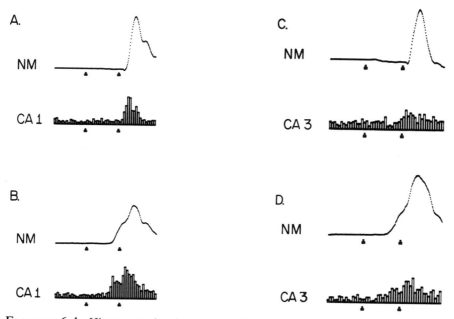

FIGURE 6.4. Hippocampal unit responses from two rabbits (left and right) given tone–corneal airpuff pairings. *Upper trace:* average nictitating membrane response for one block of eight trials. *Lower trace:* hippocampal unit poststimulus histogram (15 msec time bins) for one block of eight trials. A and C: first block of paired conditioning trials, Day 1. B and D: last block of conditioning trials, Day 1. First cursor indicates tone onset. Second cursor indicates airpuff onset. *Total trace length:* 750 msec. (*From* Berger and Thompson 1978)

pocampal activity serve as a sign that the animal has detected a contingency between CS and UCS and predict the eventual appearance of the eyelid CR.

A second dissociation between hippocampal activity and the eyelid response is that the activity, although it models the time course of the behavioral response, precedes its onset. This may be illustrated by considering an experiment by Hoehler and Thompson (1980) in which the CS-UCS interval was varied between three values—50, 150, and 250 msec. Previous work had shown that the optimal CS-UCS interval for eyelid conditioning is approximately 200–400 msec, and that neither very short nor very long interstimulus intervals (ISIs) support conditioning (Gormezano 1972). When the short (50 msec) interval was used, Hoehler and Thompson found that no CR developed, and no change in hippocampal activity was seen (further confirmation of the link between hippocampal activity and effective learning). Both the longer intervals supported CR acquisition, and in each case a hippocampal model developed that paralleled the temporal and amplitude characteristics of the eyelid response. Test CS-alone trials showed that the mean peak latency of the behavioral CR differed between the 150- and 250-msec conditions, being 197 msec in the former and 266 msec in the latter. The peak hippocampal latencies similarly differed between the groups, being 146 msec for the 150-msec condition, and 208 msec for the 250-msec condition. In each case, then, hippocampal activity preceded corresponding eyelid activity by some 50–60 msec.

Evidence already discussed has shown that unless learning occurs, no hippocampal model develops. It is also the case that in trained animals, increased hippocampal activity is seen only in trials in which the animals respond to the CS. Activity increases are not seen when "spontaneous" intertrial eyelid responses occur (Berger and Thompson 1978), nor are they seen during presentations of the negative stimulus of a discrimination—except when, as occasionally happens, the animal "erroneously" responds to the negative stimulus (Berger, Berry, and Thompson 1986). Using a detection paradigm in which CSs were so weak that they were successfully detected on only 50 percent of trials, Kettner and Thompson (1982) found that hippocampal responses were seen in trials in which eyelid CRs occurred and not in trials in which they did not (trials in which, presumably, the CS was not detected).

The formation of hippocampal models during conditioning is not peculiar to rabbits, and not peculiar to eyelid conditioning. Patterson, Berger, and Thompson (1979) have shown similar increases in hippocampal activity during eyelid conditioning in cats, and increases have been seen in rabbits associated with conditioned leg-flexion responses (Thompson et al. 1980) and in an appetitive paradigm using a saccharin solution as UCS, in which the target response was jaw movement (Berger, Berry, and Thompson 1986). Conditioned jaw movements were rhythmic (7–9 Hz), and a corresponding rhythmicity was seen in hippocampal activity, confirming the tight relationship between that activity and CR morphology.

This work has shown, then, that hippocampal activity models the form of the skeletal behavioral response (CR and UCR) evoked in animals that have detected the CS-UCS contingency. It should be noted (as it was in chapter 5, when cerebellar neuronal models were discussed) that the neuronal activity does not correlate with nonskeletal CRs, such as changes in heart rate, whose time courses differ considerably from that of the eyelid response. The close parallels with skeletal responses serve, then, to emphasize the fact that the hippocampal responses are *not* tied to other responses that are known also to be conditioned in these paradigms. As was the case with the cerebellum, we see here further support for a distinction between systems mediating acquisition of preparatory (primarily autonomic) and skeletal consummatory CRs. It is also of interest to consider the possibility that hippocampal activity may not model all that is learned with respect to the skeletal response: explicitly unpaired presentations of CS and UCS would be expected, for example, to turn the CS into a conditioned inhibitor, a stimulus whose presentation would decrease the eyelid CR otherwise obtained by presentations of an excitatory CS (Rescorla 1969). But there is, it appears, no change in hippocampal unit activity consequent upon unpaired presentations of CS and UCS.

Models Originate from Pyramidal Cells

Work using single-cell recording techniques has established that the cells primarily responsible for the increased activity are CA1 and CA3 pyramidal cells—the major output cells of the hippocampus. Berger et al. (1983) recorded from forty-eight identified hippocampal pyramidal neurons during rabbit eyelid conditioning. Forty (83 percent) of the cells showed significant increases in firing rates as a consequence of conditioning: in most of these cells, increases were seen during both CS and UCS periods, but in some cells increases were seen in only the CS or in only the UCS periods. Thirty-seven cells (77 percent) showed a within-trial pattern of response that closely matched the behavioral response (CR and UCR). In other words, neuronal models of the response were seen in the majority of individual cells; figure 6.5 shows examples taken from two such cells. However, the latency of onset of the neuronal model varied between cells: in some cells, the increase in firing rate preceded the initiation of the eyelid CR, in others the increase began after initiation of the CR. The neuronal model observed in multiple-unit recordings (whose onset consistently precedes CR initiation) therefore reflects the summed activity of a number of types of pyramidal neuron: some of these neurons do not exhibit a complete neuronal model, and those that do, show a range of onset latencies.

Models Are Elaborated in the Hippocampus Proper

An important question is whether the model is elaborated in the hippocampus proper or whether hippocampal activity simply reflects increases in its input. One approach to this question is to investigate learning-related activity in the major sources of input to the pyramidal cells.

Multiple-unit recordings from the entorhinal cortex (source of the perforant path to dentate gyrus) find in fact that activity does increase as a consequence of pairings. However, the magnitude of the increase is smaller than that seen in the hippocampus proper, and the increase reaches an asymptote early in training, within approximately twenty trials, whereas hippocampal activity continues to grow for another forty trials or so (Berger and Weisz 1987). Single-unit recordings from dentate gyrus granule cells, the target of the entorhinal cortex axons and the source of the major input to the CA3 pyramids, also show marked differences from the pattern seen in the hippocampus proper (Berger and Weisz 1987). These cells show learning-related increases in activity but, as was found in the entorhinal cortex, these increases reach asymptote very rapidly. Granule cells, moreover, do not exhibit a model of the behavioral response (whose latency changes as training proceeds) but respond at a constant fixed latency (which varies from cell to cell) from CS onset. Neither the entorhinal cortex nor the dentate gyrus cells appear, then, to follow the development of the CR in the same way as the pyramidal cells of the hippocampus proper.

A further important input to the hippocampus (one whose significance will be considered further in chapter 7) derives from the medial septal nucleus. Multiple-unit recordings from cells in this nucleus fail to find any

---

FIGURE 6.5. Responses of individual hippocampal pyramidal neurons during paired or unpaired presentations of tone and corneal airpuff. The upper traces show the time course and amplitude of the averaged nictitating membrane response for all trials during which a given cell was recorded. The bottom traces show the peristimulus time histogram produced by the response of the recorded neuron during the Pre-CS, CS, and UCS periods, respectively. Total trial length of traces: 750 msec. First arrow, tone onset; second arrow, airpuff onset. NM, nictitating membrane response; H, hippocampal pyramidal neuron response. Figures 6A and 6B show examples of responses during paired conditioning of two pyramidal neurons recorded from two different animals. Note that the conditioned nictitating membrane response in figure 6A is monophasic, and the histogram of pyramidal cell firing parallels the time course and amplitude of the nictitating membrane response with a unimodal within-trial distribution of action-potential discharges. The conditioned nictitating membrane response shown in figure 6B is triphasic, and again the histogram of pyramidal cell activity parallels the nictitating membrane response but with a trimodal distribution. The bottom four figures provide evidence that the responses seen in figures 6A and 6B are a consequence

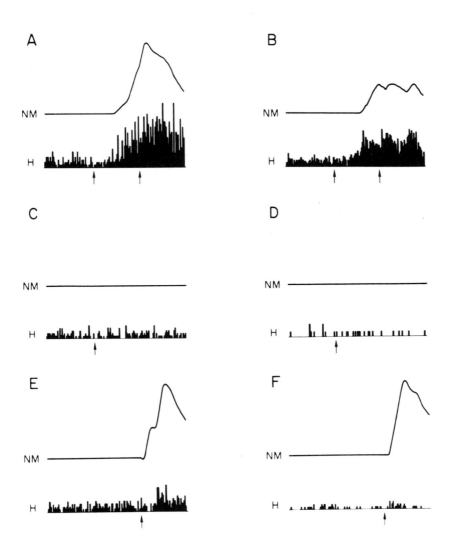

of conditioning. Figures 6C and 6E show the response of a hippocampal pyramidal neuron recorded from an animal given tone alone (figure 6C) and air puff-alone (figure 6E) presentations. Figures 6D and 6F show the response of a pyramidal neuron recorded from a different animal given, similarly, tone alone (figure 6D) and air puff-alone (figure 6F) presentations. (*From* Berger et al. 1983)

learning-related change in activity (Berger and Weisz 1987). Medial septal cells show transient short-latency responses to both CS and UCS onset, but these responses are indistinguishable between paired and unpaired conditions. They may therefore supply information about the occurrence of CS and UCS, but they do not appear to contribute to the development of the hippocampal model.

Contrasts Between Hippocampal and Cerebellar Neuronal Models

The available evidence indicates that during the course of acquisition of a discrete skeletal CR using classical training techniques there develops within the hippocampus proper a neuronal model of the behavioral response. The hippocampal neuronal model differs in two important respects from the cerebellar model discussed previously. First, the hippocampal model, unlike the cerebellar model, begins to develop well before any overt CR is seen; second, the hippocampal model mirrors the total behavioral response—CR and UCR—whereas the cerebellar model mirrors only the CR. The role played by the hippocampal model in association formation has, of course, to be assessed in the light of the fact that hippocampal ablation does not prevent acquisition of the eyelid CR using the standard (delay) procedure; this is a topic to which we shall return following consideration of a further learning-related electrophysiological phenomenon seen in the hippocampus.

Long-Term Potentiation: A Mechanism of Association Formation?

Until recently, proposals for cellular changes involved in association formation in vertebrates had been entirely speculative. This was true, for example, of Hebb's influential postulate, according to which (as will be recalled from chapter 4), the synapse between two cells would be strengthened when firing of the presynaptic cell was consistently followed by firing of the postsynaptic cell.

Stent (1973) proposed a rather complicated mechanism, which supposed that a subclass of synapses ("plastic synapses") possessed postsynaptic receptors that were unstable. Stent proposed that at plastic synapses receptors were dislodged if spike activity occurred in a postsynaptic cell in the absence of a spike in the presynaptic cell. Thus if a postsynaptic cell was activated without synchronous activity of a presynaptic cell, the synapse connecting those cells would weaken. This mechanism does not in fact envisage strengthening of connections as a consequence of synchronous activity, but a weakening as a result of asynchronous activity. It has therefore never seemed an attractive candidate as a mechanism for standard conditioning, which surely involves the selective strengthening of connections involving a particular stimulus rather than the weakening of connections of many stimuli. Stent's proposal was made in the light of observations made on plasticity in the visual cortex (a topic to which we shall return), and there was for many years no direct physiological support for Stent's specific proposals as a potential account of synaptic plasticity in general. There is now, however, evidence that asynchronous activity in two inputs (one weak, one strong) to hippocampal cells may lower the efficacy of the synapses carrying the weak input (the phenomenon of long-term depression: Stanton and Sejnowski 1989). One attractive possibility is that this mechanism may play a role in such phenomena as extinction and inhibition; but there is currently no direct evidence for the involvement of long-term depression in associative learning.

A further proposal, due to Eccles (e.g., 1953), was based on physiological findings. Work on spinal cord preparations had shown that a rapid train of impulses in a presynaptic cell, which obtained spikes in a postsynaptic cell, resulted in a facilitation of the synapse between the cells, so that presynaptic stimulation became more effective in obtaining postsynaptic spikes. This effect is known as posttetanic potentiation (PTP), and subsequent work has shown that PTP is due to enhanced transmitter release from the presynaptic terminals, caused in turn by an accumulation of intracellular calcium. But the decay of PTP, which persists for only a few minutes, seems too rapid to provide a lasting substrate for learning, and there is no evidence either that association formation does obtain PTP in any cell, or that prevention of PTP may interfere with learning.

In 1973, however, Bliss and his colleagues (Bliss and Lømo 1973; Bliss and Gardner-Medwin 1973) reported a series of studies on a phenomenon (originally discovered by Lømo 1966) that has excited much interest as a potential physiological mechanism of learning. Using rabbit subjects, Bliss stimulated fibers in the perforant path, which carries afferents from the entorhinal cortex to the hippocampus, and recorded the potentials evoked postsynaptically in the granule cells of the dentate gyrus. He found that, following a brief (3–20 msec) burst of high-frequency (10–100 pulses per sec) stimulation, there was a long-term potentiation (LTP) of the response evoked by subsequent test stimulation of the perforant path. The time course of LTP indicated that the phenomenon should be distinguished from PTP since the LTP observed by Bliss and Gardner-Medwin (1973) persisted for at least three days and, in some experiments, for as long as sixteen weeks. Subsequent work has confirmed that LTP may persist for two weeks and more (Barnes 1979; Staubli and Lynch 1987). It should, nevertheless, be noted that LTP does decay. Bliss and Gardner-Medwin, for example, found that LTP induced by a single train of 15–20 sec never lasted more than three days, although longer-lasting LTP was observed after multiple trains.

A number of features besides the long-lasting nature of the effect encourage the belief that LTP may be involved in learning. First, its discovery in the hippocampus is suggestive, since there is, as we shall see in chapters 7 and 8, good evidence for the involvement of the hippocampus in some types of learning and memory. Second, the effect is selective to synapses that are active during the induction of LTP: stimulation of one set of afferent fibers produces LTP of response evoked by test stimuli delivered to that set, but not to other sets of fibers (in which, nevertheless, LTP can be induced in a similar way). Third, despite the selectivity, it is the case that there is a degree of what is commonly called "co-operativity" (e.g., Lynch 1986): weak stimulation of separate groups of afferents that activate an overlapping set of target cells may obtain LTP when stimulation of either group alone does not.

Selectivity and cooperativity are properties that are well suited to a form of association formation. Consider, for example, a number of afferent inputs converging on a single output node. Activity in some input channels might be subthreshold for activation of the output, while activity in others was suprathreshold. If activation of a subthreshold input channel (A) was paired with activation of a suprathreshold channel (B), then because of cooperativity, LTP might enable subsequent stimulation of A alone to activate the output; because of selectivity, the facilitation of input A would not spread to other subthreshold channels. And if A is taken to represent a CS, and B a UCS, it can be seen that a mechanism is available that might permit classical conditioning. Figure 6.6 provides a diagrammatic representation of this associative property of LTP.

We shall consider somewhat more direct evidence for a link between LTP and learning at the end of this section. One final piece of indirect evidence for such a link will be introduced here, partly because it serves also to illustrate nicely the properties of selectivity and cooperativity. The work was reported by Larson and Lynch (1986) and involved the use of the hippocampal slice. The slice preparation (some 600 μm thick) not only preserves the functional trisynaptic pathway, but shows other major

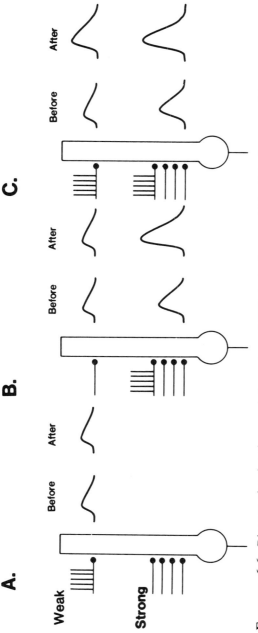

FIGURE 6.6. Diagram showing the associative nature of LTP. A single pyramidal cell is shown receiving a weak and a strong synaptic input. A: Tetanic stimulation of the weak input does not cause LTP in the pathway (compare the EPSP before and after tetanus). B: Tetanic stimulation of the strong input alone does cause LTP in the strong pathway but not in the weak. C: Tetanic stimulation of both the strong and the weak pathways together causes LTP in the weak pathway. (*From* Nicoll, Kauer, and Malenka 1988)

phenomena observed in the intact hippocampus, including LTP. These properties have encouraged the widespread use of the hippocampal slice as an *in vitro* preparation that allows precise detailed investigation of cellular events involved in normal hippocampal function, and many of the results to be described in the following paragraphs were obtained with the use of slices.

Larson and Lynch stimulated independently two separate groups of afferents (both Schaffer collaterals and commissural projections) that converged on a common set of pyramidal cells (but on different sets of synapses) in the CA1 region of the hippocampus. Figure 6.7A is a diagrammatic representation of the design of this experiment. Short (40 msec) bursts of high-frequency stimulation were delivered asynchronously to the two stimulation sites; the interburst interval at each site was 2 sec. The onset of each burst to one set of afferents (S1) preceded that of each burst to the other set (S2) by 200 msec, and Larson and Lynch reported (see figures 6.7B and 6.7C) that whereas LTP developed in the S2 fibers, it did not develop in the S1 fibers. Since stimulation of the S2 fibers alone did not produce LTP, the induction of LTP here demonstrates not only selectivity (to the S2 fibers) but also cooperativity. Larson and Lynch took advantage of the fact that afferents from different sources may terminate in different dendritic zones to show that the same result was obtained when the S1 fibers terminated at synapses on the apical dendrites of pyramidal cells, and the S2 fibers terminated at synapses on the basal dendrites. This result demonstrates that cooperativity may be obtained even when there is a considerable spatial separation between the synapses concerned.

Larson and Lynch (1986) did not, then, obtain LTP in S1 fibers when stimulation of S2 fibers preceded S1 stimulation by approximately 2 sec, and they found also that simultaneous bursts failed to obtain LTP in either set. Other experiments (e.g. Larson, Wong, and Lynch 1986) have shown that repetitive bursts of high-frequency stimulation to a single set of fibers are maximally effective in obtaining LTP at an interburst interval of 200 msec. The fact that brief bursts of synchronous activity at a frequency of 5 Hz are effective in obtaining LTP is of particular interest since rhythmic slow activity (the theta rhythm, which may range from 3–12 Hz, depending on the species) occurs in the hippocampus: theta activity may be presumed to reflect the synchronous firing of large numbers of neurons and can be recorded using gross electrodes from the hippocampus of free-moving animals. Theta activity (which will be discussed further in chapter 7) is reliably elicited from many mammals when they are actively exploring their environment. These findings suggest, then, that LTP could

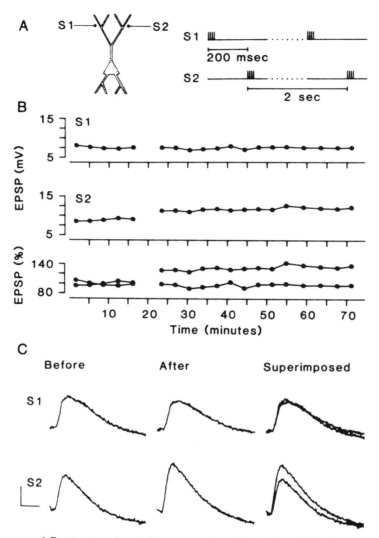

FIGURE 6.7. At top, fig. 6.7A summarizes the design of the Larson and Lynch (1986) experiment (see text for further details). Fig. 6.7B shows data obtained from one neuron in which intracellular EPSPs were recorded alternately on each input at 10-sec intervals before and after the burst-stimulation episode. The upper panel shows the amplitude of the EPSPs evoked by S1, the middle panel those evoked by S2 (each point is an average of six successive responses). Burst stimulation was applied at the gap in the graphs, and the graphs show that LTP occurred only on the input in which bursts occurred 200 msec after a burst on the other input. The bottom panel shows the EPSP amplitudes for both pathways expressed as a percentage of their respective mean sizes before the burst episode. (*From* Larson and Lynch 1986)

be triggered by natural events, and that one behavior that may induce it is exploration, an activity with clear links to learning.

The potential importance of LTP has triggered a huge number of physiological experiments focused on such questions as: What physiological events trigger LTP? What persisting physiological changes underlie LTP? Is LTP a pre- or postsynaptic phenomenon? Since LTP is currently the most promising candidate available for a physiological mechanism that may underlie learning in vertebrates, these questions merit discussion here in some detail.

A Postsynaptic Site for Induction of LTP

There are grounds for believing that the induction of LTP is dependent upon postsynaptic events. Much of the evidence in support of this conclusion is provided by the discovery of a class of receptors in hippocampal cell membranes whose properties do much to explain the phenomenon of cooperativity. The principal excitatory transmitter within the hippocampus is generally believed to be the amino acid, glutamate. Glutamate acts upon a number of receptor types, probably at least five (Young and Fagg 1990). Three of these receptor types are of particular interest here and are distinguished pharmacologically according to their optimal agonists or antagonists. One receptor is readily activated by kainic acid, another by α-amino–3-hydroxy–5-methyl–4-isoxazolepropionic acid (AMPA), and the third by N-methyl-D-aspartate (NMDA). The AMPA receptor was originally named the quisqualate receptor, since it is in fact readily activated by quisqualate; it has recently been renamed because AMPA shows more selectivity than quisqualate. Of the final two known receptor types (which will not be discussed further here), one is characterized by the antagonist action of AP4 (2-amino–4-phosphonobutyric acid), and the other (metabotropic) receptor is linked to phosphoinositol metabolism. Activation of the kainate or AMPA receptors results in a rapid transient opening of ionic channels, which obtains depolarization through the influx of sodium ions; these receptors are, then, typical fast "gate-opening" receptors. The NMDA receptor is distinguished from them in a number of ways. First, its activation opens a channel that remains open appreciably longer. Second, the open channel allows influx of both sodium and calcium ions. Third, its activation is voltage-dependent: when the cell is at resting potential, NMDA receptors are to a large extent "blocked" by extracellular magnesium ions, which are removed by depolarization of the cell. Fourth, the dendritic activity induced by NMDA receptor activation increases with the level of depolarization. The contrasts between the NMDA and the AMPA/kainate receptors are summarized on figure 6.8.

The voltage-dependence of the NMDA receptor could provide a ready account of the cooperativity seen in the induction of LTP. Glutamate released by a brief burst of presynaptic activity in afferent fibers would activate kainate and AMPA receptors, but would obtain relatively little activation of NMDA receptors because the depolarization obtained by activation of kainate and AMPA receptors was insufficient to remove the Mg^{2+} block from the NMDA receptors. Added activity in other afferents,

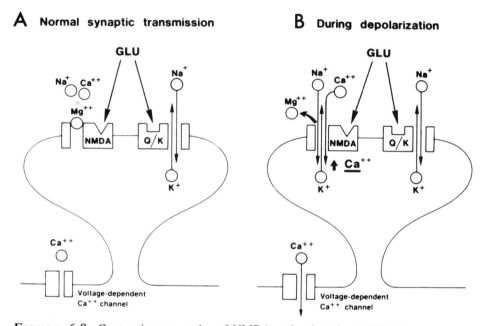

FIGURE 6.8. Contrasting properties of NMDA and quisqualate(AMPA)/kainate receptors. Fig. 6.8A shows the events occurring during low-frequency synaptic transmission. Glutamate (GLU) is released from the presynaptic terminal and acts on both the NMDA and the quisqualate(AMPA)/kainate (Q/K) type of receptors. Na^+ and K^+ flow through the Q/K receptor channel but not through the NMDA receptor channel, due to Mg^{2+} block of this channel. Fig. 6.8B shows events occurring when the postsynaptic membrane is depolarized, as would occur during a high-frequency tetanus. The depolarization relieves the Mg^{2+} block of the NMDA channel, allowing Na^+, K^+, and, most importantly, Ca^{2+} to flow through the channel. The figure also shows voltage-dependent Ca^{2+} channels on the dendritic shafts; this source of Ca^{2+} does not, however, have access to the spines on which the synapses responsible for the induction of LTP are located, and is not involved in the induction of LTP. (*From* Nicoll, Kauer, and Malenka 1988)

despite activating quite different synapses, could obtain sufficient overall depolarization of the postsynaptic cell so that the Mg^{2+} block was removed, and the NMDA receptors could then be readily activated at the synapses of any active sets of afferents. The capacity of the voltage-dependence of the NMDA receptor to explain cooperativity in LTP depends of course, on evidence that NMDA receptors are involved in the induction of LTP. Specific antagonists of the NMDA receptor have been found, and administration of these antagonists has been shown to block the development of LTP both *in vitro* (Collingridge, Kehl, and McLennan 1983; Harris, Ganong, and Cotman 1984) and *in vivo* (Morris et al. 1986). It is important to note that NMDA receptor antagonists do not affect kainate or AMPA receptors, so that their administration does not affect normal, unpotentiated synaptic transmission; the responses initially evoked by afferent stimulation are not affected by NMDA receptor antagonists, whose selective effect is simply to block the development of LTP.

If NMDA receptors do play a critical role in the induction of LTP, then they provide a mechanism for a modified type of "Hebbian" synapse. A synapse between two cells is strengthened if the presynaptic cell successfully activates NMDA receptors; whether a presynaptic spike obtains NMDA activation depends upon preceding activity in itself or in other presynaptic cells. So, the Hebbian principle of the successful activation of pre- and postsynaptic cells as a condition for increased synaptic efficacy is maintained, with the modification that the postsynaptic activity is not simply impulse generation but activation of a specific class of receptor.

The fact that activation of NMDA receptors allows calcium influx suggests that an increase in intracellular calcium may play a role in induction of LTP, and direct evidence for such a role is available. Turner, Baimbridge, and Miller (1982) found that exposure of hippocampal slices to solutions containing twice the normal concentration of calcium led of itself to an increase in synaptic efficiency, which persisted for at least three hours and so resembled LTP. And Lynch et al. (1983) have shown that intracellular injection of a calcium chelator (EGTA) into a postsynaptic cell prevents induction of LTP.

A Postsynaptic Site for Maintenance of LTP? The Lynch-Baudry Hypothesis

The steps by which an increase in intracellular calcium might lead to a sustained increase in synaptic efficacy remain the subject of much controversial speculation. One specific proposal is due to Lynch and Baudry

(1984), who suggested a chain of events that could lead to permanent structural changes in the postsynaptic membrane.

Changes in Glutamate Receptor Binding

Work on hippocampal slices in Lynch and Baudry's laboratory indicated that high-frequency stimulation obtained an increase in glutamate binding when the stimulation led to the induction of LTP. This increase in binding was dependent on the availability of calcium and appeared to reflect an increase in the number of glutamate receptors. The essence of Lynch and Baudry's 1984 proposal was, then, that an increase in intracellular calcium led to an increase in the number of glutamate receptors in the postsynaptic membrane.

The notion that the basic mechanism for maintenance of LTP is an increase in postsynaptic sensitivity to glutamate has received strong (but indirect) support from more recent experiments that have exploited the discovery of drugs that selectively block the AMPA/kainate receptors. The use of these drugs has achieved the separate measurement of components of the postsynaptic response mediated, respectively, by the NMDA and non-NMDA glutamate receptors. These experiments have shown that the induction of LTP obtains an increase in the non-NMDA component only; LTP does not obtain an increase in the NMDA component (Kauer, Malenka, and Nicoll 1988; Muller, Joly, and Lynch 1988). It had previously been shown (Bliss et al. 1986) that the induction of LTP is accompanied by increases in glutamate release; but if increased transmitter release was responsible for the phenomenon of LTP, it would, of course, be expected that the currents mediated by the NMDA and the non-NMDA glutamate receptors would both increase. Direct support for this latter supposition is provided by the demonstration that PTP (believed to be mediated by increased transmitter release) does increase both NMDA and non-NMDA components (Kauer, Malenka, and Nicoll 1988); a parallel finding has been reported for paired-pulse facilitation, another phenomenon believed to be mediated by increased transmitter release (Muller, Joly, and Lynch 1988). Furthermore, induction of LTP does not attenuate the degree of facilitation obtained by procedures that yield either PTP or paired-pulse facilitation (Muller and Lynch 1989; Zalutsky and Nicoll 1990); had LTP shared with PTP and paired-pulse facilitation a common mechanism yielding increased presynaptic release of transmitter, some interference with those phenomena by the induction of LTP would have been expected.

The discovery that LTP is maintained solely through increases in the non-NMDA current is, of course, readily accommodated within the Lynch and Baudry scheme by the not implausible assumption that only non-NMDA glutamate receptors increase in number as a consequence of the induction of LTP. These findings therefore provide indirect support for the hypothesis.

A Role for Proteolysis in LTP

The induction of LTP is a rapid process, and Lynch and Baudry did not suggest that new receptors were created by high-frequency stimulation. Their proposal was rather that they were "uncovered" as a result of structural changes obtained by cleavage of a membrane protein. Disruption of proteins is mediated by enzymes, and Lynch and Baudry reported the identification of a calcium-dependent proteinase (calpain) in rat brain synaptic membrane fractions. Finally, Lynch and Baudry suggested that the protein upon which calpain acted was fodrin, a protein that is concentrated in postsynaptic membranes, and for which indirect evidence suggests a role in control of receptors and in cell shape. Indirect support for this aspect of the Lynch and Baudry hypothesis is available from evidence suggesting an important role for proteolysis in LTP: Seubert et al. (1988) have shown that stimulation of NMDA receptors in hippocampal slices does indeed lead to proteolysis and that leupeptin, a drug that inhibits calpain activity, disrupts the development of LTP (Oliver, Baudry, and Lynch 1989).

Summary

According to Lynch and Baudry (1984), high-frequency stimulation obtains an increase in postsynaptic intracellular calcium; the calcium activates calpain, which disrupts fodrin; the disruption of fodrin uncovers more glutamate receptors, and although the temporal dynamics of the system are not understood, it seemed possible that sufficient disruption of fodrin could lead to permanent structural changes in membrane shape, allowing permanent exposure of larger numbers of glutamate receptors. Figure 6.9 provides diagrammatic representations of the various stages proposed by Lynch and Baudry in the induction and maintenance of LTP.

Broader Implications of the Lynch-Baudry Hypothesis

Not the least of the attractions of the Lynch and Baudry hypothesis was the fact that it carried a number of far-reaching implications for behavioral psychology. Work in Lynch and Baudry's laboratory had shown that al-

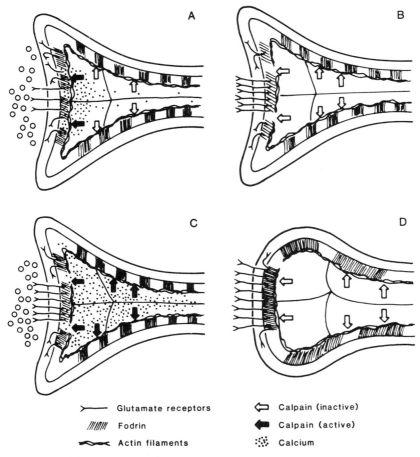

>—	Glutamate receptors	⇦	Calpain (inactive)
////////	Fodrin	⬅	Calpain (active)
∿	Actin filaments	∴	Calcium

FIGURE **6.9.** Diagrammatic representation of the Lynch and Baudry (1984) hypothesis concerning mechanisms of induction and maintenance of LTP. A: Transmitter release causes an increase in calcium in the subsynaptic zone activating calpain, which degrades fodrin and uncovers occluded glutamate receptors. B: Calcium is removed from the spine, inactivating the calpain. C: Subsequent episodes of high-frequency activity produce a larger influx of calcium because of the greater number of receptors. This stimulates calpain throughout the spine and leads to widespread disruption of the fodrin network, permitting shape change to occur. D: Calcium is again eliminated from the spine, but the structural and receptor changes produced by transient activation of calpain remain. (*From* Lynch and Baudry 1984)

though calcium obtained increases in glutamate binding with comparable efficiency in all major telencephalic areas, very little increase in binding was found in brainstem regions. They argued therefore that the calpain-fodrin mechanism was not available to extratelencephalic regions and that learning that took in the absence of telencephalon (classical conditioning, for example) involved a qualitatively different type of memory from that involved in "telencephalic" learning.

The calcium-induced stimulation of glutamate binding was found to be temperature dependent, being essentially absent at room temperatures, and maximal at 35–40°C. This suggested that poikilothermic animals might not use the calpain-fodrin mechanism, and Lynch and Baudry reported failures to find calcium-stimulated binding of glutamate in amphibians or reptiles. Since they found no calcium-stimulated binding in birds either, they suggested that the mechanism·"may be a mammalian invention" (Lynch and Baudry 1984:1061). The proposal was, then, that the calpain-fodrin mechanism was involved in a memory system that stood apart from the "simpler forms of memory" mediated by extratelencephalic regions in mammals and by nonmammalian nervous systems. We have seen that conditioning in mammals is possible in the absence of the telencephalon, but will see in chapters 7 and 8 that mammalian telencephalic damage can cause severe disruption of learning involving tasks that go beyond standard habituation and association-formation designs; it is therefore not unreasonable to suggest that the nature of learning supported by the mammalian telencephalon might differ in substantive ways from that supported by nonmammalian telencephalic (and mammalian extratelencephalic) structures. But it is also worth pointing out here one problem for this intriguing proposal, which is that efforts to establish qualitative differences in learning between mammals and nonmammalian vertebrates have met with little success (Macphail 1982, 1987).

We shall see in the following section that serious technical problems have emerged concerning Lynch and Baudry's work on glutamate binding, so that the specific implications drawn from that work do not justify further consideration here. But their exploration of the potential implications of the findings for comparative work nicely illustrates an important principle—namely, that work on the physiological psychology of one species may carry important implications for the behavior of other species that differ in some physiological respect. The potential value of comparative work in physiological psychology is an issue that will be taken up in more detail in chapter 9.

A Presynaptic Site for Maintenance of LTP?

There is general agreement that postsynaptic events are critical to the induction of LTP, so that proposals (such as the Lynch and Baudry hypothesis) that attribute the maintenance of LTP to a postsynaptic locus have an immediate advantage in plausibility over those that suppose a presynaptic locus. The two principal strands of the Lynch and Baudry (1984) hypothesis were, first, that the maintenance of LTP involved an increase in postsynaptic sensitivity to glutamate, and second, that that increase was dependent upon an increase in postsynaptic proteolysis. We shall see that challenges to both these propositions have emerged, and that it is the challenge to the first strand—the notion of increased postsynaptic sensitivity—that poses the most serious difficulty for the hypothesis.

Assessment of Postsynaptic Sensitivity Following Induction of LTP

The first problem to emerge was the discovery that there had been a flaw in the interpretation of the technique used by Lynch and Baudry to assess changes in glutamate binding. It has become clear that the increased "binding" that was observed was not in fact binding of glutamate to receptors but an increase in the sequestration of glutamate in vesicles in the plasma membrane (a component of a chloride-dependent glutamate exchange system) (Pin, Bockaert, and Recasesn 1984; Kessler, Baudry, and Lynch, 1987).

Early efforts to measure directly changes in sensitivity of cells to administration of glutamate following induction of LTP provided no support for the notion that sensitivity increased following induction of LTP (Lynch, Gribkoff, and Deadwyler 1976; Schwartzkroin and Taube 1986). A more recent report suggests that one reason for those negative results might lie in the temporal parameters of the change in sensitivity. Davies et al. (1989) measured the sensitivity of CA1 cells to iontophoretically applied glutamate before and after the induction of LTP. Their results showed that sensitivity did increase, but that no change was detectable for at least 15 min after induction of LTP, following which interval there was a gradual increase in sensitivity over a period of approximately two hours. Since LTP is demonstrable 30 sec after its induction, Davies et al. (1989) suggested that there may be two components to LTP—an early component lasting an hour or two, and a later component; the later component might be mediated by a change in postsynaptic sensitivity and the earlier component by a presynaptic change (presumably an increase in transmitter release). The notion that LTP may consist of two temporally separable components is one to which we shall return.

At this point we shall consider two studies that have used the only technique that enables uncontroversial determination of the existence or otherwise of changes in postsynaptic sensitivity, namely quantal analysis. This technique was introduced in chapter 2, and it will be recalled that it involves the statistical analysis of EPSP magnitudes, an analysis that, inter alia, allows the determination of the magnitude of the postsynaptic response elicited by the presynaptic release of a single quantum, or packet, of transmitter.

Two recent reports (Manilow and Tsien 1990; Bekkers and Stevens 1990) have employed novel physiological recording techniques (whole-cell voltage-clamp recordings) that reduce background noise (in cells in hippocampal slices) to a level sufficiently low that quantal analysis of EPSPs to minimal stimuli is possible. Both reports agree that the induction of LTP does not alter the magnitude of the postsynaptic response to a single quantum: postsynaptic sensitivity, in other words, is not changed by LTP. The reports agree also that LTP does result in an increase in presynaptic transmitter release, and an experiment that used cultured neuron pairs pinpointed the source of that increase to an increased probability of release of transmitter in response to an action potential (rather than to an increase in the number of presynaptic release sites) (Bekkers and Stevens 1990).

Although both reports caution that some small fraction of LTP might be postsynaptic in origin, their general import is quite clear: it seems now beyond dispute that the induction of LTP is accompanied by an increase in presynaptic transmitter release, along with no (or, at least, no detectable) change in postsynaptic sensitivity. It should be noted here that these findings are not easily reconciled with the Davies et al. (1989) compromise proposal, that there is an early presynaptic and a late postsynaptic component to LTP: both of the quantal-analysis reports studied changes seen during LTP that was maintained for an hour or more, and neither found any increase in postsynaptic sensitivity over that period. Since Davies et al. reported changes in sensitivity that appeared to begin some 15 min after the induction of LTP, similar changes should have been anticipated within the periods of observation used in the quantal-analysis reports.

It is not currently possible to guess how the contradiction between the Davies et al. findings and those of the reports of quantal analysis will be resolved. The demonstration of increases in transmitter release accompanying LTP raises other difficult questions also.

How does LTP succeed (as it apparently does) in increasing presynaptic transmitter release without increasing the NMDA as well as the non-NMDA current? One distinctly post hoc possibility is that induction of LTP may result in a persistent down-regulation of NMDA receptor function (Bliss 1990).

A second question arises from the fact that induction of LTP is dependent upon postsynaptic events: how, then, is information about these events conveyed back to the presynaptic site of maintenance of LTP? Two potential messengers between the post- and the presynaptic zones have been proposed. One is arachidonic acid (or some derivative), the other the diffusible molecule nitric oxide. Empirical support for each of these candidate messengers will now be briefly outlined.

There is evidence that activation of NMDA receptors (but not of AMPA/kainate receptors) does stimulate release of arachidonic acid (Dumuis et al. 1988), and evidence also that arachidonic acid does obtain LTP when (and only when) it is administered along with weak trains of stimulation of presynaptic fibers (Williams et al. 1989). The trains used in this latter report were too weak to obtain LTP in the absence of arachidonic acid, and LTP could be obtained by this technique even when the NMDA receptors were blocked by the NMDA receptor antagonist APV (2-amino–5-phosphonovalerate), suggesting that the critical effect of NMDA receptor activation might indeed be the release of arachidonic acid. It is interesting, given the Davies et al. result, to note that the LTP obtained in the Williams et al. report grew gradually to a plateau some one to two hours after the arachidonic acid was washed out. Although this finding points to the possibility of temporally separable components of LTP, it suggests (in contrast to the Davies et al. proposal) that the late component involves a presynaptic effect.

A number of lines of evidence support the notion that nitric oxide might be a retrograde messenger involved in the induction of LTP. First, intracellular synthesis of nitric oxide is dependent upon a calcium/calmodulin-dependent enzyme. Second, inhibition of nitric oxide synthesis disrupts the induction of LTP but does not alter synaptic responses to low-frequency stimulation (Haley, Wilcox, and Chapman 1992). Third, there is evidence that nitric oxide is synthesized in the same postsynaptic neurons that (unless intracellular nitric oxide synthesis is inhibited) show LTP (Schuman and Madison 1991). Fourth, induction of LTP is attenuated by administration of hemoglobin, a molecule that sequestrates nitric oxide in the extracellular medium (Schuman and Madison 1991; Haley, Wilcox, and Chapman 1992); this finding supports the view that the intracellularly synthesized nitric oxide takes its effect after diffusing out into the extracellular space, as would be expected of a retrograde messenger.

A Role for Protein Phosphorylation in LTP

The second strand of the Lynch and Baudry (1984) hypothesis was that breakdown of postsynaptic membrane proteins was the physiological mechanism responsible for the relatively permanent changes underlying the maintenance of LTP. We shall now consider a rival proposal—namely, that phosphorylation of presynaptic membrane proteins is critical for the development of virtually permanent LTP; interestingly, this proposal will also incorporate the idea that there are two temporally distinct components of LTP.

The notion that phosphorylation is involved in LTP is supported by the work of Routtenberg and his colleagues (for reviews see Routtenberg 1985; Linden and Routtenberg 1989) on a protein (of 47,000 daltons molecular mass) labeled F1, which is concentrated in presynaptic membranes. Routtenberg, Lovinger, and Steward (1985) studied the effect of stimulation of the perforant path in intact rats on the phosphorylation of F1 in the dorsal hippocampus (rapidly extracted either 1 or 5 min after stimulation). The results showed that F1 phosphorylation was increased by stimulation that induced LTP, but not by control stimulation, and that there was a highly significant positive correlation between the amount of phosphorylation observed in hippocampi excised 5 min after induction of LTP and the size of the pre- versus post-LTP change in magnitude of the response evoked by test stimuli; there was not, however, a significant correlation between phosphorylation and magnitude of LTP in hippocampi excised 1 min after induction of LTP.

The phosphorylation of F1 is dependent upon the protein kinase PKC, which activates the F1 phosphatase. PKC occurs in both the cytoplasm and the membranes of neurons, and Akers et al. (1986) have reported that 60 min (but not 1 min) after induction of LTP membrane PKC activity is enhanced, and that cytoplasmic PKC activity is correspondingly reduced. Akers et al. reported a high correlation (.85) between membrane PKC activity and the persistence of LTP (this last being measured by the percentage change in evoked spike amplitude in the period between 1 and 60 min following induction of LTP). These results suggest, then, that F1 phosphorylation, stimulated by PKC, is involved in the maintenance of

LTP; since no significant correlations were observed between the magnitude or persistence of LTP and either F1 phosphorylation or PKC activity 1 min after induction of LTP, the results suggest also that phosphorylation is not involved in the induction of LTP.

Further support for a role of PKC in the maintenance of LTP is provided by reports of the effects of PKC inhibitors on LTP. Lovinger et al. (1987) found that microinjections of PKC inhibitors into the rat hippocampus 15 min before induction of LTP did not prevent normal induction; but the LTP obtained returned (unlike that of controls) to baseline levels within 60 min of induction. Injection of PKC inhibitors 10 min after the induction of LTP similarly resulted in decay of LTP within 60 min of its original induction. LTP was, however, wholly unaffected by administration of PKC inhibitors four hours after induction. These findings suggest that PKC activation is not necessary for the induction of LTP, nor for an early component of the maintenance of LTP that decays within an hour or so; PKC activation is necessary for the transition to a later, more permanent component of LTP, but permanent activation of PKC does not seem to be required for long-term maintenance of LTP.

A more recent report implicates phosphorylation of proteins other than F1 in the maintenance of LTP. Nelson, Linden, and Routtenberg (1989) induced LTP in rat hippocampus and measured its persistence over a 10-min interval from 3 min to 13 min after induction. They found that the degree of persistence showed a significant correlation across animals with the amount of phosphorylation of not only protein F1 but also two proteins that were indistinguishable from proteins known to be associated with synaptic vesicles. These latter proteins are phosphorylated by a Ca^{2+} / calmodulin-dependent kinase, and Nelson and his colleagues (1989) suggest that activation of PKC leads to a phosphorylation cascade in which phosphorylation of F1 leads to the release of bound Ca^{2+}/calmodulin-dependent kinase, which in turn phosphorylates the synaptic vesicle proteins. What is interesting about this proposal, of course, is that it provides a route through which, perhaps, increased presynaptic release of transmitter might be mediated.

There is, then, evidence for a role in LTP of protein phosphorylation, and that evidence also supports the notion that there may be more than one component in maintained LTP. But it is clear that we are currently very far from having a precise picture of the physical basis of the maintenance of LTP. We have, after all, seen evidence in a preceding section for a role of proteolysis in LTP, and although the respective protagonists have pointed to a presynaptic site (for phosphorylation) and to a postsynaptic site (for proteolysis), almost all the evidence for either process is in fact quite neutral concerning the issue of a pre- versus a postsynaptic locus. The evidence currently available may, in other words, just as well be interpreted as supporting the view that there are presynaptic proteolytic and/or postsynaptic phosphorylation processes in LTP. Similarly, although we have seen a number of sources of support for the view that there may be temporally distinct components to the maintenance of LTP, it is difficult at present to bring those sources together to provide a unified account of such a multicomponent system: in particular, it should be emphasized that the data from quantal analysis, data that provide the most unambiguous account of the mechanism of LTP, do not suggest any fractionation into component processes, at least over the first hour or so following induction.

LTP Is Associated with Morphological Changes

Like Lynch and Baudry (1984), Routtenberg (1985) proposes that his LTP mechanism may result in permanent structural change and cites what he calls "circumstantial" evidence linking the PKC/F1 mechanism to growth. There is in fact good evidence that LTP is associated with structural changes, but precisely what changes occur may vary with the area concerned. Lee et al. (1980), for example, reported that the induction of LTP in CA1 pyramidal cells led to an increase of approximately 33 percent in the number of shaft synapses seen in electron microscopy of the dendritic field. But Desmond and Levy (1986) found that induction of LTP in the dentate gyrus was associated with a selective increase in the number of one type of dendritic spine synapse (the concave spine), there being no change in the number of shaft synapses. Changes in synaptic morphology inevitably involve both pre- and postsynaptic membranes, and it is quite feasible that changes in the postsynaptic membrane are induced by and secondary to changes in the presynaptic membrane (and vice versa). At present, then, the morphological changes observed do not specifically support either a pre- or a postsynaptic locus for the maintenance of LTP, nor do the types of changes seen encourage any particular account, such as those of Lynch and Baudry (1984) and Routtenberg (1985). But these changes do confirm that it is rational to seek a mechanism that can bring about relatively permanent structural changes in response to brief and transient stimulation; the calpain/fodrin and PKC/F1 mechanisms are plausible candidates in the search for explanation of these changes.

Different Types of LTP

LTP Also Occurs Outside the Mammalian Hippocampus

Most research on LTP has concentrated on the hippocampus, an emphasis reflected in the discussion here. This has been due partly to its original discovery in the hippocampus, partly to the convenience of the hippocampal slice, and perhaps mainly to the fact that hippocampal damage is known to have profound effects on learning and memory. LTP—defined as a relatively long-term (more than 30-min) increase in synaptic efficacy—has been reported from other brain structures. Racine, Milgram, and Hafner (1983), for example, reported LTP in the amygdala, the septal area, the subiculum, and the entorhinal cortex (all structures associated with the hippocampus). There have been reports also of LTP in neocortex (Lee 1982; Wilson and Racine 1983; Artola and Singer 1987). Outside the forebrain, LTP has been observed in, for example, cerebellar nuclei (Racine et al. 1986), and in the superior cervical ganglion of the sympathetic division of the peripheral autonomic nervous system (Briggs, Brown, and McAfee 1985). The phenomenon has also been observed in nonmammalian vertebrates—in, for example, the hippocampus of the song sparrow (Wieraszko and Ball 1991), the bullfrog sympathetic ganglion (Koyano, Kuba, and Minota 1985), and the goldfish optic tectum (Lewis and Teyler 1986), as well as in invertebrate preparations (Byrne 1987). But LTP does not occur at all synapses: although Racine et al. (1986) found LTP in the cerebellar interpositus and vestibular nuclei, they reported that they had been unable to demonstrate LTP of the Purkinje cells of the cerebellar cortex.

Not All Forms of LTP Employ the Same Mechanism

There is, of course, no need to suppose that all instances of LTP involve comparable mechanisms. Although it is interesting that LTP in the rat sympathetic cervical ganglion is due to increased presynaptic release of transmitter (Briggs, Brown, and McAfee 1985), this does not necessarily mean that a similar mechanism is responsible for all forms of LTP; the transmitter concerned is certainly not the same for all forms (being acetylcholine in the sympathetic ganglion and glutamate in the hippocampus).

Even within the hippocampus, it is clear that not all instances of LTP have similar causes: in experiments using guinea pig hippocampal slices, Harris and Cotman (1986) found that whereas the NMDA receptor antagonist APV blocked LTP in the CA1 region (elicited by stimulation of

Schaffer collaterals), it did not block LTP in the CA3 region (elicited by stimulation of mossy fibers). This finding has recently been followed up in an elegant series of experiments by Zalutsky and Nicoll (1990), who studied the characteristics of LTP elicited in the same CA3 cells by stimulation of either associative-commissural fibers (that terminate on distal zones of CA3 apical dendrites) or mossy fibers (that terminate on proximal dendrites). Zalutsky and Nicoll (again using guinea pig hippocampal slices) first confirmed the Harris and Cotman (1986) finding and showed that mossy-fiber LTP was not blocked by APV; LTP induced by associative-commissural stimulation was, however, completely blocked by APV. Zalutsky and Nicoll went on to show: that administration to a CA3 cell of a calcium chelator blocked the induction of associative-commissural LTP but not of mossy-fiber LTP; that depolarization of a CA3 cell facilitated the induction of LTP by associative-commissural stimulation but not by mossy-fiber stimulation; that hyperpolarization of a CA3 cell prevented the induction of LTP by associative-commissural stimulation but not by mossy-fiber stimulation; and that the magnitude of paired-pulse facilitation was not reduced by LTP induced by associative-commissural stimulation but was reduced by mossy-fiber stimulation. Thus the associative-commissural mechanism requires free calcium in the postsynaptic cell, is highly dependent upon the voltage of the postsynaptic cell, and does not interact with the mechanism (believed to involve increased presynaptic transmitter release) of paired-pulse facilitation. These are precisely the characteristics that we would expect of cells demonstrating the type of NMDA-mediated LTP that has been discussed in some detail. The characteristics of the mossy-fiber LTP indicate that its induction is quite independent of events taking place in the postsynaptic cell, and that it probably does involve an increase in transmitter release that employs the same mechanism as that activated by paired-pulse stimulation. What is important to note is that mossy-fiber LTP lacks those properties of NMDA-mediated LTP (selectivity and cooperativity) that make it so promising a candidate for an association-forming mechanism. It seems likely that repetitive stimulation of a mossy fiber potentiates all the synapses made by the fiber (and not simply those that terminate on a cell that is currently depolarized), and that that potentiation is not facilitated by activity in other sets of fibers. It is not easy currently to speculate on the functional implications of the very different properties of mossy-fiber LTP. In the words of Zalutsky and Nicoll: "An understanding of the consequences of increasing activity in these different sets of synapses must await a better understanding of the information processing functions of the hippocampal circuitry" (Zalutsky and Nicoll 1990:1623).

Just as there is no reason to suppose that all types of LTP employ the same physiological mechanism, there is no reason to suppose that the behavioral role of LTP is comparable in all cases: the attribution of a key role in learning to hippocampal LTP does not imply that a similar role (or indeed any role) in learning is to be attributed to sympathetic ganglion LTP. What little evidence there is on the behavioral significance of LTP refers to hippocampal LTP, and the interpretation of that work has no necessary implications for the role of LTP in other structures.

A Role in Memory for LTP?

We have seen a number of reasons for the current lively interest in LTP as a candidate mechanism of memory. LTP occurs in the hippocampus, and hippocampal damage profoundly affects certain types of learning and memory. LTP involves alterations in efficacy of specific synapses, and has associative characteristics that may be due to the properties of the NMDA receptors concentrated in the hippocampus. LTP is a long-lasting effect of a relatively brief event (or set of events) and is associated with morphological changes that could plausibly be permanent. There have, of course, been candidates other than LTP advanced as potential mechanisms of synaptic plasticity underlying learning and memory (we have encountered, for example, the phenomenon of long-term depression); but in no other case have there been so many features suggesting a link between the physiological mechanism and learning in the intact organism. A full discussion of all potential mechanisms is currently of restricted interest to physiological psychologists, since there are generally no clear psychological implications associated with one mechanism or another. In the sections that follow, we shall assess evidence derived from experiments on learning in intact animals and attempt to answer such questions as: Is there evidence that LTP is obtained by learning in the intact animal? Is learning affected by drugs that block the development of LTP? Does the induction of LTP by physiological means affect subsequent learning? One important byproduct of the sections in which these questions are considered is that it will become clear that it is in fact extremely difficult to show a convincing relationship between a relatively low-level physiological phenomenon like LTP and behavior in the intact organism. We shall see that, despite the immense research effort that has been made, it is still in fact not certain that LTP is (or is not) involved in learning and memory. Before, however, any alternative candidate for a physiological mechanism of learning could be taken seriously, experiments analogous to those described in the following sections will have to be conducted; until then, alternative proposals will remain entirely speculative.

Does Learning Obtain LTP?

We may consider first the question whether learning obtains LTP. A number of reports suggest that it may. Sharp, McNaughton, and Barnes (1985) found that rats exposed to an enriched environment (a large chamber filled with a variety of novel objects) showed as a consequence a potentiated dentate gyrus response to stimulation of the perforant path. Sharp, Barnes, and McNaughton (1987) replicated that result, using separate groups of young (14-month-old) and old (32-month-old) rats and found in both groups substantial increases in the dentate population spike evoked by perforant path stimulation after eleven days' exposure to the enriched environment. Although both old and young rats showed comparable increases in spike amplitude, the potentiation decayed more rapidly in old than in young rats, once they had been returned to their home cages. The time constant of the decay of potentiation for the young rats was thirty days, and for the old rats eleven days. This is of interest since old rats forget spatial information more rapidly that young rats, a point to which we shall return.

Increased excitability of hippocampal cells has also been reported in experiments in which hippocampal slices were obtained from rabbits 24 hours after classical eyelid conditioning; it is not, however, clear that the results reflect induction of LTP by learning. When compared to responses obtained in slices from control rabbits (given either no behavioral training or unpaired presentations of the white-noise CS and the eyeshock UCS), trained rabbits showed enhanced responses in single CA1 pyramidal cells to high-frequency stimulation of Schaffer collaterals (LoTurco, Coulter, and Alkon 1988). But no potentiation was seen when single-action potentials were elicited in CA1 cells (Disterhoft, Coulter, and Alkon 1986; LoTurco, Coulter, and Alkon 1988). The implication, therefore, appears to be either that trained rabbits develop LTP to appropriate eliciting stimuli more efficiently than control rabbits, or that a mechanism distinct from LTP is involved. Support for this latter possibility is provided by the observation (Disterhoft, Coulter, and Alkon 1986) that trained rabbits showed a reduction in the after-hyperpolarization that is elicited by a series of action potentials in hippocampal CA1 pyramidal cells. One role of this after-hyperpolarization is to allow cells to adapt to a sustained train of depolarizing inputs, and reductions in after-hyperpolarization result in higher rates of response to sustained input trains (Nicoll 1988). The after-hyperpolarization is in turn believed to be mediated by a calcium-dependent potassium channel and can be blocked by neurotransmitters that act through second-messenger systems (involving protein kinases) to phosphorylate that channel (Nicoll 1988). It will be recalled from chapter 4 that Alkon proposes that conditioning in *Hermissenda* is mediated by the phosphorylation of a calcium-dependent potassium channel. Such findings suggest that there may be important parallels between conditioning mechanisms in *Hermissenda* and in mammals, and we may expect to see vigorous investigation of the changes induced by training in the hippocampal slice preparation. For the present we should note that these changes may be quite independent of LTP, and that reservations concerning a causal role for LTP in learning will apply equally to any proposed role for reductions in after-hyperpolarization.

In contrast to the above reports, Hargreaves, Cain, and Vanderwolf (1990) have reported a failure to detect any change in response of dentate gyrus cells to perforant path stimulation following learning of either of two tasks (a radial maze task and a simple escape task). Hargreaves and his colleagues did, however, note that there were large differences in the responses evoked, according to whether or not the animals were moving when the responses were measured. Controlling for mobility of subjects is clearly an important issue: if some learning experience led to a tendency to higher mobility, that might be reflected in enhanced evoked responses.

Also relevant here are reports of the uses of perforant path stimulation as a conditional stimulus. Matthies et al. (1986) used perforant path stimulation as a CS in a shuttle-box avoidance task and found potentiation of evoked dentate gyrus responses in rats for which the CS was an effective CS, and not in those for which it was not. Weisz, Clark, and Thompson (1984) paired perforant path stimulation with a tone CS in a classical-conditioning task using the rabbit eyelid preparation, finding that once stable responding was established, the response evoked in the dentate gyrus by perforant path stimulation was enhanced. A failure to find an enhanced response to perforant path stimulation has, however, also been reported. Skelton, Miller, and Phillips (1985) used low-frequency stimulation of the perforant path as a discriminative stimulus for the availability of a food pellet for a bar-pressing response. The stimulation served as an effective CS, but no potentiation of the response evoked in the dentate gyrus occurred as acquisition proceeded (in fact, there was a slight depression).

A more general difficulty for all the positive reports described above is that there is no evidence that the effects obtained are specific to hippocampal pathways. The findings could reflect a general facilitation of telencephalic responsiveness obtained, perhaps, by an increase in some tonic excitatory input; such a mechanism would be quite different from the synapse-specific potentiation seen in LTP. It is clearly difficult to circumvent this problem, and at present it is safest to conclude that changes have been observed that could be due to the induction of LTP by behavioral events but that those changes are currently open to other interpretations.

Effects on Learning of NMDA Receptor Antagonists

A second approach to the involvement of LTP in learning is to use drugs that block the development of LTP. Studies using this technique have provided evidence that learning in tasks that are sensitive to hippocampal damage is disrupted when LTP is blocked.

Morris et al. (1986) tested the effects of intraventricular infusion of APV on two types of behavioral task. It will be recalled that APV is an NMDA receptor antagonist that blocks the development of LTP but does not appear to affect normal (non-NMDA) synaptic transmission. The apparatus used was the Morris water maze, which, as it has been widely used in investigations of hippocampal function, merits a brief introduction.

The maze (Morris 1981) consists of a large circular bath (filled with water made opaque by the addition of milk), which may contain one or more small platforms, large enough for a rat to sit on. In the standard "spatial" version of the task, the bath contains one platform situated just below the water surface. The rat is dropped into the water from various starting points around the perimeter of the bath and gradually learns to escape from the water by finding the hidden platform rapidly. Performance relies on orientation to a constellation of distal cues and not on approach to specific proximal cues.

Rats with hippocampal damage are severely disrupted in acquisition and retention of the Morris maze task (Morris et al. 1982). Morris et al. (1986) found that APV also severely disrupted performance in this task: figure 6.10 shows the striking difference between the performance of a control and an APV-treated rat on a transfer test (in which there was in fact no platform present in the maze) conducted after fifteen training trials.

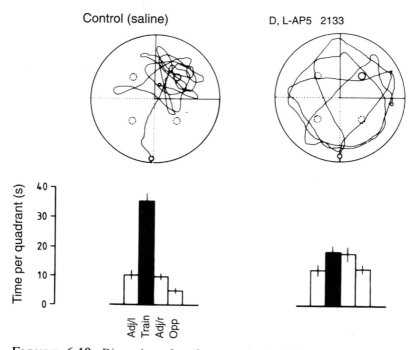

FIGURE 6.10. Disruption of performance in the Morris water maze by intraventricular infusion of APV. The bottom part of the figure shows mean time spent in a 60-sec posttraining transfer test (with no platform present) in the original training quadrant (Train), the opposite (Opp), and the two adjacent quadrants (Adj/L and Adj/R); control (saline-infused) group performance is shown on the left, and the group having APV infusion, on the right. The top part of the figure shows the swimming path taken by the individual rat closest to the group mean (calculated according to the distribution of time spent per quadrant) of each group (Control on the left, APV-infused on the right). (*From* Morris et al. 1986)

Morris and his colleagues showed also (in anesthetized rats) that intraventricular infusion of APV did block the development of LTP. The second task used by Morris et al. (1986) required the animal to discriminate between two visually discriminable platforms that projected above the surface of the water; one of these platforms was in fact floating and sank when the rat put any weight upon it, and the rat's task was to learn to swim to the stable platform. APV did not disrupt performance on this task, and a similar lack of effect of hippocampal damage on visual discriminations has commonly been reported (O'Keefe and Nadel 1978). Subsequent work (Morris 1988) has shown that similar results are obtained when APV is injected directly into the hippocampus and so is better localized within the brain, and that APV when injected into visual cortex still has no effect on visual discrimination learning.

Studies of the effects on learning of NMDA receptor antagonists are still at an early stage, and alternative accounts of the effects obtained are available. Chronic ventricular infusion of APV, for example, causes weight loss in rats (Tonkiss, Morris, and Rawlins 1988), and this raises the possibility that these antagonist drugs may result in motivational disruption. It is also the case that APV (and other NMDA receptor antagonist drugs) have disruptive effects on sensorimotor pathways and induce sensorimotor deficits such as ataxia (Mondadori et al. 1989). The side effects of these drugs have led Keith and Rudy (1990) to argue that the disruptions seen in learning tasks by Morris (and others) following infusion of NMDA receptor antagonists are disruptions, not of learning, but of performance, and due to nonassociative factors. There is evidence that runs counter to the notion that all the deficits induced by NMDA receptor antagonists should be attributed to their motivational or sensorimotor effects: the specificity of the deficit reported by Morris et al. (1986), in which spatial maze-learning was disrupted and visual discrimination learning was not, argues, for example, against motivational interpretation of the maze-learning deficit; and Morris (1990) cites evidence that supports the independence of sensorimotor and learning deficits. The potential role of the side effects of NMDA receptor antagonists is, however, a complicated issue that cannot yet be said with confidence to have been resolved.

A further problem noted by Keith and Rudy (1990) is that although water-maze performance in the Morris et al. (1986) study was disrupted by infusion of APV, there was in fact in that report evidence that the rats could learn at least something about the location of the hidden platform. Following the transfer test in that study, the rats were given eight further training trials, and then trained using a new location in the quadrant opposite that used in original training (a reversal test). The performance of the APV-infused rats was (like that of controls) markedly disrupted by the change in location of the platform. Thus although performance in the transfer test suggested that little if anything had been learned about the location of the platform, performance in the reversal test showed that, at least after further training, APV-infused rats had learned something about the platform's location.

A less serious difficulty arises from the fact that there have been reports of tasks that are not disrupted by hippocampal lesions but are disrupted by APV infusion (e.g., taste-potentiated odor-aversion learning: Willner et al. 1992). Intraventricular infusion of APV results in a spread of APV throughout the forebrain (Morris 1989), and although NMDA receptors are most highly concentrated in the hippocampus they occur also in other forebrain areas (Monaghan and Cotman 1985). It is, therefore, not surprising that tasks other than those susceptible to hippocampal damage are disrupted by infusions of NMDA receptor antagonists.

On a similar cautionary theme, it should be noted that the fact that APV is an NMDA receptor antagonist does not necessarily imply that its effects are due to the disruption of LTP. Leung and Desborough (1988) have reported that APV disrupts the hippocampal theta rhythm in rats, and we shall see (in chapter 7) grounds for supposing that disruption of theta rhythm of itself may be sufficient to reproduce many of the learning deficits induced by hippocampal damage.

NMDA Receptors and Plasticity in Visual Cortex

Evidence of a quite different kind provides a further link between NMDA receptors and neuronal plasticity. The great majority of cells in the primary visual cortex of newborn kittens at the time of first opening their eyes respond to stimuli delivered to either eye; the same is true of normal adult cats (Hubel and Wiesel 1962, 1963). But if a kitten is exposed to a brief period (as little as three or four days) of monocular deprivation during a critical period from four to twelve weeks after birth, a shift in the properties of the cortical cells occurs so that physiological investigation finds that the majority of cells now respond selectively to stimulation only of the eye that remained open (Hubel and Wiesel 1970).

A series of ingenious experiments has suggested that plasticity in geniculo-cortical synapses depends upon a threshold level of postsynaptic activity in cortical cells. This threshold may in fact be the level of depolarization required to activate NMDA receptors (which are widely distributed in visual cortex). Kleinschmidt, Bear, and Singer (1987) have shown that intracortical administration of APV blocks the neuronal plasticity normally induced by monocular deprivation; and Artola and Singer (1987), using a visual cortex slice preparation, have shown that LTP can be induced in visual cortex cells by high-frequency stimulation of geniculo-cortical afferents, and that that LTP is also blocked by APV. A further parallel with hippocampal work is provided by evidence that dendritic uptake of calcium may be necessary for geniculo-cortical plasticity (Singer 1987). Geniculo-cortical synaptic modification is a complex issue and involves weakening as well as strengthening of synapses (Bear,

Cooper, and Ebner 1987). For our present purposes it will be sufficient to note the likely involvement of NMDA receptors in a form of neuronal plasticity concerned essentially with the detection of congruence of inputs from two sources (the two retinae) onto a common cell. It is clear that the NMDA receptor–mediated "Hebbian" synapse is well suited to such a role, and clear also that detection of congruence of disparate inputs is precisely what association formation involves.

Effects on Learning of the Calpain Inhibitor Leupeptin

Further evidence for a role of LTP in learning is provided by a series of experiments using leupeptin, a drug that inhibits the activity of calpain, an enzyme believed by Lynch and Baudry (1984) to be involved in the sequence of steps leading to the maintenance of LTP. It will be recalled that administration of leupeptin does prevent the induction of LTP (Oliver, Baudry, and Lynch 1989).

Staubli, Baudry, and Lynch (1984) investigated the effect of intraventricular infusion of leupeptin on performance in the radial maze, a task that, like the Morris maze, has been used extensively by hippocampal investigators.

The radial maze, introduced by Olton and Samuelson (1976), consists of a central platform from which radiate a number of arms (typically eight). At the end of each arm is a goal-box, and all the goal-boxes are baited with food at the beginning of a trial. A hungry rat is placed on the central platform and allowed to explore the maze freely, consuming the food (which is not replaced during a trial) in each goal-box. Rats perform remarkably efficiently in the radial maze: Olton and Samuelson (1976), for example, found that rats in an eight-arm maze averaged 7.6 choices of previously unentered arms in their first eight choices within a trial. Since efficient performance requires rats to remember which arms have been visited within a trial, the radial maze provides a test of spatial memory.

Staubli, Baudry, and Lynch (1984) found that leupeptin severely disrupted performance in the radial maze but did not disrupt either active or passive avoidance learning. Staubli, Baudry, and Lynch (1985) showed that a simple olfactory discrimination task was disrupted by leupeptin. The pattern of findings once again parallels that seen after hippocampal damage, which disrupts performance in the radial maze (e.g., Olton, Walker, and Gage 1978) and in olfactory discrimination (e.g., Staubli, Ivy, and Lynch 1984) but does not disrupt active avoidance (and has variable effects on passive avoidance) (O'Keefe and Nadel 1978).

Effects on Learning of Prior Induction of LTP

Induction of LTP by physiological means prior to behavioral training has been shown to affect subsequent learning. Berger (1984) induced LTP to perforant path stimulation in the dentate gyrus of rabbits on five consecutive days. The rabbits were then exposed to a frequency discrimination in which one of two tones preceded an airpuff in an eyelid conditioning task. Rabbits given LTP training acquired the discrimination more rapidly than rabbits given control stimulation that did not obtain LTP. In contrast, a series of experiments reported by McNaughton et al. (1986) found that the induction of LTP in rats severely disrupted acquisition of spatial information in a circular maze: this maze (Barnes 1979), like the Morris water maze, involves reliance on a constellation of distal cues rather on any specific proximal cue. LTP did not disrupt retention of established memories. McNaughton and his colleagues (1986:563) suggest that "spatial information must be temporarily stored at modifiable synapses at the input stage to the hippocampal formation," and that saturation of those synapses by prior induction of LTP would interfere with the storage capacity. Why, then, did Berger (1984) find a facilitation of eyelid conditioning by prior LTP? One possibility (McNaughton and Morris 1987) is that, since spatial information is irrelevant to acquisition of the eyelid CR, an animal that is prevented from acquiring spatial information will direct more of its processing capacity to events that are relevant. But hippocampal lesions, while they do not disrupt eyelid conditioning, do not facilitate it either (e.g., Solomon 1977). Another possibility is that LTP "primes" hippocampal transmission and so facilitates activity of hippocampal cells that, as we have seen, "model" the CR in the sense that their activity corresponds closely to the amplitude of the CR observed. But again, if this is so, it is odd that hippocampal damage does not disrupt acquisition of the eyelid CR. While the effects of prior induction of LTP may indicate an involvement of LTP in learning, they do not do much to clarify the question what that role might be.

LTP and Forgetting

A final link between LTP and learning consists in the observation of correlations between parameters of LTP and the acquisition and forgetting of spatial information. Barnes (1979) found positive correlations between the percentage increase in amplitude of dentate gyrus responses evoked by a series of perforant path stimulations and asymptotic level of performance in her circular spatial maze. The correlations were significant both within and between groups of young and old rats. The critical difference in LTP between young and old rats appeared to lie in the buildup and persistence of LTP over a series of inductions. Although old rats showed smaller evoked potentials than young rats, figure 6.11 shows that the relative increase in response magnitude and its rate of decay were not different in young and old rats after one induction of LTP: but figure 6.11 also shows that after a series of four inductions, younger rats showed a larger increase in evoked potential, as well as slower decay of the potential. Similarly, Barnes and McNaughton (1985) found parallels between rates of acquisition and forgetting in the circular maze and rates of growth and decay of LTP in young and old rats.

It will be recalled that Sharp, Barnes, and McNaughton (1987) reported that LTP induced by exposure to an enriched environment also decayed more rapidly in old than in young rats. There are, then, impressive parallels between the LTP and the behavioral data obtained from young and old rats. It is, however, notoriously difficult to establish causal links from purely correlational data. It remains possible that some very general alteration in neuronal function is responsible for both the changes in LTP and the behavioral differences. Given the fact that these parallels all involve spatial tasks, it would be interesting to know whether characteristics of LTP established in some nonhippocampal region would or would not show parallels with hippocampal LTP and behavioral tasks in young and old rats.

LTP: An Associative Mechanism Involved in Spatial Learning?

The work reviewed above shows support from a number of sources for the notion that LTP is involved in learning. Certain types of experience lead to changes that are at least consistent with the idea that LTP has been obtained by them; induction of LTP prior to learning does affect acquisition; spatial learning is disrupted by a selective block of LTP; and there are correlations between growth and decay of LTP and acquisition and forgetting of spatial information. Much of the evidence—including what is perhaps the single most compelling piece of evidence (the disruption induced by manipulations that block LTP)—refers to the processing of spatial information. While this is encouraging since hippocampal damage is known to disrupt performance in spatial tasks, it is not necessarily what might have been expected from the characteristics of LTP itself. One of the reasons for the great interest in LTP has been its associative characteristics, the demonstration that the mechanism of LTP may involve "Heb-

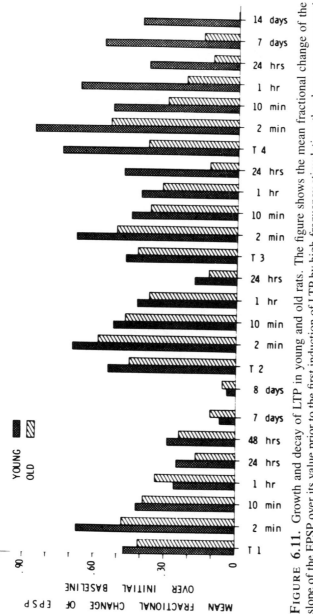

FIGURE 6.11. Growth and decay of LTP in young and old rats. The figure shows the mean fractional change of the slope of the EPSP over its value prior to the first induction of LTP by high-frequency stimulation; the slope was measured between two fixed latency points and hence was equivalent to an amplitude measure. T1, T2, T3, and T4 represent the first through the fourth time that the rats were given high-frequency stimulation. The time points shown represent the time elapsed between the end of each stimulation episode and the beginning of the test pulse measurements for that given time point. (*From* Barnes 1979)

bian" synapses. Such a mechanism might be expected to be involved in association formation, and so, to be critical for conditioning. This expectation leads naturally to an interest in a more detailed analysis of the effects of hippocampal damage on classical conditioning, and that will be the subject of the following section. We shall return to the question of hippocampal involvement in spatial processing in chapter 7; at this stage we should note that a number of lines of evidence suggest that a behavioral role for LTP may be found in the learning and forgetting of spatial tasks.

Effects of Hippocampal Lesions on Association Formation

Excitatory and Inhibitory Conditioning Using the
Standard Delay Paradigm

Hippocampal lesions do not disrupt standard delay conditioning; hippocampectomized animals are, then, able to detect a positive contingency between a CS and a UCS. And hippocampectomy does not disrupt conditioned inhibition either; that is, hippocampectomized animals can also detect negative contingencies between CSs and UCSs. Both of these points may be illustrated by considering a report by Solomon (1977) on eyelid conditioning in rabbits. Experiment 1 of that report found no effect of hippocampectomy on acquisition of eyelid CRs to either a tone CS or a compound tone plus light CS; in each case, CS onset preceded UCS onset by 450 msec in a standard delay design. Experiment 2 found that hippocampectomized rabbits showed no disruption in acquisition of a discrimination in which a light alone CS was followed by the UCS, and a light plus tone compound CS, by no UCS. This is a procedure used to develop conditioned inhibition to the unique element of the compound CS—in this case, the tone. To demonstrate that the tone was now a conditioned inhibitor, Solomon conducted a "retardation test" (Rescorla 1969) in which the tone (alone) was now followed by the UCS. The rate of acquisition of CRs to the tone was significantly slower than that seen to the tone alone CS in Experiment 1 (and there was, again, no disruption of acquisition by hippocampal damage). Thus hippocampectomized rabbits, like controls, detected the negative contingency between the tone CS and the UCS, the fact that the reinforcer was less likely in the presence of the tone than in its absence.

There have, however, been reports of the disruption of acquisition by hippocampal damage in two other classical-conditioning paradigms—sensory preconditioning and taste-aversion learning. Before discussing those reports, we should consider in more detail the disruption of eyelid trace conditioning by hippocampal damage, since that disruption may have much in common with the effects seen in the sensory preconditioning and taste-aversion studies.

Trace Conditioning

A number of reports have shown disruptions by hippocampal damage of trace conditioning, although the nature and degree of the disruption found has varied somewhat.

A recent report (Moyer, Deyo, and Disterhoft 1990) found that hippocampal damage almost totally abolished the ability of rabbits to acquire an eyelid CR to a relatively brief (100 msec) tone CS whose offset preceded the onset of an airpuff UCS by a trace interval of 500 msec; but when the trace interval used was 300 msec, acquisition proceeded normally in hippocampectomized animals. A consideration of earlier reports of the effects of hippocampal damage on trace conditioning will serve further to emphasize the importance of temporal parameters.

Moyer and his colleagues removed virtually all the hippocampus, whereas other investigators have used subtotal lesions, confined to dorsal hippocampal regions. We shall see that the effects of dorsal hippocampal lesions on trace conditioning using a 500-msec interval have generally been less striking than those reported by Moyer and colleagues. This may have been due to the use of smaller lesions, but may also have been because Moyer and colleagues used a short-duration CS, a procedure likely to have increased the difficulty of the task and so, perhaps, to have exaggerated the lesion-induced disruption.

Solomon et al. (1986) explored the acquisition of trace conditioning of the eyelid response in rabbits. In their study, CS (a tone) duration was 250 msec; this was followed by a 500-msec (trace) interval, and then by the UCS, an airpuff to the eye. Two discrete categories of eyelid CRs were observed. One type (figure 6.12, top) consisted of CRs that occurred toward the end of the CS period and were of small amplitude and short duration; these Solomon et al. designated short-latency CRs. The other CR type (figure 6.12, bottom), designated long-latency CRs, consisted of CRs whose peak amplitudes occurred within 100 msec of UCS onset and which were continuous with the UCR.

Control rabbits showed only long-latency CRs, whose probability (see figure 6.13) grew as training proceeded (occurring on about 70 percent of trials by the end of training). Figure 6.13 shows that hippocampectomized

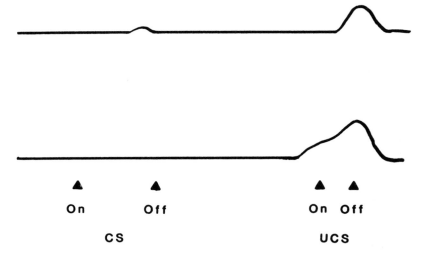

Trace Period

FIGURE 6.12. Polygraph traces of typical instances of the two types of CR observed by Solomon et al. (1986). *Top:* Short-latency CR. *Bottom:* Long-latency CR. (*From* Solomon et al. 1986)

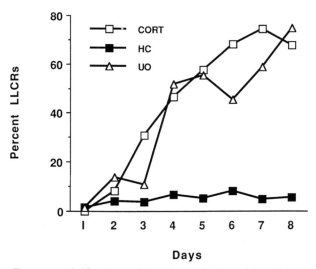

FIGURE 6.13. Disruption of acquisition of long-latency CRs by hippocampal damage. The graph shows mean percentage of long-latency CRs over 8 days of trace conditioning in hippocampal rabbits (HC), in control rabbits having damage to neocortex overlying the hippocampus (CORT), and in unoperated controls (UO). (*Data from* Solomon et al. 1986)

rabbits showed virtually no long-latency CRs throughout training. Hippocampectomized rabbits did, on the other hand, produce short-latency CRs, and the frequency of these (see figure 6.14) increased up to something over 20 percent of trials by the end of training. This pattern of results suggests that although hippocampectomized rabbits detected the CS-UCS contingency they could not translate that information into an effective response: the timing of the CR was not matched to the time of UCS onset.

Other investigations of trace conditioning following hippocampal lesions have found less dramatic deficits in operated animals, but generally agree in showing alterations in timing of CRs. James, Hardiman, and Yeo (1987), for example, found no differences in percentage of CRs between normals and hippocampal rabbits in a trace conditioning task (the trace interval was again 500 msec), but reported that hippocampectomized animals showed shorter CR onset latencies than controls over the period during which CRs were becoming firmly established. Hippocampectomized rabbits did not show shorter latencies at asymptote, and their CRs were neither smaller nor of reduced duration compared to those of controls. Port et al. (1986), using a trace interval of 500 msec, reported that when

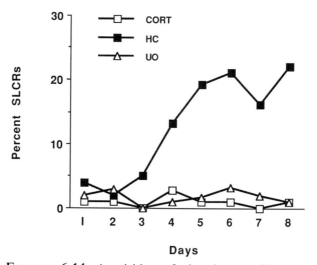

FIGURE 6.14. Acquisition of short-latency CRs by hippocampal rabbits. The graph shows mean percentage of short-latency CRs over 8 days of trace conditioning in hippocampal rabbits (HC), in control rabbits having damage to neocortex overlying the hippocampus (CORT), and in unoperated controls (UO). (*Data from* Solomon et al. 1986)

a periorbital shock UCS was used, onset latencies of hippocampectomized subjects were longer than those of controls, whereas using an airpuff UCS, shorter latencies were observed in hippocampal as compared to control rabbits; those results are summarized in figure 6.15. Finally, one investigation of eyelid trace conditioning using a 1-sec trace interval (Port, Romano, and Patterson 1986) found no change either in rate of acquisition of CRs (in a stimulus-duration discrimination task) or in onset latencies following hippocampectomy.

It is difficult to produce a unitary account of these effects, which may reflect disruptions that are not peculiar to trace conditioning: for example, Port, Mikhail, and Patterson (1985) found, using standard delay procedures, that hippocampectomized rabbits acquired an eyelid CR at the same

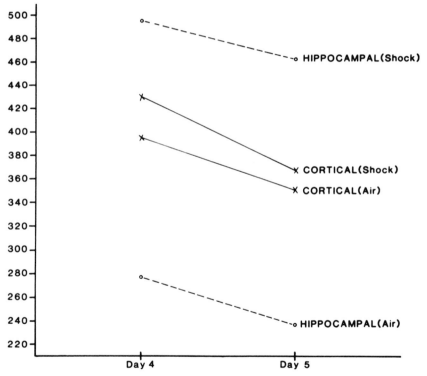

FIGURE 6.15. Effects of hippocampal damage on onset latencies of conditioned nictitating membrane CRs established using two types of UCS. The figure shows mean onset latencies (msec) for the final two days of training; for further details, see text. (*From* Port et al. 1986)

rate as controls when ISI was 300 msec, but significantly more rapidly than controls when ISI was either 150 or 600 msec. A 300-msec ISI is in the optimal range for eyelid delay conditioning (e.g., Gormezano 1972), so that it may be that whenever the temporal relationship between CS and UCS is not optimal, hippocampal performance deviates from normal— although the direction and nature of that deviation is currently neither easily predicted nor explained.

Sensory Preconditioning

Sensory preconditioning is a technique that permits the assessment of an animal's ability to detect a contingency between two neutral stimuli. There are typically three stages in sensory preconditioning experiments. In Stage 1 two stimuli, S1 and S2, are paired (S2 following S1). In Stage 2, S2 is paired with a UCS so that a CR appropriate to the UCS is established. In Stage 3, S1 is presented alone: if S1 elicits the CR established to S2 in Stage 2, then it may be inferred that an association was formed between S1 and S2 in Stage 1.

Two reports have suggested that hippocampal damage may disrupt sensory preconditioning (Port and Patterson 1984; Port, Beggs, and Patterson 1987). Each of these studies found that hippocampal damage virtually eliminated sensory preconditioning. But both studies suffer from the difficulty that the temporal relationship between S1 and S2 in Stage 1 of the design used was far from optimal.

Port and Patterson (1984) presented S1 (a tone) and S2 (a light) simultaneously, with complete overlap (each lasting 500 msec) in Stage 1. In Stage 2 the light was paired with periorbital shock, and in Stage 3 hippocampectomized rabbits showed very few eyelid CRs to the tone stimulus. But total overlap of stimuli is not optimal for association formation, since neither stimulus serves as a signal that the other is imminent, and in fact the controls in this experiment also made very few eyelid CRs in Stage 3, responding to the tone on only 11 percent of trials.

Stage 1 of the Port, Beggs, and Patterson (1987) report used as S1 a light of 500 msec duration which preceded onset of S2 (a 250-msec tone) by 250 msec. In Stage 2, the light (S1) was paired with the UCS, and responding to the tone (S2) was tested in Stage 3; the conventional design, it will be recalled, pairs S2 with the UCS in Stage 2, and tests S1 in Stage 3. Since S1 onset preceded S2 onset in Stage 1, any association between S2 and S1—the association assessed in Stage 3—must have been mediated by either backward or simultaneous conditioning: once again,

S1 was clearly not a satisfactory signal for S2, and this was reflected in the performance of controls, which showed CRs on only some 30 percent of trials to the tone in Stage 3.

The work on sensory preconditioning may, therefore, reflect a genuine difficulty for hippocampectomized animals in the association of neutral stimuli; alternatively, it may reflect a disruption of association formation seen when the temporal relationship between the stimuli to be associated is less than optimal.

Taste- and Odor-Aversion Learning

A further associative procedure that has been reported to be affected by hippocampal damage is taste-aversion learning. Krane, Sinnamon, and Thomas (1976), for example, gave rats access to a novel saline solution (0.9 percent NaCl) and injected apomorphine either during saline consumption or 15 min after the solution had been withdrawn. Apomorphine gives rise to internal discomfort and rats subjected to pairings of apomorphine with consumption of a specific taste rapidly develop an aversion to that taste. Krane and his colleagues found that rats with extensive hippocampal damage showed, compared to controls, a much attenuated aversion to the saline solution in both the simultaneous and the delayed pairing conditions. Other workers have shown that attenuation is found in odor-aversion learning also (Miller et al. 1986), and that deficits are seen not only in measure of total consumption but also in measures of preference between two tastes, only one of which has been paired with an aversive UCS (Miller, Elkins, and Peacock 1971).

A study by Nachman and Ashe (1974) found that if the hippocampus was damaged after the pairing of a taste and an aversive UCS (a lithium chloride injection) then performance in a postlesion consumption test was unaffected. If lesions were made before the pairings, however, the aversion was attenuated. It is clear, therefore, that hippocampal damage affected the formation of the relevant association and was not an effect on performance alone.

In the light of the previous discussion of the relevance of temporal parameters to the effects of hippocampal damage on association formation, disruption of taste- and odor-aversion learning is not, perhaps, surprising. Temporal parameters do, after all, differ considerably from those typically seen in eyelid conditioning: CSs are of longer duration, and UCS delivery is typically either simultaneous with CS representation or follows after a trace interval that may be many minutes long. Moreover, it is far from clear that the delivery of the UCS by the experimenter constitutes the time at which the effective UCS occurs: the aversiveness of poisons presumably begins at the point at which they begin to create the internal disturbance induced by them.

Investigations of the consequences of hippocampal damage on taste-aversion learning in fact have reported a range of effects, from no effect (e.g., Murphy and Brown 1974) to total abolition of taste-aversion learning (e.g., Miller, Elkins, and Peacock 1971), so that it is not a topic about which confident conclusions may be drawn. In the present state of knowledge it is best to note that most workers have found a disruption, and to entertain the hypothesis that the disruption obtained may reflect a further instance of disruption by hippocampal damage of a task in which CS-UCS onset asynchrony differs markedly from the range that is optimal, at least for eyelid conditioning.

Neophobia

Before leaving this topic it is worth introducing one finding that emerges from a number of the taste-aversion learning reports. When exposed to a solution having a novel taste, rats typically show an initial wariness and consume less on initial exposure than on subsequent exposures. This neo-phobic reaction is reduced by hippocampal damage (e.g., Krane, Sinnamon, and Thomas 1976; Miller et al. 1986). It will be recalled that in the discussion in chapter 3 of the effects of hippocampal lesions on habituation of the orienting response, it was suggested that hippocampectomy might selectively impair the process of recognition. Thus all stimuli appear relatively novel, and genuinely novel stimuli may therefore not be effectively classified as novel. This account can readily accommodate reduced neophobia in hippocampectomized animals. Consumption is reduced in intact animals by the contrast between a novel taste and familiar tastes: animals with a disrupted capacity for recognition should not experience such a contrast and should therefore display less marked neophobia.

Phenomena Attributed to Selective Attention

The studies considered thus far have pointed to the conclusion that hippocampal damage does not disrupt standard eyelid conditioning when temporal parameters are optimal. The standard eyelid-conditioning procedure involves the presentation of a single CS; but it has been suggested that when more than one CS is presented simultaneously (when, that is, a compound CS is used), hippocampal damage does disrupt learning. Disruptions of conditioning to compound stimuli have led to the proposal that the primary role of the hippocampus is the control of selective attention, more specifically, "that the hippocampus is responsible for tuning out stimuli that have no motivational significance to the organism" (Solomon 1977:416). The principal support for this proposal comes not only from experiments concerning compound conditioning but also from work (introduced in chapter 3) that has shown hippocampal involvement in latent inhibition. The assessment of the selective attention hypothesis of hippocampal function will begin by looking at the effects of hippocampal damage on latent inhibition and will then proceed to discuss effects of hippocampal damage on two phenomena—overshadowing and blocking—that involve conditioning to compound stimuli.

Latent Inhibition

It was noted in chapter 3 that there have been a number of reports confirming the disruptive effect of hippocampal damage on latent inhibition, and we shall give some details here of one study, involving eyelid conditioning in rabbits. Solomon and Moore (1975) exposed rabbits to 450 presentations of a tone before pairing the tone with a periorbital shock UCS. Control (cortex-lesioned and unoperated) rabbits were, as expected, slower to acquire the CR to the tone following preexposures than rabbits that had experienced comparable previous experience of the apparatus but had not received preexposures: hippocampal rabbits acquired the CR at the same rate as the nonpreexposed control animals—but this was true for hippocampal rabbits whether or not they had experienced preexposures. Table 6.1 summarizes the results of the experiment.

Overshadowing

Overshadowing is, like blocking (a phenomenon introduced in chapter 4), a phenomenon observed in tasks involving compound stimuli. Typically, a compound stimulus consisting of two stimuli, one of which is more salient than the other, is paired with a UCS. After CRs are well established, the two component stimuli of the compound are tested separately, in the absence of UCS deliveries. Overshadowing is said to have occurred when the level of responding to the less salient stimulus is less than that found following a comparable number of pairings of that stimulus alone with the UCS. The salient stimulus overshadows the less salient stimulus, but the less salient stimulus does not normally overshadow the salient stimulus (Mackintosh 1975).

TABLE 6.1
Effect of Hippocampal Lesions on Latent Inhibition in Rabbits

Preexposure Condition	Lesion Group		
	Hippocampal	Cortical	Unoperated
Apparatus only	260.6	293.6	264.0
450 tone preexposures	283.2	201.8	181.8

SOURCE: Solomon and Moore 1975.
NOTE: Mean number of CRs as a function of lesion group and number of CS exposures.

There are currently no reports available on the effects of hippocampal damage on overshadowing in rabbits, but there are two reports of the attenuation of overshadowing by hippocampal damage in rats (Rickert et al. 1979; Schmajuk, Spear, and Isaacson 1983). Each of these studies used a somewhat complicated design involving acquisition of discriminations, and we shall describe the simpler of the two here. Rickert and his colleagues (1979) employed the conditioned-suppression technique, in which the strength of fear conditioned to a CS is assessed by presenting the CS to an animal that is performing an instrumental response (lever-pressing, for example) at a relatively steady rate for reward. The degree to which the ongoing instrumental behavior is suppressed is taken to reflect the strength of conditioned fear aroused by the CS. In the Rickert et al. (1979) study, rats were exposed to a discrimination between two tones of different frequencies (500 versus 2,000 Hz), one of which (CS +) was consistently followed by a footshock UCS; the other tone stimulus (CS −) was never followed by the UCS. A light stimulus was presented in compound with each tone, so that it was followed by the UCS on 50 percent of the presentations of the compound stimuli. Once the discrimination had been established, test presentations of each of the components of the compound stimulus were carried out in the absence of UCS delivery. Both sham-operated and hippocampal-lesioned rats showed conditioned suppression (of food-motivated bar pressing) to the tone CS + , but not to the tone CS − ; but whereas the control rats showed no suppression to the light stimulus, the hippocampal rats showed suppression to the light also.

The standard interpretation (Wagner et al. 1968) of the control rats' failure to suppress to the light stimulus is that conditioning to it was overshadowed by stimuli (the tone CS + and CS −) that were better predictors of delivery or nondelivery of the UCS; thus the fact that hippocampal rats learned about the contingency between the light and the UCS indicates a failure of overshadowing in those animals. There was also a control condition run in which the same two compound stimuli were each followed by the shock UCS on a random 50 percent of trials; in this condition, both sham-operated and hippocampal rats showed suppression to all three elements of the compounds when tested alone. It appears, therefore, that it was indeed the case (for the sham-operated rats) that the light stimulus was overshadowed in the experimental condition by stimuli that were more consistent predictors of reward.

Blocking

It will be recalled from chapter 4 that blocking consists in the observation of weaker conditioning to an element of a compound stimulus when the other element of the compound has previously been paired with the UCS. The phenomenon of blocking has been explored in the rabbit eyelid preparation by Solomon (1977), who used three groups of animals (hippocampal-lesioned rabbits, cortex-lesioned controls, and unoperated controls). Rabbits in the blocking condition were initially given pairings of tone and periorbital shock, until CRs were reliably elicited by the tone (after 300 or 400 trials). Rabbits in the control (no blocking) condition were given equivalent amounts of exposure to the apparatus, but received neither tones nor UCSs. All rabbits then experienced 500 pairings of a compound stimulus consisting of a tone plus a light. There then followed test presentations of the light and the tone stimulus (50 of each), neither now being followed by the UCS. Table 6.2 summarizes performance in the test presentations and shows that whereas unoperated and cortex-lesioned control subjects in the blocking condition showed a much smaller number of CRs to the light than that obtained in the control condition, the reverse was the case for the hippocampal animals. The ratio data in the right-hand column of the table allow for differences between the groups in overall rates of CR

TABLE   6.2
Effect of Hippocampal Lesions on Blocking in Rabbits

Lesion Group	Preexposure Condition	Light CRs	Tone CRs	Light/Total CRs
Hippocampal	Tone + shock	60.4	69.6	.46
	Apparatus only	44.6	50.0	.47
Unoperated	Tone + shock	24.0	82.6	.23
	Apparatus	52.2	58.8	.47
Neocortical	Tone + shock	13.0	81.0	.14
	Apparatus	40.2	65.2	.38

NOTE: Mean number of CRs to light and to tone, and the ratio of light CRs to total (light plus tone) CRs.
SOURCE: Solomon 1977.

and confirm that the number of responses made to the light was just below 50 percent of the total number of CRs for the unoperated subjects in the control condition, and for the hippocampal subjects in both conditions, but was less than 25 percent for the unoperated subjects in the blocking condition. Disruption of blocking by hippocampal damage has been reported also in rats, using light and tone CSs in the conditioned-suppression paradigm (Rickert et al. 1978; Rickert et al. 1981).

Assessment of the Selective Attention Hypothesis

Latent inhibition, overshadowing, and blocking are three phenomena that are of considerable importance in contemporary behavior theory because they are compelling demonstrations of the fact that the strength of conditioning that accrues to a stimulus is not determined simply by the number of pairings of the stimulus and a UCS. All three phenomena have attracted explanations in terms of selective attention. In each case, it is assumed that conditioning is weaker because the to-be-conditioned stimulus obtains less attention, that the stimulus has been "tuned out."

In the course of latent-inhibition training, an animal learns that the stimulus is not followed by an important consequence, and therefore pays less attention to it. Overshadowing occurs because an animal diverts attention to a stimulus that is either more salient or a better predictor of reward. Blocking occurs because the added stimulus does not predict any consequence not already predicted by the pretrained stimulus and therefore fails to sustain attention. The disruption of the three phenomena by hippocampal damage, then, does support the notion that they may indeed be reflections of the operation of a single common mechanism. And to the extent that at least some rival theories (e.g., Wagner and Rescorla 1972) suppose that the explanation of latent inhibition is different from that of overshadowing and blocking, the pattern of effects of hippocampal damage supports an interpretation of those phenomena in terms of selective attention.

There are other findings that may also be accommodated within a selective attention framework. A number of studies have found that although the acquisition of discriminations may proceed normally in hippocampal animals, reversal of those discriminations (so that the former CS + becomes CS − , and vice versa) is severely disrupted. We shall consider here an example using once again the rabbit eyelid-conditioning paradigm. Berger and Orr (1983) compared the performance of hippocampal and control rabbits in a task in which presentations of a tone of one frequency (CS +) were consistently followed by an airpuff UCS, and presentations of a tone of a different frequency (CS −) were never followed by the UCS.

The discrimination was acquired (see figure 6.16) at the same rate by the control and the hippocampal-damaged rabbits. Figure 6.16 shows, however, that when the significance of the stimuli was subsequently reversed so that the former CS − was now followed by UCS delivery, and the former CS + had no consequence, the hippocampal animals were much impaired in their ability to switch CRs between the stimuli. Analysis of the pattern of performance during reversal learning showed that the hippocampal deficit lay in excessive responding to the former CS + during reversal: they learned as rapidly as controls to show CRs to the new CS + (the former CS −).

One general point that should be made about the selective disruption by hippocampal damage of reversal—as opposed to acquisition—of discriminations is that it implies that reversal learning involves some process that is not engaged in acquisition. To the extent that behavioral theories do not anticipate any major difference between the mechanisms involved in the two tasks (and the major behavioral theories of learning do not), this in turn implies that those theories are incomplete. And analysis of the nature of the disruption may point to some of the characteristics of a process that should at some point be incorporated into those theories. How, then, may the selective disruption of reversal learning be understood?

The selective attention account of hippocampal function could argue that the nature of the deficit in the hippocampal animals reflects a further failure to gate out an irrelevant stimulus: having learned during original acquisition to attend to the CS + , the hippocampal rabbits find it difficult in reversal learning to ignore the now irrelevant former CS + . Since their difficulty lies precisely in being unable to ignore stimuli, they do, of course, learn as rapidly as controls to attend to the new CS + , and show, therefore, normal acquisition of CRs to the former CS − .

The interpretation of reversal disruption in terms of impaired selective attention does, however, run into difficulties, which may be illustrated by considering another result obtained by Berger and Orr (1983). Control and hippocampal rabbits first acquired an eyelid CR to a single tone that was invariably followed by an airpuff UCS. That response was then subjected to an extinction procedure in which the CS was repeatedly presented and no UCS presentations occurred. Figure 6.17 shows that, as expected, there was no difference between the groups in rate of acquisition of the CR; figure 6.17 also shows there was no difference between the groups in rate of extinction of the CR. If hippocampal animals cannot gate out irrelevant stimuli (stimuli not associated with important consequences), why do they not persist in showing CRs during the extinction procedure? And

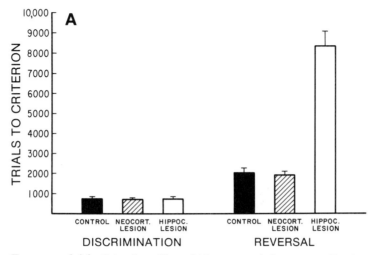

FIGURE 6.16. Selective effect of hippocampal damage on discrimination reversal in rabbits. The graph shows mean total trials required by control animals that had received sham operations involving no brain damage (solid bars), animals with lesions of neocortex overlying the hippocampus (striped bars), and animals with hippocampal lesions (open bars) to reach two-tone discrimination and reversal criteria; also indicated are standard errors of the means. (*From* Berger and Orr 1983)

if, as seems quite reasonable, it is argued that extinction occurs not because the animals ignore the CS but because they learn that it is no longer followed by the UCS, then why do they not learn similarly to withhold CRs to the former CS + in a reversal task? The fact that hippocampal damage does not lead to a general difficulty in reducing CR output is, then, a problem for the selective attention account of hippocampal function.

Two other problems—one specific, one general—have combined to rule out widespread current acceptance of the selective attention hypothesis. The specific problem is posed by a report (Garrud et al. 1984) of failures to obtain disruption of either blocking or overshadowing by hippocampectomy in rats; there is even a report (Winocur and Gilbert 1984) of the occurrence of overshadowing (of visual by tactile cues) in hippocampal rats in a procedure in which normal rats did *not* show overshadowing. Garrud et al. used the conditioned-suppression paradigm, as did Rickert and his colleagues in their investigations of the effects of hippocampal damage on overshadowing and blocking. In discussing the dis-

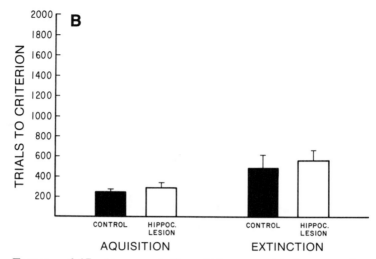

FIGURE 6.17. Absence of effect of hippocampal lesions on extinction in rabbits. The graph shows mean total trials to criterion of sham-
operated controls (solid bars) and of rabbits having hippocampal damage (open bars) in acquisition and extinction of an eyelid CR to a tone
CS; also indicated are standard errors of the means. (*From* Berger and
Orr 1983)

crepancy between their findings and those obtained by other workers, Garrud and his colleagues were able to point to a number of weaknesses in all
the earlier reports in which rats were used. And although they did not see
any problem with Solomon's (1977) demonstration of the abolition by
hippocampal damage of blocking in rabbits, it appears that there is a serious weakness in that report also. In Solomon's experiment, control (unoperated and cortex-lesioned) rabbits learned less about a light presented
in compound with a tone when the tone had previously been presented in
pairings with the UCS; hippocampal rabbits learned as much about the
light whether or not prior tone-UCS pairings had been given. But in the
control condition, animals were simply exposed to the apparatus cues and,
in particular, no UCSs were delivered. This control provides no evidence
that the blocking effect seen in the control groups was in fact due to the
tone-UCS pairings; it may be that presentations of the UCS alone would
have had a similar disruptive effect on subsequent conditioning to the
light. Such a possibility in effect supposes only that a preexposed UCS is
a less effective reinforcer than a novel UCS, a possibility that is hardly
implausible, given the existence of the UCS-preexposure effect (intro-

duced in chapter 4). This alternative account is of particular importance in the context of hippocampal damage since we know that hippocampal animals, unlike controls, continue to investigate stimuli that have been presented repeatedly (e.g., Kaye and Pearce 1987; see chapter 3). Probably the best control condition for a blocking experiment is one in which animals are preexposed to pairings of the UCS with a CS that is not reused as one of the two stimuli in the compound stimulus of the second stage of the experiment. This control (used in the Garrud et al. 1984 report) allows the conclusion that any blocking effect seen is due specifically to pairings with the UCS of the stimulus re-presented as part of the compound, rather than to any nonspecific effect of pairings per se, or of exposure to the UCS.

The basic findings on which the selective attention theory rests are therefore not as solid as it once appeared. There is good support for the conclusion that hippocampal damage does disrupt latent inhibition in rabbits and in rats. But there is—to put it at its best—only equivocal support for the view that either overshadowing or blocking is disrupted by hippocampal damage in rats.

A more general cause of dissatisfaction with the selective attention interpretation of hippocampal function is that there are very many tasks in which performance is disrupted by hippocampal damage, and those disruptions do not seem readily amenable to interpretation in terms of selective attention deficits. Relevant examples will be found in the following two chapters, which will consider interpretations of hippocampal function in terms of contextual processing and of memory processes.

No single theory of hippocampal function currently seems capable of handling all the known effects of hippocampal damage, and we shall consider the best supporting evidence for each type of theory as it is discussed. But it will be the case for all these theories that the evidence that provides the strongest support for one theory inevitably poses problems for a rival theory. Although we shall avoid the tedious exercise of showing how each set of data provides problems for rival theories, when any attempt is made to weigh up the relative strength of the rival theories it is clearly necessary to consider all the available data. So that when the effects of hippocampal damage on, say, maze learning are introduced, we should consider their relevance not only to the theories (of contextual processing, in the case of maze learning) with which they are most congruent but also to rival theories, such as the selective attention theory which has been under consideration here. Similarly, when considering theories of hippocampal involvement in contextual processing and memory, we should bear in mind the deficits discussed above, which gave rise to theories of involvement in selective attention.

Conclusion

The effects of hippocampectomy on eyelid trace conditioning, along with those on eyelid delay conditioning using nonoptimal ISIs, indicate that temporal relationships between CSs and UCSs are critical to the occurrence of performance changes in simple conditioning procedures following hippocampal damage. It is parsimonious currently to assume that reports of the disruption of sensory preconditioning and taste-aversion learning could be due to nonoptimal CS-UCS parameters. Most of the eyelid trace conditioning studies suggested that hippocampal lesions did not so much affect association formation as performance, in that CRs typically were obtained but had a different latency in hippocampectomized animals. Although the two sensory preconditioning studies found a virtual absence of CRs in hippocampal subjects, there was in controls also a low level of CRs. And although the Nachman and Ashe (1974) report indicated a clear disruption of association formation by hippocampal damage, the taste-aversion learning studies as a whole have produced a wide range of outcomes. In general it still seems reasonable, therefore, to conclude that given optimal temporal parameters for simple classical conditioning, hippocampal lesions are without effect; where those parameters are not optimal, hippocampal damage does disrupt performance although it is not clear that this disruption in every case reflects an impairment of association formation.

Conclusions are less easily reached concerning the role of the hippocampus when the standard procedures are complicated by, for example, CS preexposure or the use of compound stimuli. There is general agreement that hippocampal damage disrupts latent inhibition, but no consensus yet concerning effects on blocking and overshadowing. Given that other evidence currently available does not seem readily amenable to interpretation in terms of the notion that the hippocampus is involved in selective attention, it is clear that that hypothesis now enjoys very weak support: further rival accounts of the effects of hippocampectomy on latent inhibition will be discussed in chapters 7 and 8.

Neocortex and Conditioning

Investigations of the mechanisms of association formation in vertebrates have found only one site, the cerebellum, that is essential for the acquisition and retention of CRs. Even this claim has to be restricted to skeletal CRs and has to be qualified by the observation that skeletal CRs can in fact be established in the isolated spinal cord.

No other vertebrate brain locus with so general a role in conditioning has yet been identified; no region, for example, has been found that is essential for the establishment of preparatory as opposed to consummatory CRs. Areas are known, damage to which disrupts certain classes of CR. Amygdalar lesions, for example, disrupt the conditioning of fear. But amygdalar damage also impairs unlearned fear responses—in other words, reduce the UCR—and does not produce a general disruption of appetitively motivated CRs. It seems most likely, then, that the amygdala is critically involved in motivation and that the failure to develop conditioned fear following amygdalectomy reflects not a failure of association formation but a disruption of the motivational system necessary for the expression of fear CRs. The potential role of the amygdala in motivation will be taken up in more detail in chapter 8, when its role in memory will be the primary focus of interest.

Damage to sensory systems may also, of course, disrupt the formation of CRs, and it may be that sensory pathways do contain synapses whose strengths are altered during the course of normal conditioning. But the fact that conditioning is disrupted by damage does not require any such conclusion, since it is clear that sensory information must be allowed to reach whatever site or sites are involved in association formation. It is nevertheless appropriate to consider here reports of electrophysiological investigations of plasticity in the auditory pathway during conditioning, if only because it will allow a discussion of the role of the neocortex in conditioning.

It will be recalled from chapter 3 that Willott, Schnerson, and Urban (1979) found that cells in the various subdivisions of the inferior colliculus reacted differently to the repetition of a tone. Cells in the pericentral and external nuclei showed plasticity: their responses to the tone declined in parallel with behavioral habituation. Cells in the central nucleus, on the other hand, responded throughout a series of tone presentations in a way that reflected the physical parameters of the stimuli and so did not show plasticity. The latter nucleus forms part of the classical lemniscal auditory system, and the former nuclei part of the extralemniscal or lemniscal adjunct system (e.g., Graybiel 1972). A similar division between regions that show plasticity and regions that do not is found when correlates of classical conditioning are explored at the thalamic and cortical levels.

The ventral division of the medial geniculate nucleus represents the lemniscal pathway at the thalamus: input to the ventral division derives from the lemniscal zone of the inferior colliculus, and individual cells in this division are "tuned" to respond to a narrow range of frequencies. The various other divisions of the medial geniculate (the magnocellular, dorsocaudal, and ventrolateral regions) receive input from both lemniscal and extralemniscal divisions of the inferior colliculus; all show broadly tuned units and form part of the extralemniscal system.

Weinberger has recorded from cells in the lemniscal and extralemniscal systems at thalamic and cortical levels during classical conditioning of a preparatory response in cats (for an account of this work see Weinberger and Diamond 1987). An aversive shock delivered to forelimb skin served as the UCS, and tones served as CSs. The CR measured was pupillary dilation, a nonspecific autonomic response that typically develops very rapidly (within two to five trials).

When multiple-unit recordings were taken from the lemniscal zone of the medial geniculate (the ventral division), no systematic changes in response to a tone CS were seen as the CR developed. When recordings were taken from an extralemniscal site (the magnocellular region), there were marked increases in the responses elicited, and those increases paralleled the growth of the behavioral CR. Subsequent recordings from single units in the magnocellular region found that although most (71 percent) units showed a change in tone-elicited activity as conditioning proceeded, a sizable proportion (29 percent) showed a decrease.

Although the primary auditory cortex is the lemniscal neocortical zone, it receives afferents from not only the lemniscal region of the medial geniculate but also from neighboring extralemniscal cortical regions. It is, therefore, perhaps not surprising that the primary auditory cortex does, in contrast to the thalamic and midbrain lemniscal zones, show a degree of plasticity. When multicellular recordings were taken, sites in primary auditory cortex showed increased responding to the CS as the CR developed. Single-unit recordings found, however, that of nineteen cells studied, six showed an increase, six a decrease, and seven no change in response as conditioning proceeded.

Single-unit recordings from an extralemniscal neocortical area, the secondary auditory field (AII), found, as might be expected, a marked degree of plasticity. Of twenty-two cells, twenty-one showed plasticity—eleven showing increases in response, and ten decreases—as CRs became established. Thus, whereas 27 percent of AI cells showed plasticity, 95 percent of AII cells did so.

It appears that the subcortical auditory lemniscal system projects information about the physical properties of stimuli, independent of the "significance" of the stimuli. This may, then, provide an answer to the dilemma posed in chapter 3, in which evidence was found to show that transmission in S-R pathways became progressively less effective with repetitions of a stimulus, a finding that raised the question how a stimulus could be used effectively to elicit learned responses across a series of presentations. There are, at least in vertebrates, multiple routes along which auditory information may be transmitted in parallel; at least one of those routes, the lemniscal route, preserves information up to the primary cortical area (and beyond, given that 73 percent of AI units did not exhibit plasticity). And although analyses of plasticity in other sensory systems have not yet provided as clear a picture as is available for audition, it seems reasonable to assume that the principles found from consideration of audition will find application in other sense modalities.

The significance of the plasticity seen at thalamic and cortical sites during conditioning of pupillary dilation is not easily determined. Although studies of the effects on pupillary CRs of lesions in those areas have not been reported, we do know that eyelid conditioning is obtained in both cats and rabbits following decerebration, and LeDoux, Sakaguchi, and Reis (1984) have shown that fear conditioning to acoustic stimuli in rats is not disrupted by destruction of the auditory cortical regions. Moreover, Diamond and Weinberger (1984) found no relationship in individual cats between the course of development of electrophysiological plasticity at cortical sites and the course of acquisition of the pupillary CRs. These sites are, then, not essential for the formation of those associations that their activity reflects. It seems that information concerning the significance of stimuli is available to thalamic and cortical sensory regions that may in turn transmit that information on to other brain areas. But those areas are not necessary for the detection of contingencies: the primary alterations in transmission that underlie conditioning occur elsewhere.

Vertebrate and Invertebrate Mechanisms Compared

This chapter concludes the survey of mechanisms of conditioning in vertebrates that began in chapter 5, and a brief discussion of similarities and differences between the vertebrate mechanisms discussed in these two chapters and the invertebrate mechanisms discussed in chapter 4 is now appropriate.

As might have been anticipated, vertebrate conditioning has proved much less amenable to physiological analysis than invertebrate (or, at least, mollusk) conditioning. No account of any instance of conditioning in vertebrates is yet available that provides the amount of detail offered in current proposals for conditioning in *Aplysia* and *Hermissenda*. On the other hand, it is equally clear that significant progress has been made recently. We have in the cerebellum a site at which "closure" between CS and UCS pathways does appear to occur, and so, the promise that with further work it should be possible to establish the nature of that closure. We might then possess a relatively detailed account of the physiological nature of the change underlying one type of conditioning in vertebrates. And the discovery of LTP has provided at last a mechanism that can be demonstrated to exist in vertebrates and that could plausibly be involved in learning. The physiological analysis of LTP is proceeding very rapidly—largely as a result of the hippocampal slice preparation—and a major task for the future will be to establish the nature of the connection between LTP and behavior.

The survey of invertebrate conditioning provided two models for synaptic changes that might underlie conditioning. One, derived from the *Aplysia* work, suggested that activity-dependent facilitation of presynaptic transmitter release might occur; the other, derived from the *Hermissenda* work, suggested that postsynaptic membrane currents might be modified (according to a Hebbian principle). The cerebellar work has to date not progressed far enough to provide clear-cut support for either pre- or postsynaptic conditioning-induced changes (although difficulties for the operation of the Hebbian principle were seen).

We have seen that conditioning may reduce after-hyperpolarization of hippocampal cells, and have noted the suggestion that this may reflect the modification of a postsynaptic membrane current comparable to a current modified in *Hermissenda*. At present, however, little is known of the mechanisms involved in conditioning-specific after-hyperpolarization, and there are few concrete grounds for supposing that they will parallel the mechanisms proposed for conditioning in *Hermissenda*. It will be recalled (from chapter 4) that those mechanisms depended heavily for their activation on the cotermination of CS and UCS, a requirement that does not seem likely to be central to mammalian conditioning.

The induction of LTP (of the type mediated by NMDA receptors) depends upon both pre- and postsynaptic events, and LTP is a mechanism that acts according to a Hebbian principle. In that respect LTP differs from the activity-dependent presynaptic facilitation found in *Aplysia,* since that facilitation is independent of the activity in the postsynaptic cell (see chapters 2 and 4); it may, however, be worth recalling in this context that Glanzman, Kandel, and Schacher (1990) could not obtain morphological changes in response to serotonin application in cultured *Aplysia* sensory cells unless those cells were paired with motor neurons. There is, on the other hand, now good support for the view that LTP involves facilitation of presynaptic transmitter release so that there is at least one major parallel with the mechanism of conditioning in *Aplysia*.

Mossy-fiber LTP appears to involve facilitation of transmitter release and to be independent of events in the postsynaptic cell, and in those respects it does resemble the mechanisms identified in *Aplysia*. But there is no evidence of the involvement of any other (pre- or postsynaptic) cell, so that the effect is, unlike facilitation in *Aplysia*, homosynaptic. Mossy-fiber LTP shows neither the cooperativity nor the selectivity of NMDA-receptor-mediated LTP; its properties therefore show no congruence with those that might be expected to be found in mechanisms involved in association formation. It would, however, be premature at this stage to conclude that the type of plasticity demonstrated in this type of LTP plays no role in learning or memory.

In summary, work on mammalian (NMDA-receptor-mediated) LTP agrees with the work in *Aplysia* in finding a modification of activity at specific synapses rather than a modification of whole-cell excitability; the work agrees also that an increase in release of transmitter is involved. But it seems currently that the mechanisms underlying mammalian LTP are very different from those involved in activity-dependent presynaptic facilitation in *Aplysia*.

Final Comment: Neuronal Models, LTP, and Theories of Hippocampal Function

In this chapter we have seen two of the reasons for the current emphasis by neuroscientists on the hippocampus: the elaboration there of neuronal models during classical conditioning and the discovery there of LTP. But we have seen also that to unravel the significance of those phenomena will not be simple, since in at least some conditions conditioning may proceed quite normally in the absence of the hippocampus. Much of chapters 7 and 8 will be devoted to attempts to explain the role of the hippocampus in tasks other than simple conditioning, and those chapters will detail a wide range of tasks (involving spatial information and demands on a variety of hypothetical memory stores) that are disrupted by hippocampal damage. One concern that should be carried forward from this chapter to the next two is the question whether theories of hippocampal function based largely on the disruptive effects of lesions can provide plausible functional roles for hippocampal neuronal models and for hippocampal LTP.

7. Contextual Learning

Physiological Analysis of Nonassociative Learning

The preceding five chapters have reviewed physiological analyses of what are widely regarded as simpler forms of learning—habituation, sensitization, and association formation. It has become clear that all those forms of learning can proceed in the absence of the telencephalon, although the data have also pointed to the unsurprising conclusion that those simpler forms of learning may be modulated by telencephalic influences. It is time now to turn to more complex aspects of learning, and this will involve consideration of tasks in which telencephalic structures clearly do play a critical role. Before considering the relevant data, some reconsideration of the rationale and potential advantages of physiological intervention is appropriate.

Behavioral psychologists have found it extremely difficult to demonstrate that there do exist types of learning distinct from the simpler types enumerated above and to show, for example, that problem-solving, however complex it may appear, is *not* mediated simply by the formation of associations. They have also found it difficult to characterize theoretically the nature of those aspects of intelligence that (if they exist) do not depend simply upon the use of a general association-formation system.

It was argued in chapter 1 that one of the potential advantages of physiological intervention is that the syndromes generated by selective brain damage might suggest ways in which the structure of normal behavior could be conceptualized. By seeing which types of learning or problem-solving go together and which appear to be dissociable, it might be possible to gain insights into the functional organization of intelligent behavior. There have been, since Lashley's day, numerous reports of telencephalic damage that has resulted in disruption of some relatively complex task; the very fact that such disruptions are obtained when we know that telencephalic structures are not necessary for simple association formation is prima facie support for the notion that not all complex learning can properly be analyzed in terms of a general process of association formation. But just as behavioral psychologists have found difficulty in characterizing the nature of nonassociative learning, so physiological psychologists have found it difficult to characterize the nature of lesion-induced deficits—to characterize them so that it will be possible to predict which hitherto untested tasks will be disrupted by the lesions, and which will not. This is hardly surprising, since a successful characterization would in effect be the characterization of some presumably nonassociative mechanism of intelligence—the solution of the very problem that has presented behavioral psychologists with so much difficulty. What is clear, however, is that the successful analysis of a lesion-induced syndrome must inevitably constitute an important contribution to our understanding of intelligence.

It is of course not possible to review here all the deficits induced by lesions in complex tasks, and in this and the following chapter, we shall concentrate on deficits that are currently attracting a concentrated research effort, and that have led to theoretical proposals that would require major modifications to traditional associative theories of intelligence. In this chapter, we consider physiological evidence supporting the notion that learning about contextual information (and about spatial information in particular) proceeds in a very different way from learning about discrete stimuli; in chapter 8, we will consider evidence for the view that there exist multiple memory systems and that, in particular, associative memory may differ from other forms of memory.

As is implicit in these introductory remarks, the primary emphasis of these chapters will be upon the interpretation of the effects of lesion damage, and although data gained by other techniques will be used widely, their role will be largely the subsidiary one of strengthening (or weakening) hypotheses that will stand or fall according to their success or failure in providing a satisfactory account of lesion effects. The central position of the hippocampus as a topic of interest to neuroscientists has been alluded to in previous chapters, and we have seen (in chapter 6) findings from electrophysiological explorations of the hippocampus that account for that strong interest. We saw also that although hippocampal damage does not prevent association formation, it does result in disruption of normal performance in associative tasks if the design of those tasks varies from the standard delay paradigm, using optimal interstimulus intervals. And in fact the greatest single stimulus for the interest of psychologists in the hippocampus is the dramatic effect that hippocampal damage does have on a wide variety of tasks that do not appear to be simply associative. One hypothesis concerning hippocampal function—the notion that it is critically involved in selective attention—was discussed in chapter 6. Although that hypothesis was rejected, it is important to bear in mind the findings associated with it when considering the merits of rival theories.

Contextual Processing and the Hippocampus

There are a number of theories that suppose that the hippocampus is in some way concerned with processing information about the context in which learning takes place. The most influential of these theories has been that proposed by O'Keefe and Nadel (1978), which was briefly introduced in chapter 3. The essence of their theory is the notion that the hippocampus contains what amounts to a map on which is represented an animal's knowledge of the context in which it is placed, and of its own spatial position relative to other features of the context. This theory will be evaluated primarily through consideration of the effects of hippocampal damage on performance. But important support for the theory is derived from electrophysiological investigations of the hippocampus, and consideration of those findings is probably the best way in which to grasp the nature of the mapping notion.

Two types of electrophysiological investigation are relevant here. The first concerns recordings (widely referred to as electroencephalographic or EEG recordings) obtained using gross electrodes that record the pooled activity of many hundreds of cells in the vicinity of the electrode; the second involves the activity of single cells.

Classification of Hippocampal EEG Records

Hippocampal EEG records may be assigned to three general classes: desynchronized or irregular activity showing a predominance of low-voltage, small amplitude waves (SIA); irregular activity involving large amplitude waves (LIA); and regular (synchronized) activity in the frequency range 3–12 Hz, this third type of activity being generally known as theta activity. A considerable research effort has focused on the question whether behavioral correlates of the various EEG patterns may be established, and in particular, on the correlates of theta activity.

The Hippocampal Theta Rhythm

Two Types of Theta

One early proposal (Grastyán et al. 1959) was that theta waves occurred during orienting responses and reflected a general inhibition of hippocampal activity. Another proposal (Gray 1971) was that theta waves of a particular frequency (7.7 Hz) occurred when an animal experienced frustration. But there has by now emerged a general consensus that there are two types of theta activity, having different behavioral correlates.

The first type of theta is associated with what Vanderwolf (e.g., 1969) originally called "voluntary" movements but now refers to "type 1" movements. Such movements include "walking, running, swimming, rearing, jumping, digging, manipulation of objects with the forelimbs, isolated movements of the hand or one limb and shifts of posture" (Bland 1986:30). This theta activity is, accordingly, known as movement-related theta, although it is important to note that not all movements are accompanied by theta. Another class of movements, originally called "automatic" but now referred to as "type 2" movements, includes "licking, chewing, chattering the teeth, sneezing, startle responses, vocalization, shivering, tremor, face-washing, scratching the fur, pelvic thrusting, ejaculation, defecation, urination and piloerection" (Bland 1986:30–31); type 2 movements are associated with LIA in the hippocampus.

The second type of theta, immobility-related theta, occurs in the complete absence of movement and is most readily elicited by the presentation of sensory stimuli. This fact has led to the suggestion that the immobility-related theta might be associated with arousal and attention. One major difficulty with this proposal is, however, that this type of theta may be observed despite the administration of a variety of anesthetics.

In rats and rabbits, movement-related theta has a frequency range of from 7–12 Hz; immobility-related theta shows a lower frequency range, of from 4–9 Hz. Other differences between the two types of theta are that movement-related theta is (unlike immobility-related theta) abolished by anesthetics, and that immobility-related theta is abolished by cholinergic receptor antagonist drugs such as atropine.

Origins of Theta

Both types of theta appear to originate and spread from each of two "generator regions," one in the CA1 region, and one in the dentate gyrus. These generators are in turn driven by pacemaker cells in the medial septal region: destruction of the medial septal region abolishes both types of theta, and stimulation there with pulses of a given frequency within the theta range obtains hippocampal theta activity of the same frequency (a phenomenon known as "theta-driving"—e.g., Gray and Ball 1970). The medial septal nucleus contains cholinergic cells that project diffusely throughout the hippocampal formation, and it seems likely that these cells are responsible for the induction of the immobility-related (atropine-sensitive) theta rhythm. It is also assumed that medial septal cells using some other neurotransmitter are responsible for the induction of movement-related theta (which is not abolished by atropine). What that transmitter might be is not yet known for certain, although there is evidence that either serotonin or GABA (or both) might be involved (Bland 1986; Freund and Antal 1988).

Inter- and Intraspecies Differences in Theta

The dominant frequency of movement-related theta varies systematically with brain size in mammals, being slower in mammals with larger brains (Blumberg 1989); since theta frequency increases with body temperature within individuals (Whishaw and Vanderwolf 1971), and since smaller brains show higher brain metabolic rates, Blumberg suggests that both between- and within-species differences in theta frequency reflect differences in brain metabolic rate.

There are also interspecies differences in the probability of occurrence of the different types of hippocampal electrical activity. One of the most striking of these (Bland 1986) is that cats, unlike other mammals that have been tested (these include rats, gerbils, guinea pigs, rabbits, and dogs) may show only immobility-related theta. A second difference is that SIA is seen relatively rarely in rats, for periods of only a second or so, but is more readily observed in cats and rabbits. The significance of these differences is currently obscure: most of the findings concerning theta have been obtained using either rabbits or rats, the animals for which the most information on lesion effects is available.

Theta Reflects Hippocampal Activity

We have seen that Grastyán interpreted theta activity as indicating a general inhibition of hippocampal activity, and the notion that synchronized activity is associated with minimal participation in information processing makes good intuitive sense: an entire population of cells firing in synchrony could hardly be contributing to complex analysis, an intuition supported by the fact that deep "inactive" sleep is dominated by neocortical synchronized slow-wave activity. But it now appears that, however plausible Grastyán's view may be, hippocampal theta occurs when the hippocampus is actively involved in information processing. This conclusion derives basically from the fact that there are extensive parallels between the effects of septal damage and the effects of hippocampal damage (for a review see Gray and McNaughton 1983). If we make the not unreasonable assumption that these parallels are found because septal damage prevents the occurrence of hippocampal theta, we are led to conclude that loss of theta is functionally similar to loss of the hippocampus: in other words, to the conclusion that the theta rhythm reflects active participation by the hippocampus in information processing. We shall return to the question of what functional role the theta rhythm might play when results obtained from unit recordings in the hippocampus have been introduced.

Hippocampal Single-Unit Activity

We saw in chapter 6 the effect on hippocampal cell activity of a classical-conditioning procedure. The majority of those data were obtained in experiments in which the subjects were rabbits, held relatively immobile in a restraining apparatus. A very different picture of hippocampal cell activity is obtained when recordings are made from animals allowed to move freely within a relatively extended environment.

Place and Displace Cells

O'Keefe and Dostrovsky (1971) were the first to discover cells in the hippocampus that fire selectively when an animal is in a particular spatial location within an environment. O'Keefe refers to such units as "place cells," and to the area in which a place cell's firing rate changes as its "place field." Place cells have been found in both CA1 and CA3 of the hippocampus proper, in the dentate gyrus, and in the entorhinal cortex. It is now clear that in the hippocampus proper, place cells are pyramidal cells, and there is evidence that the great majority (95 percent or more) of spontaneously active pyramidal cells are place cells (O'Keefe 1979).

Numerous subsequent reports have confirmed the existence of place cells (O'Keefe 1979; Best and Ranck 1982; Muller, Kubie, and Ranck 1987) and have shown also that the place field of a given cell remains stable over long periods (up to at least 153 days, the longest time over which a single unit has so far been held successfully: Thompson and Best 1990). The field associated with a given place cell does not depend upon previous experience with the environment in which the field is found, since most hippocampal place cells show specific fields immediately on being transported into an entirely novel environment (Hill 1978).

A second type of cell encountered in the hippocampus fires independently of spatial location but is correlated with movement; O'Keefe (1979) refers to cells of this type as "displace" cells. Displace cells have been found to fire in phase with the theta rhythm whenever theta activity (either movement- or immobility-related) occurs; they are accordingly also known as theta cells. The physiological properties of theta cells strongly suggest that they are hippocampal interneurons, and it appears that virtually all nonpyramidal hippocampal cells are theta cells (Kubie, Muller, and Bostock 1990).

Both place and displace cells were observed in an experiment (O'Keefe 1976) in which rats with implanted unit electrodes roamed around freely on a 3-arm elevated maze in an experimental room. The maze had no walls and permitted observation by the rat of a variety of extra-maze cues such as windows, lights, and the door. Figure 7.1 shows recordings made from a rat in the maze. The recordings are from a place cell, with activity of a displace cell (which yielded smaller spikes) in the background.

Properties of Place Cells

The fact that a cell fires when an animal is in one part of an environment but not another might have a number of explanations. It might, for example, be that the animal engages in some motor activity in that place and not elsewhere; or that the cell is sensitive to some sensory modality, input from which is maximal in that location; or that the animal has associated that place with reward or punishment, and experiences a particular emo-

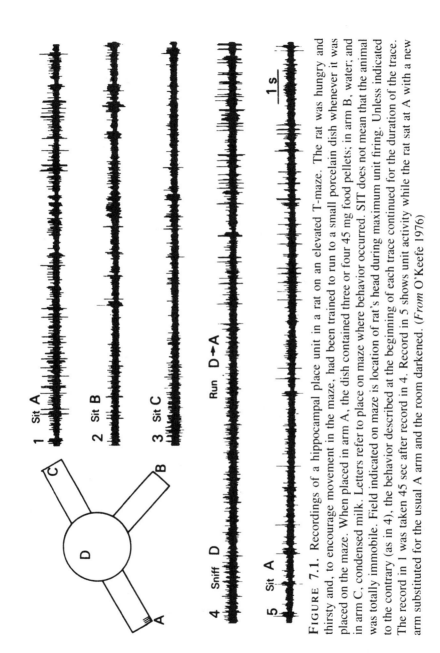

FIGURE 7.1. Recordings of a hippocampal place unit in a rat on an elevated T-maze. The rat was hungry and thirsty and, to encourage movement in the maze, had been trained to run to a small porcelain dish whenever it was placed on the maze. When placed in arm A, the dish contained three or four 45 mg food pellets; in arm B, water; and in arm C, condensed milk. Letters refer to place on maze where behavior occurred. SIT does not mean that the animal was totally immobile. Field indicated on maze is location of rat's head during maximum unit firing. Unless indicated to the contrary (as in 4), the behavior described at the beginning of each trace continued for the duration of the trace. The record in 1 was taken 45 sec after record in 4. Record in 5 shows unit activity while the rat sat at A with a new arm substituted for the usual A arm and the room darkened. (*From* O'Keefe 1976)

tion there. Control experiments (e.g., O'Keefe 1976; O'Keefe and Conway 1978) have shown that no such simple explanation is tenable. In the O'Keefe (1976) study, for example, the place cell did not increase its firing rate when the animal either ate or drank, and its firing persisted when the original arm (A) was substituted with a new arm and when the main lights were switched off (see figure 7.1).

Clearly, an animal is dependent upon sensory stimulation to establish its location; but the implication is that no single one of the constellation of cues that are correlated with a given location is essential to the firing of a place cell. Provided that the sensory information available is adequate to allow the animal to determine its location within the environment, place cells continue to fire within their appropriate fields despite substantial changes in sensory input.

Further work on place cells has inevitably complicated our view of them without, however, altering the basic notion that their firing is sensitive to spatial location. O'Keefe (1979), for example, reported that some place cells fire only when the animal is oriented in a particular direction within its place field; some fire only when the animal is moving in its place field; some cells show a decrease in spontaneous firing rate when in their place fields; and that when tested in two distinct environments, some cells show place fields in each environment, and some in only one environment. A subclass of place cells (which O'Keefe calls "misplace" cells) fire maximally when as a result of some change having been made within the place field (the absence of customary food, for example) the animal shows exploratory sniffing.

Place Cells and Anticipated Action

One striking finding (Foster, Castro, and McNaughton 1989) suggests that place cells fire only if an animal is prepared for movement. These workers first identified place fields for hippocampal cells in rats moving freely in a test environment. They then manually transported and placed rats in preestablished place fields under one of two conditions: in one condition, the rats were unrestrained and could therefore move if they so chose; in the other condition, the rats were restrained by a towel wrapped round the body. In fact the unrestrained rats remained relatively immobile, and the behavior of the rats in the two conditions was similar, involving head movements and myostatial sniffing. Despite the similarity of behavior in the two conditions, the activity of place cells was considerably affected by restraint, the effect of which was virtually to abolish the responding of place cells (which fired reliably in their place fields—but not elsewhere—

in the unrestrained condition). One reasonable account of this finding is that place cells become active when animals are processing information concerned with anticipated movement from one place to another.

Another finding that relates place-cell firing to anticipated action is provided by O'Keefe and Speakman (1987), who tested hungry rats in a simple cross-maze set among a collection of six controlled cues. These cues (a dim lamp, a white card, an electric fan, a towel, an aromatic pen, and a cage containing two rats) always bore the same spatial relationship to one another, but could be moved, en bloc, with respect to static background cues in the experimental room. Rats were trained to obtain food from one arm of the maze: the correct arm was determined by its spatial relationship to the controlled cues (the absolute spatial position of the correct arm, reflected in its relationship to the background cues, accordingly changed from trial to trial). Recordings were obtained from hippocampal pyramidal cells, and O'Keefe and Speakman found that most pyramidal cells had place fields that were defined with reference to the controlled cues (a minority had place fields defined with respect to the background cues). On some trials, the rats were placed in one arm of the maze (the start-arm for that trial) and restrained there for some 30–120 sec; the controlled cues were then either physically removed or (in the case of the light and the fan) switched off, and after a delay of 30–60 sec, the rat was allowed to make its choice. Of the place cells whose fields were defined relative to the controlled cues, some 90 percent maintained those fields at the time the rat made its choice. In other words, firing of those cells was maintained, not by the physical presence of the controlled cues but by the rat's memory of their location, a memory used by the rat to determine its subsequent anticipated choice.

Head-Direction Cells in the Subicular Complex

One recent report, which agrees with those previously discussed in suggesting a general role for the hippocampal formation in spatial processing, concerns cells identified in the rat postsubiculum (a part of the subicular complex that receives a major input from the subiculum and sends efferents to the entorhinal cortex). Taube, Muller, and Ranck (1990) found that 26 percent of cells identified in the postsubiculum fired whenever the rat's head was in a particular direction in the horizontal plane. The planes of preferred head direction were always parallel, whatever the rat's position in the environment, and firing bore no relation to the angle between the rat's head and its body; we are seeing, then, the output of a system that has computed the spatial direction of the head with respect to fixed features of the environment. The existence of cells having these properties in a region having intimate connections with the hippocampus clearly strengthens the case for supposing a role for the hippocampus in establishing spatial frames of reference.

Hippocampal Pyramidal Cells: Multiple Functions?

Place cells appear, superficially at least, to possess very different characteristics from those hippocampal cells investigated by Thompson and his colleagues which, as we saw in chapter 6, develop "neuronal models" of learned responses as a consequence of conditioning. It will be recalled (from chapter 6) that most hippocampal pyramidal cells form neuronal models during classical conditioning. Since we now know that most spontaneously active pyramidal cells serve as place cells, it appears that the same cells that form neuronal models also function as place cells, and this is an important point to which we shall return.

A Spatial Map in the Hippocampus: The O'Keefe and Nadel Theory

Interpretation of Electrophysiological Data

The existence of place cells has provided some of the most convincing support for O'Keefe and Nadel's (1978) spatial map theory of hippocampal function, and we shall now consider further details of that theory and of the role proposed in it for the theta rhythm in spatial information processing.

The Nature of the Hippocampal Representation of Space

The spatial map envisaged by O'Keefe and Nadel (1978) consists of representations of places in an environment and of the spatial relationships between those places. A place is represented by an array of hippocampal place cells, but it has not proved possible to specify how spatial relationships between places are represented. There does not appear to be an isomorphy between spatial relationships within the hippocampus and those in the real world: although there is a tendency for place cells with neighboring place fields to occur in local "clusters," the region served by one cluster is no more likely to be close to a region served by a neighboring cluster than to a region served by a cluster in quite another part of the hippocampus (Eichenbaum et al. 1989).

Construction of the Map

O'Keefe and Nadel (1978) suggested that the hippocampal map is formed using polysensory input derived from entorhinal cortex. The role of the dentate gyrus would be to detect regular conjunctions of stimuli; input from the dentate gyrus would be used to form a map in CA3; and the principal function of the CA1 region would be to use information derived from the CA3 region to determine whether a mismatch had occurred between the stimuli actually encountered at a given place and those that had been anticipated there. Although it originally appeared that no place cells were to be found in the dentate gyrus, the subsequent discovery of such cells in both the dentate gyrus and entorhinal cortex threw doubt on the O'Keefe and Nadel scheme; these doubts are strengthened by the demonstration (McNaughton et al. 1989) that virtually total elimination of dentate gyrus cells (by administration of the neurotoxin colchicine, to whose toxic effects dentate gyrus cells exhibit a supersensitivity) has no detectable effect on the place fields of pyramidal cells in the hippocampus proper. CA3 cells themselves receive direct input from the entorhinal cortex, and Miller and Best (1980) found that damage to the entorhinal cortex considerably reduced the percentage of cells in the hippocampus proper that were classified as place cells. It therefore appears likely that the critical input for the establishment of place fields in the hippocampus proper derives from the entorhinal cortex rather than from the dentate gyrus, and, since place cells are found in both the dentate gyrus and the entorhinal cortex, that the incremental construction of representation of place does not proceed in the manner outlined by O'Keefe and Nadel (1978).

The Role of the Theta Rhythm. According to O'Keefe and Nadel, theta activity plays a major role in the construction and use of the hippocampal map. The essential notion here is that theta cells, through their inhibitory action upon pyramidal cells, modulate the excitability of those cells in such a way that different sets of cells will be maximally excitable at different times. This is in turn because theta activity spreads spatially from its origin at one of the hippocampal generators, so that different regions of the hippocampus show different phases of the theta cycle at a given instant. There is evidence that the frequency of movement-related theta varies according to the distance that a movement covers (Morris and Hagan 1983), and O'Keefe and Nadel suggest that theta provides a mechanism whereby movements that alter an animal's spatial location may feed into the mapping domain. During map construction, theta provides a correlate of distance traversed, so that a specific set of place cells is maximally excitable (and, presumably, maximally modifiable) at a given distance from an initial location. And during movement through a known environment theta may provide a mechanism for predicting what sensory stimuli should be encountered after a given movement, and so, for enabling activation of misplace cells when mismatches occur.

Potential Importance of Lesion Data

Although the existence of place cells is not in dispute, their significance clearly is, and we have seen that some aspects of the scheme advanced by O'Keefe and Nadel (1978) are, to say the least, speculative. But the details of the O'Keefe and Nadel scheme could be incorrect even although the basic proposal was valid: we should, then, put aside reservations concerning the details of that scheme and turn instead to what is the basic issue of interest—*does* the hippocampus contain a spatial map? The view taken here is that this question is best approached by considering the ability of the spatial map hypothesis to account for the consequences of hippocampal damage. Does a hippocampectomized animal behave as though it has lost its spatial map?

Two Systems for Learning: The Locale and the Taxon Systems

The great majority of learning tasks require an animal to move within an experimental chamber so as to orient itself toward and to manipulate the experimental manipulanda—response keys, levers, and so on—by appropriately guided movements. Hippocampal animals have no difficulty with such requirements, and this raises the question how, in the absence of a spatial map, is accurate location of any kind possible for an animal?

O'Keefe and Nadel's (1978) response to this problem is to suggest that an animal possesses two systems that provide alternative ways in which movement might be guided. The first is the "locale" system, which involves the construction and use of maps, and their continual rapid updating in the light of environmental change. The second is the "taxon" system, a system that involves the learning of egocentrically referred movements such as turn left, run rapidly ahead, and so on. These responses are tied to specific (and usually proximal) stimuli or cues in the environment, and the strength of these stimulus-response (S-R) associations is modified gradually in an incremental or decremental fashion, by reward and punishment.

Before going on to consider further details of the locale versus taxon distinction, it should be pointed out that this particular distinction is one of a number of hypothetical distinctions between what might be called more and less cognitive systems that have been advanced as a result of hippocampal research. Other characterizations of the distinction between a more and a less cognitive system will be introduced in chapter 8; at this point it will be sufficient to note that the distinction drawn by O'Keefe and Nadel implies that there is, in intact animals, a very real difference between association formation and the cognitive processes involved in spatial learning. The implications of their interpretation of hippocampal function for behavioral theory are, then, profound; we shall find that this is true again of those rival interpretations that also appeal to distinctions between cognitive systems.

The locale system is more flexible than the taxon system in a number of ways. Suppose, for example, that an animal finds itself in a region that it has not previously visited and whose proximal cues are therefore unfamiliar. An animal that has formed a map of its environment may use the constellation of distal cues available to establish the relationship of that place to other places on the map, and so be able to direct itself toward any other place that is represented on its map. But an animal that is relying upon the taxon system does not learn about "places" and knows nothing of the relationship between different regions of the environment. It has learned only inflexible routes so that it will turn left on perceiving one cue, turn right on perceiving another, and so on: when placed in a region whose local cues are unfamiliar, the animal will not be able to respond appropriately.

A further example of the superior flexibility of the locale system is provided by considering the consequences of environmental alterations. An animal using the locale system would, on encountering a change at a particular place, be alerted by its mismatch system to engage in exploration so as to update the map immediately; an animal relying upon the taxon system would, on encountering change, modify its S-R bonds in a graded fashion.

An animal with hippocampal damage is assumed to possess an intact taxon system but a disrupted locale system. Its performance on tasks for which normals rely upon the taxon system should therefore be unaffected; but on tasks in which normals use the locale system, its performance should show deficits. The simplest way to assess O'Keefe and Nadel's proposal will, then, be to see whether tasks that appear to involve place learning do yield hippocampal deficits.

Spatial Learning Following Hippocampal Damage

Maze learning is an obvious example of a task that might be expected to involve place learning, and there is indeed good support for the mapping hypothesis from maze-learning studies.

Simple Mazes

Consider first the simplest form of maze, a T-maze. Hippocampectomized rats generally show no deficit in learning to find a food reward in (say) the left-hand goal-box of a T-maze. This finding may be accommodated by the spatial map theory on the assumption that the hippocampal animal solves the problem efficiently enough by using its taxon system and learning simply to turn left at the choice-point. When, however, the correct response is reversed (so that the food is now in the right-hand goal-box), hippocampals consistently show a marked deficit (O'Keefe and Nadel 1978). This deficit is taken to reflect the impaired flexibility of hippocampal animals: whereas normals that are using the locale system simply alter the information about the left goal-box on the map and so quickly abandon going to it, the hippocampals require a long series of trials to weaken the S-R bond underlying their left-turning response before they no longer turn left and can now reverse the response. Thus, hippocampal animals show normal acquisition but impaired reversal (due to response perseveration) of a simple spatial discrimination, and this pattern of results is readily accommodated by the spatial map hypothesis.

Complex Mazes

In more complicated mazes, a hippocampal deficit is reliably found. This is true for conventional mazes having multiple choice-points (O'Keefe and Nadel 1978), and for the Morris water maze and Olton's radial maze.

The Morris Water Maze. The Morris maze is particularly relevant here since the rationale for its introduction was largely that it provided a spatial learning task in which accurate performance required the use of a constellation of distal cues rather than approach to any specific local cue.

Morris et al. (1982) compared rats with total hippocampal extirpation and control rats in two versions of the water-escape maze. In the first (conventional) version, the platform onto which the rats could escape was not visible and lay 1 cm below the surface of the opaque water. Its position remained unchanged each day. Over the course of five days, animals experienced twenty-eight trials on which they were placed in the water, and the time taken to escape onto the platform was recorded. Figure 7.2 shows that hippocampal subjects performed consistently more poorly than controls and that although their performance improved, it reached a level no better than that reported by Morris (1981) for a control group of rats for which the platform was located in a different part of the bath on every trial.

The hippocampals' deficit was not due to their simply swimming more slowly: analysis of swimming patterns at the end of training in the conventional version of the maze showed that hippocampal rats swam longer, more circuitous routes to the platform. Moreover, unlike controls, hippocampal rats showed at the beginning of a trial no preferential tendency to swim toward the area in which the platform was located, as opposed to swimming toward any other region of the bath.

In the second version of the maze, the escape platform projected above the surface of the water and so provided a proximal visual cue that the rats could approach. The platform was now located in a different part of the bath and stayed at that new location throughout training. Figure 7.2 shows that hippocampal rats rapidly learned to escape onto the visible platform. When, however, the platform was replaced by the lower, invisible platform (now in the same place that the visible platform had occupied), hippocampal rats' performance once again deteriorated dramatically.

Two control tests were carried out at the end of training on each version of the maze. In each test there was no platform in the maze, and the swimming patterns of the rats were monitored. Control rats spent in both tests a significantly higher proportion of time swimming in the area in which the platform had been located than in other areas. This result indicates that they had learned the location (with respect to distal cues) of not only the invisible but also the visible platform. Hippocampal rats in both tests swam around aimlessly, spending no more time in any one part of the bath than in any other. Thus even though hippocampals learned, like controls, to approach the visible platform, they did not, unlike controls, learn *where* that platform was located.

The results of the Morris et al. (1982) study point to a total failure of hippocampal rats to learn about spatial relationships, and the analysis of swimming patterns provides detailed support for an interpretation in terms of loss of a spatial map.

The Olton Radial Maze. The involvement of the hippocampus in radial-maze performance has been explored by Olton and his colleagues,

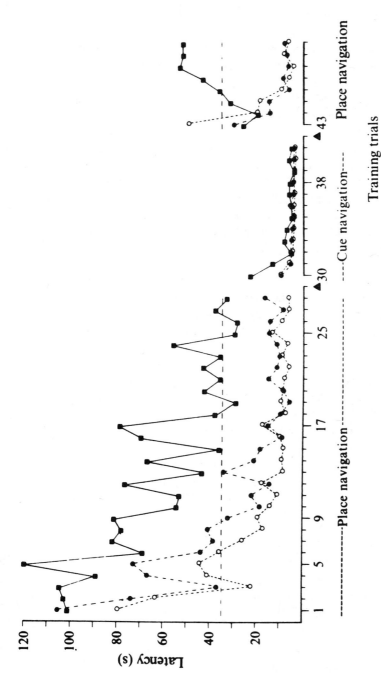

FIGURE 7.2. Effect of hippocampectomy on performance in the Morris water maze. The graph shows mean escape latencies for the 50 trials of the Morris et al. (1982) experiment. *Filled squares:* hippocampectomized rats; *filled circles:* rats having lesions of neocortex overlying the hippocampus; *open circles:* control rats that had either received sham operations involving no brain damage or had remained unoperated. The trial number of the first of each daily set of trials is shown on the abscissa. The two transfer tests are indicated by solid triangles. The horizontal broken line (trials 1–28 and 43–50) at 34.5 sec corresponds to the best performance shown by a group of normal rats trained to search in 20 trials for a hidden platform that was moved randomly from one place to another over successive trials. Twenty-eight trials of place navigation were followed by a transfer test (see text for details); there then followed 12 trials of cue navigation, followed by a second transfer test; rats were returned to place navigation for the final 8 trials. *(From* Morris et al. 1982)

who have used fornicotomized rats. The fornix is, it will be recalled, part of the Papez circuit and mediates important connections between the hippocampus and subcortical zones: it carries, for example, efferents from the hippocampus to the septal area, the thalamus, and the hypothalamus, and afferents to the hippocampus from the septal area (these latter connections being necessary for the occurrence of the theta rhythm). As a method of disrupting normal hippocampal function it enjoys the advantage that the surgery avoids damage to areas adjoining the hippocampus—for example, to the inferotemporal neocortex, a region of visual-association cortex known in primates to be critically involved in certain types of visual discrimination.

The major findings may be summarized rapidly. Fornicotomized rats showed no evidence of spatial memory in the radial maze. This was true whether the maze was relatively simple (4-arm) or more complicated (8- or 17-arm). The disruption was seen despite preoperative training to criterion, and performance remained at chance levels following extensive postoperative testing, and when several months postoperative recovery were allowed (Olton, Becker, and Handelmann 1979).

In the standard free-choice procedure, fornicotomized rats' behavior differs in the radial maze in two ways (besides the reduction in choice accuracy) from that of normals. First, they spend less time than normals in the goal-box at the end of each arm; second, they show a different pattern of response preference from normals: whereas normals show a strong tendency to enter an arm adjacent to the arm they have just visited, fornicotomized animals show their highest preference (in a 17-arm maze) for an arm separated by three intervening arms from that just visited. But neither of these factors appears to be the cause of the performance deficit: when the time spent in the goal-box was controlled (by confining rats in the goal-box of each arm for a 30-sec period), fornicotomized rats in a 4-arm maze still showed no evidence of remembering which arms had previously been entered, whereas controls showed virtually perfect performance (Walker and Olton 1979). And when systematic turning tendencies were virtually eliminated (by confining animals in the central choice area for 10–15 sec following each visit to an arm), fornicotomized animals nevertheless showed essentially no spatial memory, while controls showed high levels of accuracy (Olton and Werz 1978).

The results of the radial-maze studies do therefore provide evidence that fornicotomized rats are quite unable to discriminate between places recently visited and places not recently visited. They show, that is, poor spatial memory. This may be accounted for by the spatial map hypothesis on the assumption that efficient radial-maze performance relies upon the ready identification of the different arms, and upon updating of the significance of an arm each time it is visited: such performance would clearly require an intact locale system.

Learning in a variety of complex mazes is, then, disrupted by damage to the hippocampal system, and this provides support for the spatial-mapping interpretation of hippocampal function. The reports considered above all involved experiments on rats moving from one part of an apparatus to another. But there is good evidence for the existence of spatial deficits arising from hippocampal damage in other species and in tasks in which the animal's position in space does not change.

Spatial Tasks Other Than Mazes

Spatial Reversals. In a series of experiments using rhesus monkeys (*Macaca mulatta*), Mahut reported a selective disruption of spatial learning following hippocampal damage. In the first report of her series (Mahut 1971), monkeys with lesions of the hippocampal formation were compared to (normal and operated) controls; in subsequent reports (Mahut 1972; Mahut and Zola 1973), the fornix was transected. Mahut's experiments involved the acquisition and reversal of spatial and object discriminations in a Wisconsin General Test Apparatus (WGTA), in which animals are required to pick up three-dimensional objects from a stimulus tray (rather than to respond to two-dimensional stimuli such as keylights). In the spatial discriminations monkeys had to choose between two identical gray plaques on the stimulus tray, one of which (the left, say) was consistently associated with reward; once the original discrimination was established, the reward values of the two positions were reversed. In the object discrimination, the animals had to select between two junk objects each of which appeared equally often on the left as on the right side of the tray. Neither hippocampal damage (Mahut 1971) nor fornicotomy (Mahut 1972) affected acquisition of either discrimination. Both types of lesion did, however, severely disrupt reversals of the spatial discrimination without disrupting reversals of the object discrimination. In fact, there was good evidence that object-discrimination reversal learning was facilitated by the lesions; this appeared, however, to be a modality-specific phenomenon since the facilitation was found when fornicotomized monkeys were tested in light but not when tested in darkness (when the discrimination was based on tactile cues) (Mahut and Zola 1973; Zola and Mahut 1973). It is important, then, to note that the disruptive effect of fornicotomy was not modality dependent; spatial-reversal learning was disrupted in both light and dark (Mahut and Zola 1973).

Visuo-Spatial Conditional Discriminations. Further experiments on monkeys provide evidence of remarkable specificity in the disruptions obtained. Consider, for example, performance of fornicotomized monkeys in tasks in which each of two stimulus patterns, displayed on a computer-controlled screen, required a different response for reward to be obtained. In one study (Rupniak and Gaffan 1987) cynomolgus monkeys (*Macaca fascicularis*) had to touch the screen four times in response to one stimulus, and to withhold response to the other stimulus: performance was severely disrupted by transection of the fornix. In the second study (Gaffan and Harrison 1988), monkeys were rewarded for making sustained contact with the screen (a 2-sec press) in response to one stimulus and for tapping the screen (eight times) in response to the other: fornix transection did not disrupt performance of this task. It is important to note that in both these tasks, reward was available for the appropriate response to both stimuli. A more conventional type of successive discrimination is the go/no-go discrimination, in which reward is available for a response to one stimulus, but no reward is available for response to the other stimulus. There is evidence that conventional go/no-go discriminations are acquired normally despite interference with hippocampal function: Gaffan et al. (1984:Experiment 6) found that go/no-go discrimination was not disrupted by fornicotomy and Mahut (1971) found that hippocampal damage did not disrupt go/no-go alternation learning. These are striking findings, since the standard go/no-go task is not easily discriminated from the technique used in the Rupniak and Gaffan (1987) study, and each procedure obtains the same outcome—approach to one stimulus, withdrawal from the other. How can those contrasting effects be explained?

The conditional task that was disrupted involved the animal's learning to move its arm to one of two spatially defined positions (toward the screen, away from the screen). The conditional task that showed no disruption required the animal to make one of two responses (hold or tap) at a single spatial position. Thus the disrupted task required a spatial discrimination, the task that was unaffected did not. And despite the close similarity between the Rupniak and Gaffan (1987) procedure and the standard go/no-go task, it can be argued that the go/no-go task does not require spatial learning. For the go/no-go task can readily be acquired through simple classical conditioning: the stimulus associated with reward elicits approach (the unconditional response to rewarding stimuli); the negative stimulus, not being associated with reward, would not elicit approach. In the Rupniak and Gaffan study, because both stimuli were associated with reward no such simple mode of solution was possible: the animal in that case had to acquire a discrimination between two spatially differentiated responses.

Nonspatial Learning Following Hippocampal Damage

The effects of hippocampal damage in monkeys in a variety of discrimination tasks do, then, provide further support for the notion that hippocampal damage has a selective effect on spatial processing. There are, however, many tasks that do not show an overt spatial component but do show disruption following hippocampal damage, and the proponents of the spatial map hypothesis have shown considerable ingenuity in accounting for many of these deficits. Particularly convincing analyses have been advanced for effects seen across a range of avoidance-learning paradigms.

Avoidance Learning

Avoidance-learning tasks may be divided into active avoidance-response (AAR) tasks, in which animals have to produce a specific response in order to avoid an aversive event, and passive avoidance (punishment) tasks, in which animals have to withhold a specific response in order to avoid an aversive event.

Active Avoidance. AAR tasks may be further subdivided into 1-way and 2-way AAR tasks. In 1-way AAR tasks, an animal has to move within some specified time from the (dangerous) start region of an apparatus to some other (safe) region. In a typical experiment, a rat might be required to jump over a hurdle dividing the grid floor of one part of a box to the unelectrified other section of the floor within, say, 5 sec of the removal of a partition between the two regions. Each trial would begin with the placing of the rat onto the grid floor and would end with its removal from the unelectrified area.

In 2-way AAR, an animal must shuttle between the two halves of an apparatus in order to avoid shocks, which can be delivered in either half: typically, a rat would be required to jump a hurdle between the two halves within (say) 5 sec of the onset of a CS (a buzzer or a light, for example), and CS onsets would occur equally often with the rat in one half as in the other. Two-way AAR responding is of particular interest since it is a task that normal rats find more difficult than 1-way AAR, but that consistently shows facilitation following hippocampal damage (Black, Nadel, and

O'Keefe 1977). The potential theoretical significance of an *improvement* in learning brought about by brain damage hardly needs emphasis.

Why, then, should hippocampal damage improve 2-way AAR? Why, in particular, should loss of the locale system improve 2-way AAR? Black and his colleagues (1977) suggest that the answer is to be found in the fact that normal rats placed in a dangerous but inescapable place freeze, and that freezing is incompatible with the movement required to avoid shocks. For the normal rat, both halves of the apparatus are dangerous places, since shocks are delivered in both; a 2-way AAR therefore requires the rat to run toward a dangerous place, and this sets up a conflict that results in freezing. Consider, however, the hippocampal rat, an animal incapable of learning about places. The hippocampal rat learns simply to run on presentation of the CS—a simple S-R habit: the hippocampal rat experiences no conflict since it is not running from one place to another place, much less to a dangerous place.

The place-learning analysis of 2-way AAR provides an intuitively satisfying account of the facilitation observed following hippocampal damage. It can also, of course, explain the fact that 1-way AAR is *not* consistently facilitated. Normal rats in 1-way AAR are moving from a consistently dangerous place to a consistently safe place, and therefore experience no conflict. Most investigations of effects of hippocampal damage on 1-way AAR have found no differences between control and hippocampal performance (Black, Nadel, and O'Keefe 1977), and when any effect is seen it consists in a hippocampal *deficit*. Black and his colleagues make out the case that when deficits in 1-way AAR have been reported in hippocampals, the apparatus used favored place as opposed to cue learning. The contrasting effects on 1-way and 2-way AAR of hippocampal damage can thus be accommodated plausibly by the spatial mapping theory.

Passive Avoidance. Early reports of the effects of hippocampal damage on punishment showed a confusing picture with many contradictory findings. Black and his colleagues (1977) provided an ingenious account of the diversity seen and helped considerably to disentangle the difficulties.

Black and colleagues point out, first, that in the great majority of studies in which consummatory behavior (such as drinking from a cup) is punished, that behavior is inhibited as efficiently by hippocampals as by controls; second, that when an apparatus is used in which rats are punished for moving from some safe start region onto a clearly demarcated dangerous area (normally a grid floor), punishment is again as effective in obtaining response inhibition in hippocampals as in controls. In these simple tasks, then, most reports agree that no differences are found between normals and hippocampals.

But another simple task involves punishing rats for traversing a runway: suppose that an animal is trained initially to run for food reward at the end of a runway, and that a shock is then delivered in the goal area. Some studies find deficits in hippocampals (the animals persist in running faster than controls), others do not. Black and his colleagues surveyed the data available and found that much of the variation between the results could be accounted for by considering the response measure used. Studies that found no deficit used measures related to goal-box performance (such as latency to eat there, or number of shocks received); studies that found a deficit used a performance measure that took into account performance in the early sections of the runway, such as latency to leave the start-box, or total running time. Why should hippocampals show deficits at points somewhat distant from the site of punishment, but not close to the punishment site?

According to Black and colleagues, normal rats in a runway punishment task use their locale system and update the information about the goal area on their maps. This has the result that they withhold approach to that area from any other region represented on the map (and that, of course, includes the start-box). Hippocampal animals require only a few pairings of the local cues in the goal-box area and the aversive UCS to avoid those local cues. But cues distal to the punishment site will acquire aversive strength only gradually (as a result of generalization back through the series of cues along the runway). This account can, of course, explain also the normal performance of hippocampals in those simple punishment procedures described earlier, in which the aversive event could readily be associated with a proximal cue (the drinking cup, or the grid floor, for example).

Difficulties for the Mapping Hypothesis

The preceding sections have documented support for the spatial mapping theory from electrophysiological and lesion studies. We have seen also that the theory is of sufficient generality that it can account for deficits induced by hippocampal damage in not only spatial tasks but tasks that do not make overt demands on spatial processing. However, like all current theories that ascribe a unitary function to the hippocampus, the spatial mapping theory does have difficulty in accounting for all the available data. We shall now consider some discordant data, beginning with electro-physiological findings and going on to data from lesion studies.

Unit Recordings

Hippocampal place cells have been reliably demonstrated in tasks in which rats have been allowed to move freely in an extended environment, and control experiments have shown that their activity is not dependent on the occurrence of either specific stimuli or specific behavior patterns in those places. The existence in the hippocampus of cells having those strik-ing properties has provided strong support for the notion that the hippo-campus is involved in spatial processing. But we have already noted the fact that, just as virtually all spontaneously active hippocampal pyramidal cells are place cells, the great majority of pyramidal cells also develop neuronal models in the rabbit eyelid-conditioning paradigm. This suggests that a given pyramidal cell may serve quite different roles in different tasks, a conclusion that would clearly weaken the claim that the principal (and perhaps only) function of the hippocampus is the processing of spa-tial information. There is in fact a report (Thompson and Best 1989) showing that most hippocampal pyramidal cells are *not* spontaneously ac-tive in freely behaving rats, so that the proportion of pyramidal cells that are place cells may be lower than originally appeared to be the case. But there is, nevertheless, good evidence both that the place field of a given cell may be modified as a consequence of learning, and that one and the same cell may be a place cell in one task and show other properties in other tasks.

Place Fields Are Modifiable

A relatively simple example of the modifiability of place cells is provided by Breese, Hampson, and Deadwyler (1989), who recorded from hippo-campal cells in thirsty rats moving around an environment in which a drop of water was delivered every 30 sec to any one of a number of locations, selected at random. The purpose of this procedure was simply to encour-age movement in the environment, and Breese and his colleagues were able to identify, as expected, a large number of conventional place cells. When the procedure was modified so that drops of water were now con-sistently delivered in one place only, the place fields of the great majority of cells (more than 80 percent) now shifted to the region at which the drops were delivered. Thus, although (as we have seen) place fields are remarkably stable in a constant environment, they may change rapidly in response to a simple manipulation (with, presumably, the consequence that the quality of mapping of the environment as a whole is severely degraded).

A Single Pyramidal Cell May Serve Many Functions

Other workers have shown that the same cell may serve different functions in different tasks. Thompson and Best (1990), for example, having established place fields for hippocampal cells in one environment, subsequently exposed their rats to tone-footshock pairings in a novel environment. They reported that, as a consequence of the pairings, hippocampal cells (identified as place cells in the original environment) showed systematic changes in response rate to tone onset (most cells showed rate decreases). When returned to the original environment, it was found that place fields had been entirely unaffected by the tone-footshock pairings experienced in the novel environment. In other words, in one environment a given cell functioned as a place cell; in the other environment, it responded to a CS signaling shock.

A similar point is made by a report (Wiener, Paul, and Eichenbaum 1989) in which rats performed two different tasks in the same apparatus. One task was an analogue of the radial maze and required movement throughout the apparatus; the other task was a simultaneous odor discrimination, the stimuli being presented through two ports in a fixed location. Some 75 percent of hippocampal cells were classified, in the radial-maze analogue, as place cells. In the odor discrimination task, the rats stayed, as would be expected, in the relatively small area within which the stimuli were presented and the rewards delivered, and Wiener and his colleagues determined whether hippocampal cells fired selectively in any of three phases of each trial: cue sampling (the period between the initiation of a trial and choice); port approach (the choice phase, in which the rat chose by approaching a specific port); and cup approach (in which the rat, following its choice, moved toward the cup in which reward was delivered). Some 58 percent of hippocampal cells showed increases in firing rate that were associated with one (or more) of the phases of each trial. The great majority of those cells were classified as place cells in the radial-maze analogue, and individual cells often showed a place field in the maze task that was quite distinct from the location associated with the functional correlate identified in the odor-discrimination task.

A final example will be considered in some detail, as it gives a good flavor of the complexity of interaction of the variety of factors that are now known to influence the firing of hippocampal pyramidal cells when an element of learning is introduced.

In a study reported by Wible et al. (1986), rats with implanted electrodes ran down a runway toward two goal-boxes (one black, the other white) placed side by side. Two experiments were carried out. The first used a delayed matching-to-sample (DMTS) test procedure in which each trial consisted of two phases—a sample and a choice phase. In the sample phase, the route to one of the goal-boxes was blocked off, and the rat was then forced to enter either the white or the black box, where it obtained reward; a counterbalanced design was used so that the box was equally often black or white, equally often on the left or on the right. The rat was then replaced in the start-box of the runway, and the choice phase began. Both goal-boxes were now available, and the box that had been entered in the sample phase contained reward: on half the trials the box remained in the same position as in the sample phase, and its position was switched with that of the other (unentered) box on the other half. The animal therefore had to remember which box, black or white, had been used in the sample phase, its position being irrelevant.

Recordings were obtained from twenty-seven hippocampal pyramidal cells, and rates of firing in the goal-box were analyzed to see whether they changed reliably according to position (left or right) of the goal-box, to its brightness (black or white), or to the phase (sample versus choice) of a trial. Nineteen units showed systematic variations with one or more of those variables, and twelve of those units (less than half of the total number of units studied) showed changes in firing rate according to the position of the goal-box. There was evidence, however, that most of those twelve "place" cells were coding other aspects of the task since nine of them showed interactions with phase or goal-box brightness (or with both). One unit, for example, responded more in a goal-box on the right than on the left of the apparatus; more in the black than in the white goal-box; and more during the sample than during the choice phase. Overall, there were four units whose activity varied only with brightness, two only with phase, and three only with position; the activity of the other ten units varied according to some combination of these variables.

The second experiment of the study involved two procedures, each a straightforward discrimination between either position (with brightness irrelevant) or brightness (with position irrelevant) of the goal-boxes. So, for example, in the position discrimination, the left goal-box would contain reward on all trials, and in the brightness discrimination the black goal-box consistently contained reward. All the rats performed in both the position and the brightness discrimination. In this experiment, goal-box unit activity was analyzed according to task (position versus brightness discrimination), goal-box position, and goal-box brightness. Recordings were obtained from twenty-nine units, of which fifteen showed significant correlations between unit activity and one (or more) of the variables analyzed. None of the units responded according to position alone; six showed activity correlated with position and either task or goal-box brightness. Five units showed variation according to task alone, and ten varied significantly with combinations of task and position, brightness, or both.

Place Cells Do Not Guarantee Efficient Spatial Learning

The results surveyed above do not argue against the widespread existence of place cells in the hippocampus. But they do show that those same cells code quite other information when tasks that specifically involve learning are used. Wible et al. (1986) in fact used the different patterns of significant effects between the two experiments as support for the notion that the hippocampus plays a particular role in "working memory" (assumed to be involved in delayed matching-to-sample but not in simultaneous discrimination learning). This proposal will be discussed in some detail in chapter 8, but the point may be made here that the electrophysiological data do not provide strong support for that theory for precisely the same reason that their support for the mapping theory is weakened by Wible et al.'s findings: the hippocampus clearly receives (and, perhaps, processes) complex information of many types. The available data do not support exclusively any one interpretation of hippocampal function. Only experiments using lesions can establish the necessity or otherwise of the hippocampus to any process of learning or memory, a point that may nicely be illustrated by introducing one final report that casts some doubt on the relevance of place cells to spatial learning.

It will be recalled that selective destruction of dentate gyrus cells does not disrupt the place fields of cells in the hippocampus proper (McNaughton et al., 1989); however McNaughton and his colleagues also showed that destruction of dentate gyrus cells did disrupt spatial learning (in three mazes—the Barnes circular maze, the Morris water maze, and the Olton radial maze). Spatial learning was, in other words, disrupted by a manipulation that did not disrupt the activity of place cells and so, presumably, did not disrupt the spatial map. If the hippocampus does contain a spatial map, that map may be necessary for efficient spatial learning: but it is not sufficient for efficient spatial learning.

Lesion Data

Not All Spatial Tasks Yield Hippocampal Deficits

A number of instances in which spatial learning has proceeded normally in hippocampal animals have been reported. Some pertinent examples concern conditional discriminations in which the appropriate choice is made dependent upon an animal's location.

Murray et al. (1989) reported three experiments in which rhesus monkeys were required to choose one of a pair of objects when the monkey was in one location, but the other of the pair when in a different location. The objects used covered two food wells in a stimulus tray. In two experiments, the stimulus tray was moved between two locations; in the third experiment, the monkey had to select one object when viewing the stimulus tray from one side, and the other object when viewing from the other side. Fornix transection did not disrupt performance on any of these tasks. These same monkeys had, however, shown an impairment in postoperative retention of a spatial delayed non-matching-to-sample (DNMTS) task. This task used a T-maze, and each trial consisted of two phases. The sample phase consisted of a forced run to one goal-box in which reward was available. The choice phase, run after a 1-min delay, consisted of a choice between the two goal-boxes, and the goal-box not sampled now contained a reward. Performance in this task was severely disrupted by fornix lesions despite the fact that the control monkeys found the DNMTS task less difficult (in terms of trials to criterion) than the conditional tasks. Similar results were obtained in a companion study that explored the effect of fornix transection in rats on both spatial DNMTS and spatial conditional problems (Markowska et al. 1989). The failure of fornicotomy to disrupt these conditional tasks is particularly forceful since it is difficult to see how they could be solved with the use of the taxon system alone. The animals in these tasks could not easily base their responding on egocentric coordinates since the selection of the correct response—to the animal's left or to its right—depended precisely on the discrimination by the animal between the locations in which it found itself.

A further example of successful spatial learning despite damage to the hippocampal system has been provided by Olton and Papas (1979), in a report that will be considered in more detail in chapter 8. The aspect of their report that is relevant here may be summarized rapidly: Olton and Papas used a 17-arm radial maze, nine arms of which were never baited. Fornicotomized rats learned successfully to avoid the unbaited arms (although, as we shall see in chapter 8, they did not perform efficiently on the eight baited arms). Since learning to avoid a subset of arms appears to involve spatial learning no less than the conventional radial-maze task, one implication of the Olton and Papas (1979) finding would seem to be that fornicotomy does not result in the general disruption of spatial learning.

There is, then, evidence that although many spatial tasks are disrupted by hippocampal damage, not all spatial tasks are. If disruption of spatial learning was due to loss of a spatial mapping capacity, that disruption should clearly be general.

Some Nonspatial Tasks Do Yield Hippocampal Deficits

Chapter 8 will describe a number of deficits induced by hippocampal damage that do not seem readily explicable in terms of disruption of spatial processing. This section will discuss only deficits introduced in chapter 6, partly with a view to showing again how the spatial mapping theory of hippocampal function can be used to account for apparently nonspatial deficits, partly to show the difficulties that nevertheless remain.

Solomon has argued that "it is unlikely that spatial cues play any role in the rabbit NMR [nictitating membrane response—i.e., eyelid-conditioning] preparation. Here the animal remains virtually motionless throughout the conditioning session, and the conditioned stimuli (CS) and unconditioned stimuli (UCS) are delivered in the same spatial location at all times" (1979:1273). Nevertheless, as we saw in chapter 6, hippocampal lesions do disrupt learning under certain conditions in that preparation.

The particular task on which Solomon concentrated his attention was latent inhibition: preexposure of a to-be-conditioned CS retards rate of conditioning to that CS in normal but not in hippocampal-damaged rabbit eyelid-conditioning preparations (Solomon and Moore 1975; see chapter 6 for further discussion of the effects of hippocampal damage on latent inhibition). Can the spatial mapping theory accommodate the fact that learning may be disrupted by damage in a task to which spatial cues are not relevant?

O'Keefe, Nadel, and Willner (1979) believe that it can, and that place learning *is* involved in latent inhibition in the eyelid-conditioning preparation. Specifically, they argue that the rabbit does attend to the context in which it is restrained, and learns that certain events occur there (and not, for example, in the home cage). Applied to latent inhibition, their argument runs as follows: "pre-exposure to the specific cues will reduce their role in conditioning within that context because they will have been incorporated into the hippocampal representation of that environment, and there will be no misplace output to identify them as novel when they are reintroduced with the US" (p. 1284). In support of this account of latent inhibition, O'Keefe and his colleagues cite evidence that latent inhibition is a context-specific phenomenon: the preexposure of a stimulus in one context does not reduce ease of conditioning to that stimulus in a different context (Lubow, Rifkin, and Alek 1976).

The account proposed by O'Keefe and colleagues (1979) is ingenious and provides a plausible interpretation of the lack of effect of CS preexposure in hippocampectomized animals. It does, however, raise problems when we consider the effects of preexposure in normals. The argument of O'Keefe and colleagues suggests that the effect of CS preexposure is to deprive the CS of novelty; the absence of novelty leads to a reduced ease of conditioning. If hippocampal-damaged animals (as a result of loss of misplace cells) never experience novelty, their performance should, then, be comparable to that of normals following stimulus preexposure. But their performance is in fact equivalent to that of normals without stimulus preexposure, to that of normals for which stimuli are novel. The fact that in the standard eyelid-conditioning preparation hippocampectomized rabbits acquire the CR as readily as controls shows that if novelty is a factor in ease of conditioning, then hippocampectomized rabbits experience novelty as readily as controls. In fact it seems, at least to this writer, rather that (as suggested in chapter 3) hippocampectomized animals see all stimuli as novel rather than none as novel, and this is a point to which we shall return in chapter 8.

Other differences between control and hippocampal performance in the eyelid-conditioning preparation also raise difficulties for the mapping theory. It is, for example, very difficult to see why place strategies should not be employed under optimal conditions (where hippocampal performance is equivalent to control performance) but are employed when, for example, nonoptimal ISIs are used or when a trace procedure is introduced (see chapter 6 for details). One final example from chapter 6 may be considered here. Berger and Orr (1983) found that although hippocampectomized rabbits acquired a discrimination between two CSs at a normal rate, they showed a retarded rate of reversal of that discrimination. The source of the poor reversal performance lay in overresponding to the former CS +. Now the mapping theory can explain this finding by supposing that normals used the locale system to register that in this context the (former) CS + was no longer followed by the UCS, and so rapidly ceased to respond to it. The hippocampectomized rabbits, by contrast, were compelled to use the taxon system, which allows only gradual increments or

decrements in associative strength. The problem, of course, is that Berger
and Orr also showed that straightforward extinction was not disrupted by
hippocampal damage: why should the locale system be used in reversal
but not in extinction? We have noted previously the difficulty found for
the selective attention account by the Berger and Orr findings: those findings pose problems also for the mapping theory and, indeed, for those
early theories of hippocampal function that supposed a general role for the
hippocampus in inhibition of responding (e.g., Altman, Brunner, and
Bayer 1973).

The Hippocampus and Context Change

The discussion thus far has concentrated on one particular theory of the
involvement of the hippocampus in contextual processing—the spatial
map theory. Other theories proposing a somewhat different role for the
hippocampus—but a role involving context—have been advanced. Hirsh
(e.g., 1980) has argued that the hippocampus is essential for the appropriate retrieval of associations according to contextual cues; Gaffan (e.g.,
Gaffan and Harrison 1989) has argued that the hippocampus is involved
in "snapshot memory," a memory that preserves the entire contents of a
scene and, in particular, the spatial relationships between items within a
scene; and Sutherland and Rudy (1989) have argued that the hippocampus
plays an essential role in conditioning to configural cues, and that contextual learning is a special case of configural learning. There is not space to
review these theories in detail here (although much work that is relevant
to them has been introduced in the preceding discussion). But one issue
that is pertinent to all theories that suppose a hippocampal role in contextual processing is the sensitivity (or otherwise) of hippocampal-damaged
animals to contextual change. If the hippocampus is essential for the processing of contextual information, or for reinstating memories conditional
upon the current context, then changes in context should have less effect
on performance of learned responses in hippocampals than in normals.
The available experimental data do not, however, support that general prediction.

   Winocur and Olds (1978) trained control and hippocampal-damaged
rats on a simultaneous visual discrimination (horizontal versus vertical
stripes) in either of two readily discriminable apparatuses that were placed
in environments between which there were, again, salient differences.
There were no significant group differences in acquisition of the discriminations. Retention of the discriminations was then tested either in the same

context (that is, the same apparatus in the same environment) as the training context or in the context not previously experienced (a different apparatus in a different environment). Hippocampals showed unimpaired retention in the same context, but showed a substantial disruption of retention (compared to controls) in the novel context. In a second experiment, control and hippocampal rats acquired an orientation discrimination in one context, and a reversal of that discrimination in either the same or a novel context. As anticipated, the hippocampal animals showed a significant deficit in reversal learning when tested in the same context; but that deficit was markedly reduced (and was not statistically significant) when the rats were tested in a novel context. This result, like that of the first experiment, suggests that associations formed by hippocampal animals are more closely tied to contextual cues than is the case for normals.

The Winocur and Olds data suggest, then, that performance of learned responses by hippocampal rats in fact shows exaggerated dependence on context. There have, however, been some more recent reports that appear to conflict with this conclusion. Two studies, for example, have reported that a switch of contexts resulted in less disruption of a learned response in hippocampal than in control animals. Good and Honey (1991) found that whereas control rats showed a decrease in rate of a classically conditioned appetitive response when the CS was presented in a context in which the CS had not previously been presented, rats with hippocampal lesions showed an increase. Similarly, when Penick and Solomon (1991) presented an established CS in a novel context, they found a decrease in probability of occurrence of a classically conditioned eyelid CR in control rabbits but an increase in hippocampectomized rabbits.

A problem with these reports is that they employ as a measure not choice between responses but rate or probability of occurrence of a single response. Measures that do not employ choice are liable to contamination by the potentially sensitizing effects of novelty, effects that would counter the decrement occasioned by context change. The discussion (in chapter 3) of the reaction of hippocampal animals to novel stimuli concluded that although hippocampal animals were less likely to detect novelty, exploratory responses to novelty would be enhanced when novelty was detected. Given the not unreasonable assumption that enhanced curiosity may obtain a general sensitization of behavior, the results of these recent studies may be reconciled with those of Winocur and Olds (1978): hippocampal rats are more sensitive than normals in changes of context and are sensitized by such changes so that overall levels of response are likely to increase in spite of the decremental effects of change in the stimulus complex controlling behavior. It may be added here that similar considerations apply to recent claims (based on studies that have not used choice measures) that hippocampal damage attenuates conditioning of fear to contextual cues (Kim and Fanselow 1992; Phillips and LeDoux 1992).

Concluding Comments

We have seen in this section some of the difficulties that currently face proposals that link hippocampal function to contextual processing. It need not, however, be concluded that such proposals should now be rejected. The fact is that all current theories of hippocampal function face serious difficulties. It may be that all are invalid; or that the hippocampus serves several relatively independent functions; or that one of the current theories is basically correct and that we have yet to understand the full behavioral implications of disruption of the process in question. We have seen, for example, that disruption of spatial mapping may indeed plausibly be supposed to lead to disruption of performance in tasks to which spatial cues would appear, on the surface, to be irrelevant. At this point we should, perhaps, concentrate on the fact that evidence from a number of paradigms points to relatively selective disruption of the processing of spatial information in those paradigms. When we return to a consideration of hippocampal function in chapter 8, we shall encounter further examples of disruptions by hippocampal damage that do not appear to be attributable to impairment of spatial processing, and the possibility that the hippocampus plays a role in a specific type of memory will be assessed. The interpretation of deficits in memory (for spatial and nonspatial information) should proceed against the background of the known effects of hippocampal damage on spatial tasks.

The Role of Extrahippocampal Limbic Structures in Spatial Processing

This chapter has concentrated on the potential role of the hippocampus in spatial processing and has discussed the effects both of damage to the hippocampus itself and of fornicotomy. The effectiveness of transection of the fornix raises the question whether damage to sites outside the hippocampus but anatomically connected with it might obtain spatial deficits. Specifically, we may ask whether any of the anatomically defined systems to which the hippocampus belongs appears to act as a coordinated whole in the processing of spatial information. Such systems include the limbic system, the Papez circuit, and the hippocampal trisynaptic pathway. If damage to each of the components of any one of those systems obtains deficits in spatial processing, one implication might be that the system concerned does act as an integrated system for spatial processing, and, perhaps, that each station of the system operates sequentially on spatial information.

The Limbic System and Spatial Processing

The major extrahippocampal components of the limbic system are the septal area, the cingulate gyrus, and the amygdala. Of those structures only the septal area has attracted from physiological psychologists anything approaching the research effort devoted to the hippocampus. That research has shown that there is a good correspondence between the effects of septal lesions and of hippocampal lesions on avoidance learning (both active and passive), on reversal learning, and on maze learning (for a review see Gray and McNaughton 1983).

It will be recalled that the medial septal nucleus is the source of a major cholinergic input to the hippocampus and contains the pacemaker cells that control the hippocampal theta rhythm. There is evidence that damage to the medial septal area is primarily responsible for the deficits obtained following septal damage. Mitchell et al. (1982), for example, found that medial septal lesions disrupted hippocampal theta, obtained a reduced level of cholinergic activity in the hippocampus, and led to impaired acquisition in a radial maze. Similarly, Hagan et al. (1988) have shown that neurotoxic lesions that damaged the medial septal region but spared the lateral region disrupted acquisition of place learning in the Morris water maze.

Two reports of the effects of cingulate cortical lesions in rats suggest that the cingulate cortex may play a role in spatial processing. Markowska et al. (1989) found an impairment in a spatial DNMTS task (similar to the impairment found in fornicotomized rats), and Sutherland, Whishaw, and Kolb (1988) found an impairment in both acquisition and retention of place learning in the Morris water maze. Markowska et al. (1989) reported a further parallel between cingulate- and fornix-lesioned rats: neither lesion had any effect on three spatial conditional discriminations (modeled on those used with monkeys by Murray et al. 1989).

The final major component of the limbic system is the amygdala, and it appears that, unlike the other three, the amygdala is not essential for efficient spatial learning: Becker, Walker, and Olton (1980), for example, have reported that preoperatively established radial-maze performance was not disrupted by amygdalar damage.

Role of the Papez Circuit and the Trisynaptic Pathway

The stations of the Papez circuit outside the hippocampal formation are the mammillary bodies, the anterior thalamic nucleus, and the cingulate gyrus. We have already seen that the cingulate gyrus does appear to be involved in spatial learning. We shall see (in chapter 8) that there is evidence for the involvement of both the anterior thalamic nuclei and the mammillary bodies in memory; however, what little information there is on the subcortical stations of the Papez circuit does not suggest a critical role for them in spatial (as opposed to nonspatial) processing. Béracochéa, Jaffard, and Jarrard (1989) reported that destruction of the anterior thalamic nuclei did not affect either acquisition of radial-maze performance or spatial reversal learning. There have been reports (e.g., Rosenstock, Field, and Greene 1977; Béracochéa, Alaoui-Bouarraqui, and Jaffard 1989) of disruption of spatial memory tasks by mammillary body lesions, but there is little to suggest that the deficits that have been found are specific to spatial tasks; moreover, Jarrard et al. (1984) have reported that damage to the mammillary bodies did not disrupt preoperatively acquired radial-maze performance.

The entorhinal cortex is a major source of input to the hippocampus and forms part of both the Papez circuit and the hippocampal trisynaptic pathway; the subicular complex is the target of the trisynaptic pathway and (as the site of origin of the fornical efferents to the mammillary bodies) properly a part of the Papez circuit also. Thus if either the Papez circuit or the trisynaptic pathway must be intact to allow efficient spatial processing, damage to either of those cortical regions would be expected to disrupt spatial performance. There is evidence to support this expectation. Olton, Walker, and Gage (1978) reported that entorhinal cortical damage produced a permanent and severe disruption of preoperatively acquired radial-maze performance; similarly, Jarrard (1983) found disruption of radial-maze performance following destruction of subicular cells by injections of the neurotoxin, kainic acid.

In summary, some but not all the components of both the limbic system and the Papez circuit do appear to be necessary for efficient spatial processing; and although damage to either the input to or the output from the trisynaptic pathway (and damage to the hippocampus itself) disrupts spatial learning, structures outside that pathway are also necessary. These findings neither strengthen nor weaken the case for there being a system for spatial processing that is centered on the hippocampus. But there is one body of evidence that does pose serious problems for the notion that the hippocampus enjoys a primary role in spatial processing (and, indeed, in cognitive processing in general), and early warning of that evidence, which will be introduced in more detail in chapter 8, must be given here.

Jarrard has claimed that the effects of hippocampal damage caused by conventional techniques such as aspiration and electrolytic lesions are different in important respects from those obtained by neurotoxic lesions that destroy cells whose somata lie in the vicinity of the injection site, but do not destroy fibers of passage passing through that region. Jarrard's reservations extend even to work carried out with the neurotoxin kainic acid, since there is evidence that kainic acid may cause cellular damage at sites far removed from the injection site (e.g., Jarrard 1983). We shall see that Jarrard's recent work suggests that neither of the cortical regions critically involved in the input and output of the hippocampus—the subiculum and the entorhinal cortex—are necessary for efficient radial-maze performance (Bouffard and Jarrard 1988); not only that, but in rats given preoperative training, extensive neurotoxic damage of the hippocampus itself (including the dentate gyrus) does not prevent efficient maze performance (Jarrard 1986). Jarrard's work involves variations of the conventional radial maze that allow assessment of the contributions of different types of memory to performance, and so is best further discussed in chapter 8, after various proposals concerning a potential role of the hippocampus in specific types of memory have been introduced.

Spatial Processing and the Frontal Cortex

When deficits in spatial learning have been reported following damage to limbic forebrain structures associated with the hippocampus, those deficits have shown broad parallels to those reported following hippocampal damage. There is, however, a forebrain structure that does not belong to the limbic system (but has strong connections with it), damage to which causes selective deficits in spatial learning and memory that differ in important ways from those obtained by hippocampal damage. The structure in question is the dorsolateral frontal neocortex.

Frontal Cortex: Anatomy

Discussion of the functional role of the dorsolateral frontal cortex may be placed in context by giving a brief introduction to the anatomy of frontal neocortex (an excellent detailed discussion of frontal anatomy and physiology is to be found in Goldman-Rakic 1987; see also Pandya and Seltzer 1982). The work introduced here is based almost exclusively on data from primates, although there are data (summarized in Macphail 1982) to suggest parallels in both anatomy and function between frontal cortex in primates and other mammals.

The frontal lobes occupy the hemispheric surface anterior to the central sulcus. They consist of primary motor cortex, premotor cortex, and the (oddly named) prefrontal cortex: in primates (but not in other mammals) the prefrontal region is distinguished by a prominent layer of granule cells (layer 4) and is therefore sometimes known as frontal granular cortex. The prefrontal region of primary interest here is the dorsolateral frontal cortex, which in turn shows a number of subdivisions and, in particular, includes the lips and banks of the sulcus principalis. Figure 7.3 shows the locations of the major regions of interest in the monkey frontal lobes.

Prefrontal cortex receives sensory input from all the major senses but, as is the case with the hippocampus, that input derives not from primary sensory cortex nor from first-order parasensory association cortex: it derives from second-order parasensory association cortex and from multimodal association cortex. The implication, as for the hippocampus, is that the role of prefrontal cortex concerns highly processed information. Like the hippocampal formation, prefrontal cortex not only receives projections from association areas but feeds back projections to those same areas.

Prefrontal cortex also receives direct thalamic input from at least three thalamic nuclei: the dorsomedial nucleus (long thought to be the only source of thalamic input to prefrontal cortex), the anterior nucleus, and the medial pulvinar nucleus (which receives visual input both directly from the retina and indirectly, via the superior colliculus). All three nuclei project extensively throughout prefrontal cortex, and in each case there is a topographical organization, so that different subdivisions of the nuclei project to different regions within prefrontal cortex. For example, the medial division of the dorsomedial nucleus, which receives input from primary olfactory cortex, projects to orbitofrontal cortex; the lateral division projects to lateral prefrontal regions.

The projection from the anterior nucleus (part of the Papez circuit) is only one of many connections, direct and indirect, of prefrontal cortex

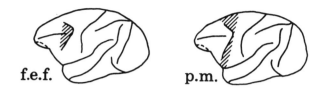

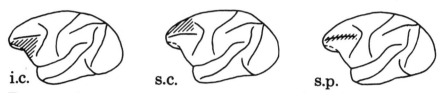

FIGURE 7.3. Locations of subdivisions of the frontal lobes in macaque monkey brain: p.m. = premotor cortex; f.e.f. = frontal eyefields; s.p. = sulcus principalis; s.c. = superior prefrontal convexity; i.c. = inferior prefrontal convexity. (*From* Passingham 1985b)

with limbic structures: the dorsolateral frontal cortex, for example, shows reciprocal connections with the hippocampal formation. There are reciprocal connections also between prefrontal cortex and the cingulate gyrus, and extensive interconnections with what Pandya and Seltzer (e.g., 1982) call "paralimbic" cortex—cortex, typically not true neocortex but transitional cortex, that shows direct connections with limbic structures.

The multiple projections to prefrontal cortex from diverse sensory association areas remain largely (but not exclusively) segregated in the frontal cortex, so that Goldman-Rakic sees the prefrontal cortex as "organized into separate territories defined by higher order inputs originating in primary sensory cortices" (1984:425). The dorsolateral frontal cortex receives a massive projection from posterior parietal association cortex, both from regions that are unimodal visual association cortex, and from regions that are unimodal somatosensory association cortex. Damage to parietal association areas in humans leads to marked disturbances of visuo-spatial function, and to disorders of body image including unilateral neglect from contralateral hemispheric damage: similar (but less severe) deficits are seen in monkeys following comparable damage (Hyvärinen 1982; Pandya and Yeterian 1984). The nature of cortical input to dorsolateral frontal cortex is therefore congruent with the notion that that region of prefrontal cortex may play a particular role in spatial processing. But the principal support for that notion derives from results obtained in lesion studies.

Learning and Memory Following Frontal Damage

Spatial Delayed Response and Delayed Alternation

It was Jacobsen who, more than fifty years ago, reported that extensive frontal lesions in primates led to severe disruption of spatial delayed-response performance (e.g., Jacobsen, Wolfe, and Jackson 1938). Typical versions of this task use the WGTA. An animal is shown the concealment of a reward under one of two identical plaques, one of which is to the left of the animal, the other to its right. An opaque screen is then lowered for, say, 5 sec, and when it is raised, the animal is allowed to select one of the two plaques. Successful performance requires, then, that the animal remembers which of the two locations, left or right, contained the reward.

A second task that has consistently been shown to be disrupted by frontal lesions is spatial delayed alternation, in which the correct spatial location on a given trial is that not rewarded on the preceding trial: in this case, again, successful performance requires the animal to remember which location contained reward (on the preceding trial).

Subsequent work has shown that these deficits are obtained only from lesions that involve damage to the sulcus principalis; lesions elsewhere in the prefrontal cortex do not selectively disrupt delayed response or spatial delayed alternation (e.g., Butters and Pandya 1969; Goldman et al. 1971). Indeed, there is evidence that the critical locus for these deficits is the middle third of the sulcus principalis (Butters and Pandya 1969).

The behavioral disruption obtained by sulcus principalis lesions is remarkably specific. The lesions have no effect on acquisition of discriminations based on visual, auditory, or tactile cues; nor do they affect acquisition of spatial discriminations (frontal monkeys can, then, learn as readily as normals consistently to select one of two spatial locations). And although conditional discrimination performance may be disrupted by damage elsewhere in the prefrontal cortex (e.g., Petrides 1985), sulcus principalis lesions have caused little or no disruption of conditional discrimination learning in a variety of tasks (e.g., Petrides 1982, 1985).

Jacobsen interpreted his findings in terms of a disruption by frontal lesions of "immediate memory." But it has become clear that this account requires modification, since monkeys with sulcus principalis lesions are able to perform normally in tasks that appear to involve immediate memory provided only that the information to be retained does not concern spatial location.

Nonspatial Tasks Involving Delays

Although monkeys with sulcus principalis lesions cannot acquire spatial delayed alternation, they can successfully perform in nonspatial delayed-alternation tasks (e.g., Goldman et al. 1971; Mishkin and Pribram 1955). Goldman et al. (1971) explored retention of a preoperatively acquired go/no-go alternation task in which a single location was used. Reward was available on alternate trials, and in such a procedure monkeys learn to make or to withhold responses depending upon the outcome—reward or nonreward—of the preceding trial. Sulcus principalis lesions had no effect on performance although the delay between trials was the same (5 sec) as that used in a spatial delayed-alternation task, retention of which was severely disrupted by smaller sulcus principalis lesions (Butters and Pandya 1969). Mishkin and Manning (1978) have, similarly, reported that sulcus principalis lesions have minimal effect on retention of a (difficult) object-alternation task in which the object (of two presented) that concealed reward was that which had not concealed reward on the preceding trial. The positions of the objects were varied from trial to trial and were irrelevant, and the delay between trials was, again, 5 sec.

Mishkin and Manning (1978) also reported that retention of delayed-matching tasks that involved visual cues was little affected by sulcus principalis lesions: in a color-matching task, animals had to remember over a 5-sec delay whether red or green had been displayed on a central sample key; an object-matching task required subjects to remember over the same delay which of two objects had been presented as a sample. A final example of successful nonspatial memory performance in monkeys with sulcus principalis lesions concerns 1-trial object-recognition memory. The task involves the use of a large pool of objects, each of which is seen on only one trial. In phase 1 of each trial, a novel object is shown over a central food well, and the monkey finds a reward on displacing the object. In phase 2, that object and an entirely new object are placed over two lateral food wells, and the monkey can obtain reward by selecting the object not presented in phase 1 (a DNMTS procedure). Monkeys with extensive dorsolateral frontal cortex damage are capable of normal performance in this task (Bachevalier and Mishkin 1986).

It seems, then, that sulcus principalis lesions disrupt performance only in tasks in which spatial information is involved. But it is clear that not all spatial tasks are disrupted. We have already seen that acquisition of spatial discriminations is not disrupted by sulcus principalis lesions. And there are reports also of successful performance in more difficult tasks having a spatial component. In an experiment of Rosenkilde, Rosvold, and Mishkin (1980), for example, monkeys learned a conditional discrimination in which the correct spatial response (left versus right) depended on the duration of the preceding intertrial interval (which might be 10 or 30 sec).

The work reviewed this far supports the generalization of Goldman et al. (1971) that deficits following sulcus principalis lesions are seen only in tasks that involve both a spatial factor and a delay factor. This in turn suggests that the sulcus principalis may be involved in a modality-specific immediate memory store.

Representation of Specific Visuo-Spatial Information in Frontal Cortex

Evidence that directly supports the notion that specific representational information may be maintained in the prefrontal cortex is provided by electrophysiological and lesion studies of Goldman-Rakic and her colleagues, using an oculomotor delayed-response task. Monkeys were trained to fixate a central test spot while a target (a small white square) was projected briefly (for .5 sec) at one of eight locations in the monkey's peripheral visual field. To obtain a reward of sweetened water, monkeys were required to maintain fixation of the central spot during a delay period (of 1 to 6 sec), and then to make a saccade to the locus at which the target had appeared. This task therefore required short-term memory for a specific location in visual space. Funahashi, Bruce, and Goldman-Rakic (1989) recorded the activity of 288 cells in the sulcus principalis during performance of this task. Eighty-seven of the cells showed a systematic change in activity (either an increase or a decrease in the resting level) during delay periods; of these cells, 69 showed a delay-related change only when the target had appeared in a specific part of the visual field; most of these cells responded maximally when the target had appeared in the contralateral visual field. These findings suggest a role for sulcus principalis cells in maintaining a representation of visual loci during a delay period. Further evidence for this proposal is provided by lesion studies that have shown that unilateral sulcus principalis lesions, which did not disrupt the accuracy of eye movements that were initiated immediately a peripheral target appeared, did disrupt performance in the delayed version of the task (Funahashi, Bruce, and Goldman-Rakic 1989). The effect of these lesions was specific to locations in restricted regions of the visual

field: deficits were found for contralateral locations only, and when small
unilateral lesions were used, for specific subdivisions (e.g., upper versus
lower) of the visual field.

Cells in the neighboring frontal eye fields (so-called because, as has
been known since the nineteenth century, stimulation there obtains eye
movements that resemble voluntary saccades) showed similar electrophysiological properties, and unilateral frontal eye field lesions also disrupt
eye movements toward remembered target locations (Deng et al. 1986).
Goldman-Rakic (1987) suggests that the frontal eye fields may in this
respect be subordinate to sulcus principalis, playing a motor role in initiating eye movements toward targets whose location is remembered by the
visuo-spatial short-term memory store located in sulcus principalis.

Two questions arise from the conclusion that sulcus principalis contains
a modality-specific short-term memory store. The first is, to what extent
do these findings suggest that the processing of spatial information is qualitatively different from that of nonspatial information? The second is,
should the spatial system suggested by these findings be identified with
the spatial mapping system that, according to O'Keefe and Nadel (1978),
has its principal representation in the hippocampus?

Spatial Versus Nonspatial Processing in Frontal Cortex

Insofar as the deficits obtained by sulcus principalis lesions appear to be
specific to spatial information, the clear implication is that that information is processed independently of nonspatial information. But there is no
necessary implication that nonspatial information is processed in a way
different from spatial information: it has been suggested, for example, that
damage to different sites within prefrontal cortex disrupts short-term retention of information from different modalities (Goldman-Rakic 1987).
According to this view, there are multiple short-term memory stores
within prefrontal cortex, each performing similar functions on different
types of information. If this account of prefrontal function is valid, then
we need not assume a special status for spatial information, a status that
might lead us to expect that the laws of spatial learning might differ substantially from those of nonspatial learning. There is, however, little direct
support for this suggestion.

Multiple Short-Term Memory Stores in Frontal Cortex?

Goldman-Rakic suggests that the inferior frontal convexity is "concerned
with memory for visual features such as form, color, or with other non-

spatial aspects of the stimulus rather than with the spatial position of stimuli" (Goldman-Rakic 1987:401). In support of this view, Goldman-Rakic cites both anatomical and lesion evidence. There are orderly projections from anterior inferotemporal cortex to the inferior convexity, and inferotemporal cortex is an important visual association area. There are, then, reasons for supposing that the inferior convexity is well-placed to analyze visual information. And lesions of the inferior convexity do disrupt tasks involving short-term retention of visual stimuli irrespective of their spatial location, such as DMTS for objects and colors—tasks that are immune to sulcus principalis damage (e.g., Mishkin and Manning 1978). There are, however, good reasons to doubt the attribution of the lesion-induced deficits to a disruption of visual memory. This is largely because lesions of the inferior convexity also disrupt nonvisual tasks, such as auditory go/no-go discrimination, spatial alternation, and spatial reversal learning (Iversen and Mishkin 1970). The deficits obtained by Iversen and Mishkin appeared to reflect an exaggeration of perseverative responding; for example, in the auditory go/no-go task (a task that did not involve short-term memory), the deficit of the monkeys with inferior convexity lesions consisted in persistent overresponding to the negative stimulus. Such observations led Mishkin and Manning to caution that, despite the deficit seen in visual memory tasks, "it would be premature to conclude from this that the lesion affected nonspatial visual memory processes per se" (Mishkin and Manning 1978:321).

A similar argument may be applied to data reported by Passingham (1978) concerning lesions of the superior frontal convexity—the region of dorsolateral frontal cortex lying medial and dorsal to the sulcus principalis. Although these lesions disrupted performance in a task in which monkeys had to remember (and to reproduce) the number of key-tapping responses (one or five) that they had made prior to keylight offset, there was no conclusive evidence that it was the *memory* demands of the task that were responsible for the deficit. Animals with superior convexity lesions showed an impairment with a 0-sec delay that was as marked as the impairment found with delays of up to 5 sec. All that may safely be concluded is that the superior convexity is involved with the analysis of information about movements.

The failure to find modality-specific memory stores for nonspatial information in the prefrontal cortex lends support, then, to the notion that the analysis of spatial information may indeed proceed in a way that differs qualitatively from the way in which spatial information is processed.

Sulcus Principalis and Hippocampus: Components of the Same System?

The most direct way to approach the question whether the spatial system implied by frontal deficits is the same as that implied by hippocampal deficits is to ask to what extent the effects of sulcus principalis lesions are comparable to those of hippocampal lesions. At this point we meet the problem that whereas most research on frontal damage has involved primates, the majority of research on effects of hippocampal damage has involved rats. Some of the best support for the O'Keefe and Nadel proposal was provided by evidence of severe disruption of maze learning by hippocampal damage in rats. Understandably, locomotor maze-learning studies in primates have been rare, and we do not know what effect either frontal or hippocampal damage would have in them. We can, however, make a beginning by asking whether the rat possesses cortical regions that are comparable to primate dorsolateral frontal cortex and whether damage to such regions does impair maze learning.

Rat Frontal Cortex and Maze Learning

It was originally believed that rats did not possess any structures that corresponded to primate prefrontal cortex. But Leonard (1969) showed that the rat dorsomedial thalamic nucleus does project to two regions of neocortex (now generally known as the medial and the ventral frontal cortex: Kolb 1986), and proposed that those areas corresponded to the primate prefrontal cortex, the cortical target of dorsomedial thalamic afferents in primates. The pattern of connectivity of the rat medial frontal cortex (with both the dorsomedial nucleus and other brain regions) supports the notion that it may be, if not homologous, then at least analogous to the primate dorsolateral frontal cortex (for a review and discussion of the relevant anatomical issues, see Kolb 1986). The anatomical parallels are supported by functional parallels: spatial delayed response and spatial delayed alternation are severely disrupted by medial (but not by ventral) frontal lesions in rats (Kolb 1986).

The parallels between rat medial frontal and primate dorsolateral frontal cortex indicate the potential relevance to primate dorsolateral frontal function of studies on rat medial frontal cortex. Of primary interest here is the effect of such lesions on maze learning, and the results obtained are unequivocal: medial frontal lesions in rats disrupt performance in conventional alley mazes, in the Morris water maze, and in the radial maze (Kolb

1986). The implication would seem to be that the spatial system disrupted by dorsolateral frontal cortical lesions in primates would—if the appropriate tests were conducted in primates—be found to be involved in maze learning. Unfortunately, this conclusion is not as helpful as might be supposed. The problem is that we have been interested in the primate work in one small subdivision of dorsolateral frontal cortex—the sulcus principalis. The analogy established between primate and rat brain concerns the entire dorsolateral frontal cortex and the rat medial frontal cortex: there are no data that allow us to determine which (if any) division of rat medial frontal cortex might correspond to primate sulcus principalis. Moreover, we do know that damage to divisions of dorsolateral frontal cortex other than sulcus principalis may severely affect performance in certain learning tasks, although having no effect of delayed spatial tasks. Damage to the superior frontal convexity does not disrupt delayed-response performance (Passingham 1975); but we have seen that superior frontal damage did disrupt performance in a task in which correct performance required retention of the number of key-tapping responses made (Passingham 1978).

There are in fact data that do suggest that although medial frontal lesions do disrupt maze learning in rats, the nature of that disruption differs from the disruption obtained by hippocampal damage and may not be a specifically spatial disruption. Winocur and Moscovitch (1990), for example, trained rats in two versions of a Hebb-Williams maze (different versions of this maze may be made by altering the positions of barriers within a square arena). One maze, Maze A, was learned initially and the second maze, Maze B, after a 30-day interval. Both hippocampal and medial frontal rats were, as would be anticipated, impaired on acquisition of Maze A. Following the 30-day interval, hippocampal rats learned Maze B at the same rate as they were relearning Maze A; they had, then, retained from their earlier training no information specific to Maze A. However, hippocampal rats that had received prior training in Maze A learned Maze B (and relearned Maze A) with fewer errors than hippocampal rats in a condition in which initial training on Maze A was not given. This latter finding indicates that hippocampal rats did benefit from their previous experience in Maze A, but the fact that they showed no fewer errors in relearning of Maze A than in learning Maze B indicates that they had retained nonspecific information appropriate to learning any maze of that type—they had, then, learned and retained some general maze-learning strategy or skill.

Rats with medial frontal lesions showed a quite different pattern of results. They relearned Maze A with many fewer errors than they learned

Maze B: they had, then, unlike the hippocampal rats, retained information that was specific to Maze A. But the performance of frontal rats on Maze B was similar whether or not they had learned Maze A thirty days previously. The frontal rats showed, then, no evidence of either acquisition or retention of a generalizable rule appropriate to different versions of the maze. A deficit in general rule-learning does not seem likely to be responsible for spatial delayed-response deficit, given the specificity of that deficit to spatial information: frontal animals appear quite able to master the rules of nonspatial tasks that differ only in the modality of the information that is relevant to their solution. It may therefore be the case that the deficit seen in the maze learning of frontal rats is independent of the frontal delayed-response deficit seen in both monkeys and rats.

The distinction between specific and nonspecific information that emerges from the Winocur and Moscovitch (1990) report will find an echo in chapter 8 in the distinction that will be introduced there between declarative and procedural knowledge. For present purposes, the results of that report serve to strengthen the argument that the deficits seen in rats with medial frontal lesions on spatial delayed tasks may be independent of those seen on maze-learning tasks and that monkeys with sulcus principalis lesions would not necessarily be expected to show deficits on maze-learning tasks.

Do Frontal Monkeys Show a Generalized Spatial-Learning Deficit?

Although no studies have been conducted using frontal monkeys in complex locomotor mazes, Passingham (1985a) has reported the use of a task devised by Collin et al. (1982) that is formally analogous to the radial maze. The monkey is faced with a board on which there is an array of 25 small doors, each of which covers a food well. The doors are sprung so that, following their being moved by the animal, they return to their original position over a well when they are released. At the beginning of a trial, all 25 wells contain a peanut, and the trial ends when the monkey has obtained all the peanuts. As in Olton's radial maze, efficient performance requires memory for locations already visited. Monkeys with sulcus principalis lesions showed a severe disruption in this task, whereas performance of monkeys with lesions of the superior frontal convexity did not differ significantly from that of controls (Passingham 1985a). This finding confirms once again, and in a novel setting, the conclusion that sulcus principalis lesions disrupt short-term retention of information about spatial locations. But it does not necessarily imply that performance in all types of maze would, as happens with hippocampal damage, be disrupted. For performance in conventional alley mazes and in the standard version of the Morris water maze does not require short-term retention of spatial information acquired within a trial—information that differs from one phase of a trial to another, and which must be erased or lost before the start of a new trial. For that reason, these tasks are conventionally known as "reference memory" tasks, while the Olton radial maze is known as a "working memory" task (a distinction that will be further discussed in chapter 8). Hippocampal rats show disruption of all types of maze learning, congruent with O'Keefe and Nadel's claim that they suffer from a loss of a general spatial mapping system. Even if we assume, as seems reasonable on the basis of Passingham's work, that monkeys with sulcus principalis lesions would show deficits on a locomotor radial maze, we need not assume that deficits would be found in mazes that impose demands on reference memory as opposed to working memory.

We have, therefore, arrived at something of an impasse in our consideration of the potential effects of sulcus principalis lesions on maze learning: frontal damage in rats does disrupt maze learning, but the disruption may be due to damage to some area other than that which corresponds to monkey sulcus principalis; sulcus principalis damage in primates does disrupt performance in an analogue of the radial maze, but there is no certainty that performance in other types of maze would be disrupted. There is, moreover, at least one example of the lack of disruption by frontal damage of a task that is arguably spatial in nature, does not involve delays, and is disrupted following hippocampal damage. The task in question is that used by Rupniak and Gaffan (1987), in which monkeys learned to make an approach response for reward in the presence of one stimulus and a withdrawal response for reward in the presence of another. Animals with fornix transections showed, as previously noted, severe disruption in this task: animals with sulcus principalis lesions performed normally.

Delayed Spatial Learning in Hippocampal Monkeys

We have seen that the evidence currently available does not allow any confident conclusion on the question whether sulcus principalis lesions disrupt spatial learning in as general a way as do hippocampal lesions. We may now pursue the question of the comparability of the deficits induced by prefrontal and hippocampal damage by asking whether hippocampal lesions in primates have effects on delayed spatial tasks comparable to those of sulcus principalis lesions.

Investigations of delayed-response performance in monkeys have generally agreed that at short delay intervals hippocampal lesions do not disrupt performance, but that deficits may be seen when longer delays are used. Zola-Morgan and Squire (1985), for example, found that monkeys with lesions that caused extensive damage to both the hippocampus and the amygdala showed normal acquisition of a delayed-response task using an 8-sec delay; their performance was, however, poorer than that of normal controls when the delay was increased to 15 or 30 sec. Monkeys with sulcus principalis lesions typically perform at chance levels when minimal delays (5 sec or less) are used (as a result of which it has proved difficult to show that the frontal impairment in delayed response varies as a function of delay: Passingham 1985a). Bachevalier and Mishkin (1986), for example, showed that monkeys with dorsolateral frontal cortex lesions learned as rapidly as normals to select a food well that they had just seen being baited; but when an opaque screen was lowered momentarily between them and the food wells (yielding an effective delay of less than 1 sec) performance fell to chance.

There have been few investigations of spatial delayed alternation in hippocampal monkeys, and although disruptions in performance following dorsolateral frontal damage have been reported (Mahut 1971), Waxler and Rosvold (1970) found that whereas some monkeys with total hippocampal removal showed deficits in spatial delayed alternation (with a 5-sec intertrial interval), others showed normal performance.

Conclusion: Spatial Mapping and the Prefrontal Cortex

We have seen that monkeys with hippocampal damage do show some disruption in the tasks most susceptible to sulcus principalis damage—delayed response and delayed alternation. But this disruption, particularly in the case of the classic delayed-response deficit, seems so much less severe that it may seem plausible to infer a different cause. We have seen also that there is currently no conclusive evidence that sulcus principalis damage has an effect on spatial learning in general comparable to that of hippocampal damage. Finally, it will be well to note that sulcus principalis deficits do appear to be restricted to spatial tasks, whereas, as we have already seen, hippocampal damage disrupts a variety of nonspatial tasks (a point that will be further emphasized in chapter 8).

These results provide little support for the notion that the deficits seen following sulcus principalis damage and those following hippocampal damage are due to disruption of the same functional system. It is worth noting here also one important theoretical consequence of our ignorance concerning potential effects of sulcus principalis lesions on maze-learning tasks, which is, that we need not assume that the spatial tasks on which deficits have been found involve the locale as opposed to the taxon system. Both the delayed-response and the delayed-alternation task can perfectly well be performed using egocentrically based responses such as choose left or choose right (as opposed to choosing different places). In other words, although sulcus principalis lesions obtain deficits in certain spatial tasks, there is currently no reason to suppose that those tasks involved the use of a spatial map in normals. It remains possible that the hippocampus does contain a spatial map, and that the deficits seen in monkeys with sulcus principalis damage reflect disruption of a system very different from the locale system that, according to O'Keefe and Nadel, is to be found in the hippocampus.

Final Comments: Contextual Learning in Hippocampal Humans and in Slugs

The principal focus of this chapter has been on the spatial map hypothesis of hippocampal function proposed by O'Keefe and Nadel (1978). We have seen that although a large body of experimental work has produced results consonant with the theory, there have been also findings that are not easily reconciled with it. Not all spatial tasks are disrupted by hippocampal damage; some tasks that do not appear to be spatial are disrupted; and hippocampal animals are surprisingly sensitive to contextual change. One further troublesome finding should also be introduced.

This book is concerned with neuronal mechanisms in animals, and so excludes detailed consideration of human data. But much of the impetus for the current interest in the hippocampus derives from the dramatic effect of hippocampal damage on memory in humans. It is appropriate here to ask whether human amnesics with hippocampal damage appear to have lost the capacity to use spatial maps. There are in fact many reports of difficulty by human amnesics in finding their way around the environment. But this difficulty is not specific to spatial information, since amnesics have equal difficulty in registering new nonspatial information. What is, however, pertinent here is the observation that amnesics do appear to be able to find their way around environments known to them prior to the onset of amnesia. A clear example of both the failure to learn novel locations and of retention of locations known prior to onset is provided by

H.M., the best-known case of a human rendered amnesic by hippocampal damage.

H.M.'s operation, which involved bilateral removal of most of the hippocampus and the amygdala, took place in 1953. In 1966, after attending hospital in Boston, he was asked for help in finding his house by the neuropsychologists who were driving him home. "He promptly and courteously indicated to us several turns, until we arrived at a street which he said was quite familiar to him. At the same time, he admitted that we were not at the right address. A phone call to his mother revealed that we were on the street where he used to live before his operation" (Milner, Corkin, and Teuber 1968:217). With instructions from H.M.'s mother, the neuropsychologists drove H.M. to his current home, but "he did not get his bearings until we were within two short blocks of the house, which he could just glimpse through the trees" (ibid.). It is also of interest to note that, at least in H.M.'s case, acquisition of novel spatial information, poor as it evidently is, may be if anything superior to acquisition of nonspatial information: Milner and her colleagues also reported that although H.M. could not describe his job after six months of working at it for five days a week, he could draw an accurate floor plan of the bungalow in which he now lived. It seems clear that H.M. still had access to a spatial map: he found difficulty in making new entries onto the map, but then he found at least as much difficulty (if not more) in making new entries into nonspatial memory stores. It does not, then, seem likely that the human hippocampus is necessary for spatial mapping.

The fact that the spatial map hypothesis cannot accommodate all the available data is a problem that it shares with all other current hypotheses. Reservations about the ability of the hypothesis to provide a complete account of hippocampal function should not obscure the fact that spatial learning does appear to be, for whatever reason, particularly susceptible to hippocampal (and to sulcus principalis) damage. This in turn should alert behavioral psychologists to the possibility that spatial information may not be processed in the same way as nonspatial information. And, indeed, the physiological work has stimulated novel behavioral work targeted at exploring that very possibility: Chamizo and her colleagues, for example, have reported behavioral studies designed explicitly to test the O'Keefe and Nadel proposal that spatial and nonspatial information are processed independently (Chamizo, Sterio, and Mackintosh 1985; Chamizo and Mackintosh 1989). The fact that there is currently widespread interest among behavioral psychologists in contextual learning (e.g., Balsam and Tomie 1985) reflects a general belief that our understanding of how contextual information is processed is currently inadequate and that theoretical accounts of learning may require substantial modification as that understanding progresses.

One final point refers back to chapter 4, which reported that context-specific learning had been demonstrated in *Aplysia*. It will be recalled that this finding led to serious difficulties for Kandel's account of association formation in *Aplysia*, an account that is readily applicable only to discrete CSs. It may, then, be that different physiological mechanisms underlie learning involving contextual versus discrete stimuli in *Aplysia*. Such a conclusion would further support the notion that there is a fundamental difference between the processing of contextual and other information, and so indirectly encourage those who believe that, despite the difficulties cited here, the hippocampus does play a role in contextual processing.

8. The Fractionation of Memory

Memory in Animals

This chapter shares with the preceding chapter the theme of seeking insights into the structure of (nonhuman) animal intelligence from breakdowns induced by telencephalic damage. In common with chapter 7, chapter 8 will focus primarily on the analysis of hippocampal damage. But whereas chapter 7 explored the notion that contextual and noncontextual information might be processed in different ways, chapter 8 will consider evidence that telencephalic damage affects memory processes, an approach that is in tune with the major effect of hippocampal damage apparent in humans.

Discussion of the various theories of hippocampal function that will be introduced in this chapter will include a number of references to memory disorders seen in humans. This chapter will not, however, survey systematically the human data, nor will there be any discussion of memory disorders induced in humans by extrahippocampal damage. There are two reasons for the relative lack of attention paid here to human findings. The first is that there already exist excellent surveys of human amnesic disorders (e.g., Parkin 1987; Squire 1987; Mayes 1988). The second and major reason, however, is that it is not clear that a detailed review of the human literature would necessarily be relevant to the main topic of this book—namely, the analysis of the cognitive processes of animals. For although it is clear (Macphail 1982) that there are extensive parallels among the cognitive processes observed in widely differing groups of non-human vertebrates, human cognition is, at least in this writer's view, distinguished from nonhuman cognition by the uniquely human capacity for language. The involvement of language in human memory processes seems likely to be so basic that interpretations appropriate to at least some human memory disorders will be quite different from interpretations appropriate to any nonhuman disorder. Accordingly, only human material that seems directly relevant to the interpretation of the nonhuman material will be introduced in this chapter, and the material that is introduced will not be subjected to detailed analysis but used instead to point rather generally to potential parallels between animal and human neurological function.

Memory in animals was a topic that attracted little attention during the long domination of comparative psychology by monolithic theories of learning. It has, however, enjoyed a considerable renaissance in recent decades, inspired perhaps by the evident success of cognitive psychologists' investigations of human memory (Macphail 1986). This has had the consequence that animal psychologists have imported into their theorizing concepts originally introduced by cognitive psychologists. We saw an example of this in chapter 4—Wagner's proposal for a short-term memory store from which items could be displaced by the presentation of distractors. One of the two principal proposals to be discussed in this chapter is that the hippocampus is the site of a short- (or relatively short-) term memory store that is not modality-specific; the second proposal is that the hippocampus is involved in a system concerned with long-term retention of information that has in some sense been subjected to high-level cognitive processing, a system that can be differentiated from a simpler, less cognitive system concerned with the storage of a different type of information.

Both the distinction between a short-term and a long-term store and the distinction between cognitive versus noncognitive processing are concepts used by cognitive psychologists. But in each case the notion that there is a valid distinction remains controversial (e.g., Mayes 1988), so that successful analysis of nonhuman data could do more than confirm what cognitive psychologists already know: it could constitute an important contribution to some of the central debates in contemporary cognitive psychology.

Working Versus Reference Memory

The term "working memory" was originally introduced by Baddeley and Hitch (1974), who were attempting to tackle problems faced by the concept of a single human short-term memory store of the type envisaged by Broadbent (e.g., 1958). One of the major difficulties was the fact that there was surprisingly little interference between tasks performed simultaneously when both tasks were believed to employ short-term memory— between, for example, reasoning tasks and list-learning tasks (e.g., Hitch 1983). Baddeley and Hitch suggested that there may in fact be a number of relatively independent short-term memory stores having different properties, but that they could be thought of as slave systems subordinated to a single central executive system, known as working memory.

Behavioral work on short-term memory in animals has not yet achieved the sophistication of work on humans, and has not provided data relevant to a choice between a single short-term memory store and a number of short-term memory stores subjected to an overall executive. Accordingly, in considering animal work, the terms "short-term memory" and "working memory" are generally taken to be equivalent (e.g., Honig and Thompson 1978). For the purposes of the experiments to be considered in this chapter, an operational definition of working memory can be provided: working memory is used when "different stimuli govern the criterion response on different trials, so that the cue that the animal must remember varies from trial to trial" (Honig 1978:213). Information that is trial-specific and not relevant to other trials is, then, held in working memory. Reference memory in animals is regarded as being comparable to long-term memory in humans (e.g., Honig 1978) and is typically used for retention of information that is relevant to *all* the trials of a given task.

Hippocampus and Working Memory

Olton, Becker, and Handelmann (1979) have proposed that the hippocampus is necessary for working memory but not for reference memory. We shall examine relevant evidence here, bearing in mind the fact that should that evidence give good support to the proposal, the case for there being in mammals functionally independent working memory and reference memory stores would thereby be strengthened. The basic evidence for this suggestion comes from experiments that have investigated the effects of damage to the hippocampal system on tasks that are presumed to tap working memory.

Working Memory Tasks Disrupted by Hippocampal Damage

The Spatial Radial Maze

We may begin consideration of the working memory notion by discussing an experiment (introduced briefly in chapter 7) whose procedures serve also to illustrate the distinction between working memory and reference memory. Olton and Papas (1979) used a 17-arm radial maze. Nine (unbaited) arms of the maze never contained food, the other eight (baited) arms each contained food at the start of a trial. Since the location of unbaited arms did not change from trial to trial, learning to avoid unbaited arms was a reference memory procedure; but since choice of a baited arm that still contained food depended on memory for visits made within each trial, successful avoidance of baited arms that no longer contained food was a working memory procedure. Reference memory was therefore assessed by scoring (over the first eight choices of a trial) the probability of choice of an unbaited arm; working memory was assessed by scoring the probability of a correct response, given that the choice made was of a baited arm.

Olton and Papas (1979) trained rats preoperatively to a criterion of seven correct choices out of the first eight choices on ten consecutive daily trials; this required some thirty to fifty trials. The effect of fornicotomy was striking: over the first ten postoperative trials, performance on both working memory and reference memory components fell sharply, to approximately the same level as seen on the first ten trials of preoperative training. The fornix-lesioned rats showed, then, no postoperative savings on either measure. Performance on the reference memory component recovered, however, relatively rapidly—at about the same rate as original acquisition—so that, after fifty trials, avoidance of unbaited arms was comparable to terminal preoperative performance. But performance in the working memory component showed little recovery with further training and, for the two rats with the most extensive lesions, remained at approximately chance level throughout the fifty postoperative trials. The apparently permanent disruption of working memory contrasted with the transient disruption of reference memory and suggested, therefore, a critical involvement of the hippocampus in working memory.

A Nonspatial Radial Maze

To see whether the working memory deficit uncovered in the Olton and Papas (1979) study was specific to spatial information, Olton and Feustle (1981) designed a maze that required working memory for visual and tactile cues but in which spatial cues were irrelevant. The apparatus was a radial maze having four detachable arms, each of which was clearly discriminable from the others: the floor and walls of one arm, for example, were of rough wood painted white, while another arm showed a diamond pattern and was smooth. At the beginning of each trial, food was placed at the end of all four arms, and the animal was placed in the central area where doors prevented access to any arm. A trial began with the raising of all four doors and the animal had to make its first choice. The rat was then placed back in the central area, and the doors were lowered once more. Before the next choice was made, the positions of the arms were changed (unconsumed food remained in the arms not yet visited). The doors were once again raised, allowing a further choice. In this task, then, the rat had to remember which arms had been visited—the arms now being differentiated not by position (which was irrelevant) but by the sensory cues associated with them.

Rats found this task difficult in comparison with the standard (spatial) radial maze, but after some 45 trials did achieve the preoperative criterion (a mean of 3.8 correct out of the first four choices of a trial for ten consecutive trials). Following fornix damage, performance remained at chance through 60 postoperative trials. Thus, although spatial cues were irrelevant (and were minimized by running the experiment in dim light and by using high walls to the maze), performance was severely disrupted. Olton, Becker, and Handelmann (1979) argue that the results of this study, taken along with those of the Olton and Papas (1979) study, indicate that disruption of spatial radial-maze performance reflects an impairment of working memory, a memory system that is not restricted to spatial (or to any other type of) information.

Nonspatial Delayed Matching-to-Sample Tasks

Further support for the working memory hypothesis is provided by a study of Raffaelle and Olton (1988) that used the nonspatial DMTS procedure employed in the Wible et al. (1986) report (described in chapter 7); the goal-boxes used in this study were distinguished not only by brightness but also by tactile cues—the white goal-box had a smooth floor, and the black goal-box had strips of carpeting glued to the floor and walls. As in the Wible et al. report, each trial consisted of a sample phase in which only one (rewarded) goal-box was available, followed a few seconds later by a choice phase in which both boxes could be entered (but food remained available only in the same box used in the sample phase). However, since the positions of the two goal-boxes were changed in a pseudorandom fashion (both between sample and choice phases and between trials), successful performance depended on the rats remembering which goal-box had been entered during the sample phase rather than where that goal-box had been located. Following extensive preoperative training, all the rats were showing choice accuracy of 80 percent or better; however, following fornix damage, performance fell to chance level and remained there throughout the 400 trials of postoperative testing.

Spontaneous Alternation

Olton, Becker, and Handelmann (1979) found another source of support for the working memory hypothesis in the effects of hippocampal damage on spontaneous alternation. If a rat is run in a T-maze in which both goal-boxes invariably contain reward, it will tend to alternate choices between the goal-boxes; a number of reports agree that this alternation is attenuated or abolished following hippocampal damage (O'Keefe and Nadel 1978; Olton, Becker, and Handelmann 1979). Whatever the correct explanation of spontaneous alternation may be, it is clear that, in common with other alternation procedures, its occurrence depends on retention across the intertrial interval of information concerning the goal-box chosen on the preceding trial. Thus the disruption of spontaneous alternation by hippocampal damage is congruent with a working memory interpretation of hippocampal function (although it will be noticed that the deficit concerns a spatial task and could equally well be accommodated within the spatial map framework).

Perception of Time

The final set of experiments to be introduced in this section concern the effects of hippocampal damage on the perception of time, and are of importance not so much because they support the working memory hypothesis (although they do, albeit in a qualified way) as because of their own intrinsic interest. Two basic procedures—the peak-trial and gap-trial procedures—are of central concern; both procedures are relatively simple, and we shall illustrate them by considering a report by Olton, Meck, and Church (1987).

The Peak-Trial Procedure. There were three groups of rats in Olton, Meck, and Church's 1987 study. One group had fornix lesions; a second group, amygdalar lesions; and the third (control) group, sham operations. All the rats were trained preoperatively to press a lever in a discrete-trial procedure in which the beginning of a trial was signaled by the onset of a white-noise stimulus. On a random 50 percent of trials, responding in the presence of the white-noise stimulus was reinforced according to a fixed-interval schedule having a value of 50 sec; food reward was, then, delivered for the first lever-press that occurred more than 50 sec after white-noise onset. The other 50 percent of trials were peak trials, during which no reward was delivered and the white-noise stimulus terminated after 130 sec. The performance of interest at this stage of training was seen on the peak (nonreward) trials: the rats showed a response rate that gradually increased to reach a peak approximately 50 sec after trial onset; the rate then declined as the trial continued. This pattern of response is taken to reflect the fact that the rats (as a result of the schedule in force on the rewarded trials) had a maximal expectation of food 50 sec after stimulus onset.

The Gap-Trial Procedure. Following training on the peak-trial procedure, operations were carried out, and the animals were returned to peak-trial training for five sessions. A second type of nonreward trial (a gap trial) was then introduced. In gap trials, a (silent) gap was introduced at some point during the white-noise stimulus. The gap could occur either 5 or 10 sec after stimulus onset, and could be either .5 or 5 sec in duration. Previous work (e.g., Meck, Church, and Olton 1984) had shown that normal rats react to the intrusion of a gap by apparently stopping their (internal) clocks during the gap: their peak response is postponed by the duration of the gap and still occurs after the white-noise stimulus has been on for a cumulative time equivalent to the value of the fixed interval in force on rewarded trials (50 sec in the Olton, Meck, and Church study).

Effects of Fornix Lesions. The principal results of the experiment are summarized on figures 8.1 and 8.2, which show that the effects of the lesions were clear-cut. In peak trials, whereas both control and amygdalar animals showed a peak response rate approximately 50 sec following white-noise onset, fornix-lesioned rats showed peak response rates much earlier, at about 41 sec. On gap trials, control and amygdalar animals showed peak response rates at a point when the total stimulus duration (excluding the gap) was approximately 50 sec (in other words, they appeared successfully to stop their internal clocks and so to time accurately the time for which the white noise had been present). The fornix-lesioned rats, on the other hand, appeared to reset their internal clocks during the gap, since their peak response time occurred some 41 sec after the end of the gap, regardless of the duration of the gap or of its temporal position within the white-noise stimulus.

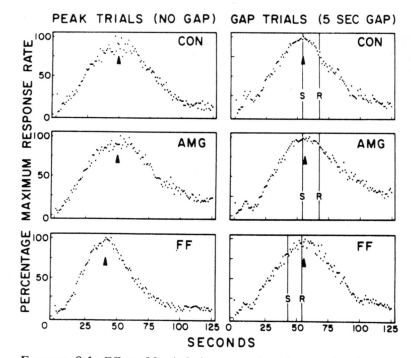

FIGURE 8.1. Effect of fornix lesions on peak- and gap-trial performance in the 1987 Olton, Meck, and Church study. The top two graphs show performance of the sham-operated controls in peak trials (left) and gap trials (right). The middle two graphs show performance of the group having amygdalar lesions; and the bottom graphs show performance of the fornicotomized group. On rewarded trials, food was delivered for the first response that occurred 50 sec or more after onset of the white-noise stimulus. For the gap trials, the white-noise stimulus was interrupted 10 sec after its original onset; the gap duration was 5 sec. The mean percentage of maximum response rate for mean responses per minute is plotted as a function of white-noise stimulus duration. The arrows indicate the observed peak time. The vertical lines labeled S and R indicate, respectively, the peak time expected if rats on gap trials stopped or reset their internal clocks. (*From* Olton, Meck, and Church 1987)

In considering the interpretation of these experiments, we shall begin with the effect of fornix damage on peak trials. Rats having fornix damage show peak response rates too early on such trials: they appear, then, to show maximal expectation of the arrival of food at a time considerably earlier than that at which food is actually delivered (on reward trials). This

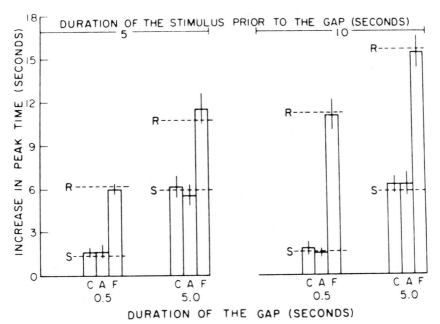

FIGURE 8.2. Mean (and standard error of the mean) increase in peak time during gap trials as compared to peak trials for the three groups in the 1987 Olton, Meck, and Church study. C = sham-operated controls; A = rats with amygdalar lesions; F = fornicotomized rats. The left and right sides present data from trials in which the white-noise stimulus duration prior to the gap was 5 and 10 sec, respectively. The horizontal dotted lines marked S indicate the results expected if rats stopped their internal clocks during the gap trials (an increase in peak time equal to the duration of the gap plus about 1 sec, an estimate of the latency to start timing after the gap). The horizontal lines marked R indicate the results expected if rats reset their internal clocks during the gap trials (an increase in peak time equal to the duration of the gap plus the 1-sec estimate of the latency to start timing after the gap plus the duration of the stimulus prior to the gap). (*From* Olton, Meck, and Church 1987)

problem does not reflect reduced sensitivity to temporal duration; when different values of fixed interval are used, fornicotomized rats show different peak times, each about 80 percent of the appropriate value (Meck 1988). There are psychophysical data also to show that fornix-damaged rats are as sensitive as normals in discriminations between CSs that differ in duration (Meck, Church, and Olton 1984). The fact that fornicotomized animals show normal sensitivity to stimulus duration suggests that the reason for their early peak response time must be that the remembered stimulus duration, stored in reference memory, is reduced (e.g., Meck, Church and Olton 1984).

The fact that control animals in the gap-trial procedure successfully stop their (internal) clocks without resetting them indicates that they retain across the gap a memory for the duration of the stimulus that preceded the gap: this clearly places demands on working memory, and the failure of fornix-lesioned rats to achieved this may well be interpreted as further evidence of disruption of working memory. The gap-trial procedure provides, then, evidence for disruption by hippocampal damage of a working memory that holds many different types of information—spatial, sensory, and temporal. It should, on the other hand, be remembered that the peak-trial procedure provided evidence for a disruption of reference memory also.

Summary

The principal support for Olton's hypothesis is derived from a series of experiments on rats: in radial mazes, fornicotomized rats reenter arms entered previously within a trial; spontaneous alternation in T-mazes and visual DMTS performance are disrupted by hippocampal damage; and fornicotomized rats fail to stop their internal clocks during gap trials. The disruptions obtained are severe and are found in tasks to which spatial information does not seem relevant. Inevitably, however, there are findings that are less easily accommodated by Olton's hypothesis, and we should now consider some of that contradictory evidence.

Difficulties for the Working Memory Hypothesis

The working memory hypothesis has two strands: the first, and most important, is that working memory is dependent upon an intact hippocampus; the second is that reference memory is not. In considering problems faced by the hypothesis, we shall discuss the latter strand first.

Some Reference Memory Tasks Are Disrupted by Hippocampal Damage

There are in the literature many reports of disruption by hippocampal damage of tasks that do not seem to involve any overt working memory component. We saw in chapter 7, for example, that both reversal learning and latent inhibition are disrupted by hippocampal damage; and we have seen in this chapter that rats show a deficit in the peak-trial procedure that implies a disruption of reference memory. Two further examples of disruption of reference memory will be introduced here, beginning with a consideration of the task that has provided the biggest single body of evidence of disruption by hippocampal damage of tasks that do not appear to involve working memory—namely, maze learning in rats.

Maze Learning

We have already noted the fact that Olton and Papas (1979) found no postoperative retention of the preoperatively acquired reference memory component of the radial-maze task. A more striking finding has been reported by Rasmussen, Barnes, and McNaughton (1989), who employed a simple procedure in which only one arm of an 8-arm radial maze contained food; the same arm contained food on every trial, so that the task was in effect a radial-maze task that tapped only reference memory. Rats with entorhinal cortex lesions were severely impaired in learning to select only the arm containing food (since the entorhinal cortex is the gateway for cortical input to the hippocampus, it may be assumed that its destruction leads to gross disturbance of normal hippocampal function). Entorhinal-lesioned rats showed no deficit in a similar task (that controls found more difficult) in which the correct arm was indicated, not by its spatial position (which varied at random from trial to trial) but by nonspatial (visual and tactile) cues. Since both of the tasks used by Rasmussen and colleagues were reference memory tasks, their results clearly support the spatial mapping as opposed to the working memory theory of hippocampal function.

There is in fact for most mazes other than the conventional radial maze no obvious reason why working memory should be involved in performance. In conventional alley mazes, the correct choice at a given junction is the same on all trials; similarly, in the Morris water maze, the location of the hidden platform is unchanged from trial to trial. Nevertheless, hippocampal damage disrupts performance in all but the simplest T- and Y- mazes. One possibility is that, although mazes conform to the formal definition of reference memory tasks, there may nevertheless be demands made upon working memory during maze learning. The existence of a covert working memory component in maze-learning could, of course, accommodate disruption of maze learning within the working memory theory of hippocampal function. Since Rawlins (1985) has in fact suggested a specific role for (a form of) working memory in maze learning, his suggestion should now be assessed.

Intermediate-Term Memory Involved in Maze Learning?

Rawlins's proposal, which amounts to a modification of working memory theory, is that the hippocampus contains, not a short-term memory store, but an intermediate-term store that is used in association formation to bridge a temporal gap between a relevant CS or response and a reinforcer. Rawlins suggests that maze learning is disrupted by hippocampal damage because "a hippocampectomized animal has a shorter span of memory for recent events, and so cannot build up an overall picture relating spatially (and hence, usually, temporally) discontiguous events to each other" (Rawlins 1985:495).

Sutherland and Rudy (1988) tested Rawlins's proposal in an experiment that minimized temporal demands in the Morris maze. In their experiment, control and hippocampal-damaged rats were trained initially to swim to a visible platform in the maze. When both groups had learned this easy task and were showing escape latencies of less than 3 sec, probe trials were introduced in which the visible platform was replaced by a hidden platform in the same location. Control rats readily found the hidden platform, but hippocampal-damaged rats showed the long latencies typically seen in such animals when a hidden platform is used in the Morris maze. It appears therefore that whereas the control rats had learned not simply to swim toward the visible platform but also its location, the hippocampal rats, although swimming rapidly to the appropriate place when the platform was visible, had learned nothing about the platform's location. It is hard to see that either the working memory or the intermediate-memory hypothesis can provide a satisfactory account of the maze-learning deficit obtained by Sutherland and Rudy (1988), and similarly unlikely that either proposal can account for the disruption of maze learning in general.

Configural Learning

A reference memory task that was severely disrupted by hippocampal damage was described in a report (Rudy and Sutherland 1989) that used a simple design. The task, sometimes called negative patterning discrimination, consisted in rewarding rats for pressing a lever in the presence of either a tone or a light stimulus, and not rewarding lever-pressing in the presence of a compound tone/light stimulus. Whereas control rats learned relatively rapidly to respond to either stimulus presented alone and not to respond to the compound, rats with extensive neurotoxic lesions of the hippocampus altogether failed to learn the discrimination. If trained preoperatively, hippocampal rats showed total loss of the discrimination and were unable to reacquire the appropriate pattern of response.

The Rudy and Sutherland (1989) report provides support for the hypothesis (Sutherland and Rudy 1989) that the hippocampus is essential for the formation of configural associations—associations that involve the recoding of representations of a number of discrete simple stimuli into a unique representation that captures the relationship between the stimuli. The predictions of this theory (as expounded in Sutherland and Rudy 1989) have much in common with those derived from O'Keefe and Nadel's spatial mapping theory (1978), so that configural theory faces many of the difficulties faced by the mapping theory. But a brief digression is in order here to point to two problems that are peculiar to configural theory, problems that derive from the fact that configural theory naturally expects disruption by hippocampal damage in most tasks involving compound stimuli.

The first problem is that configural theory expects disruption of blocking and overshadowing to follow hippocampal damage; this is so, according to Sutherland and Rudy, because: "Animals with hippocampal damage are unable to neutralize irrelevant cues" (1989:137). We have seen (in chapter 6), however, that hippocampal animals may in fact show normal performance in blocking and overshadowing paradigms.

The second problem is that there are studies using both monkeys (Saunders and Weiskrantz 1989) and rats (Whishaw and Tomie 1991; Gallagher and Holland 1992) that show that at least some forms of configural learning are immune to hippocampal damage. In the Saunders and Weiskrantz study, for example, monkeys with extensive hippocampal lesions had to learn to choose between two pairs of objects, one pair covering the left food well of a WGTA (Wisconsin General Test Apparatus), the other pair the right food well. A given object could be presented along with any of three other objects. Two identical versions of each of the four objects were available, and a set of discriminations was arranged so that each object appeared equally often as a member of a rewarded pair as of a nonrewarded pair. Thus, if the four objects are characterized as A, B, C, and D, the monkeys learned: AB+ vs. AC−; CD+ vs. BD−; AB+ vs. BD−; and CD+ vs. AC−. Accurate choice could not, therefore, be based upon selection of any one object: the reward value of an object depended upon the identity of the other object with which it was paired—upon, in other words, a compound or configural stimulus. The hippocampal monkeys nevertheless showed no deficit in acquiring the discrimination. Thus, although the Sutherland and Rudy (1989) report provides an example of a reference memory task that is susceptible to hippocampal damage, it is not clear that all configural tasks are similarly susceptible. It may be that the negative-patterning discrimination paradigm possesses some characteristic other than reliance upon configuration that renders it liable to disruption (although it is frankly difficult at present to speculate what that characteristic might be).

Not All Working Memory Tasks Are Disrupted by Hippocampal Damage

The preceding section marshaled evidence to show that at least some reference memory tasks are disrupted by hippocampal damage. But it remains possible that the working memory hypothesis is basically sound— that working memory *is* dependent upon an intact hippocampus, and that reference memory deficits reflect some other type of disruption induced by hippocampal damage. Is it, then, the case that all working memory tasks are disrupted by hippocampal damage? There is by now rather good evidence that this is not so, and the most convincing evidence comes from studies on DMTS and DNMTS tests in both monkeys and rats; but before discussing those studies, brief reference should be made to relevant work using other paradigms.

We saw in chapter 7 that delayed-response performance was little affected by hippocampal damage in primates unless long delays were involved. We saw also that the effects of hippocampal lesions on delayed alternation were inconsistent. And although there is good agreement that hippocampal damage in rats disrupts spontaneous alternation (in which all choices are rewarded), there is conflict in the literature concerning the effects of hippocampal damage on both go/no-go alternation (in which reward is available on alternate trials only) and spatial alternation (in which reward is available only for selection of the place not rewarded on the preceding trial). In his discussion of single-alternation studies in rats, Rawlins notes "the inconsistency of outcomes reported even when the experimental designs are almost identical" (Rawlins 1985:484). The fact, however, that in at least some studies rats with hippocampal damage have shown efficient performance on both go/no-go alternation (e.g., Cogan, Posey, and Reeves 1976) and spatial alternation (e.g., Jarrard 1975) clearly poses problems for the working memory theory. Finally, although Olton and Feustle (1981) found disruption by fornix lesions of a nonspatial version of the radial maze, Rasmussen, Barnes, and McNaughton

(1989), using a similar procedure, found no disruption following entor-hinal lesions, lesions that did result in disruption in a spatial radial-maze procedure.

DMTS and DNMTS Tasks: Monkey Studies

There is general agreement that monkeys with hippocampal damage show little or no deficit in conventional DMTS and DNMTS tasks in which visual stimuli are used, at least when relatively short (10 sec or so) delays are used (e.g., Gaffan 1974; Mishkin 1978; Owen and Butler 1984; Overman, Ormsby, and Mishkin 1990). Reports of the effects of hippocampal damage on DMTS and DNMTS tasks using longer delays have produced inconsistent outcomes and will be discussed further in the sections in which the recognition theory of hippocampal function is considered. But it is worth noting here that some reports find that monkeys with hippocampal damage show little or no deficit in visual matching (or non-matching) performance at relatively long delays (2 min and more) (e.g., Mishkin 1978; Owen and Butler 1984; Bachevalier, Saunders, and Mishkin 1985). And in a DNMTS task that was carried out in the dark and required tactile discrimination of objects, Murray and Mishkin (1984), using delays of up to 2 min, found that hippocampal damage had no effect on performance.

DMTS and DNMTS Tasks: Rat Studies

We have seen that the fornicotomized rats in the Raffaelle and Olton (1988) report showed severe disruption of visual DMTS, using delays of only a few seconds—a finding that contrasts with the immunity of short-delay matching in monkeys to hippocampal damage. There are, however, reports on both DMTS and DNMTS tasks in rats that agree with the monkey studies in finding no effect of hippocampal damage.

Aggleton, Hunt, and Rawlins (1986) used a Y-maze that consisted of three replaceable boxes, each of which could serve as both a start- and a goal-box. The boxes used were selected from a pool of 100 boxes, consisting of 50 pairs of identical boxes. Each pair was differentiated from all other pairs by a variety of visual and tactile cues, as well as by the presence in each box of some object, such as a plastic cup or a wooden block. At the beginning of a trial, the rat was placed in one of the boxes; of the other two boxes, one was identical to the start-box, while the other was drawn from a different pair. The rat was rewarded for choosing the goal-box that differed from the start-box. When an error occurred, the trial was repeated until the correct box was selected. The animals were confined in the correct goal-box for 20 sec, and that box then served as the start-box for the following trial. There were ten trials each day, so that a given pair of boxes was seen on average every fifth day of training; boxes were not reused within a session. This is, then, a running recognition task in which the rat has to select the goal-box that is novel (in the sense that the goal-box that matches the start-box is familiar owing to its being experienced as the start-box). Figure 8.3 summarizes the design of the trials.

Aggleton and colleagues reported that large hippocampal lesions had no effect on either acquisition or retention of their DNMTS task. The delay involved was, of course, minimal, although memory did appear to be involved since "previous observations have shown that rats rarely attempt to make a direct comparison of all 3 boxes" (Aggleton, Hunt, and Rawlins 1986:134).

Another version of the task explored the effect of increasing the delay. To achieve this, animals were again confined in the correct goal-box for 20 sec at the end of each trial; that box was then replaced by a blank featureless box in which the rat was confined for a further 20 or 60 sec.

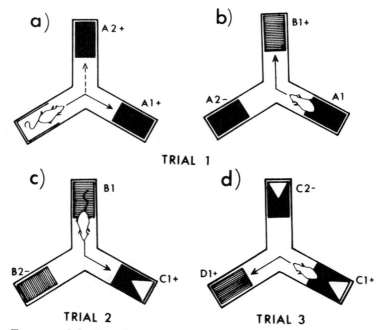

FIGURE 8.3. Representation of the delayed non-matching-to-sample procedure used by Aggleton and colleagues (1986). Arrows indicate direction of correct response. (*From* Aggleton, Blindt, and Rawlins 1989)

At the end of the 20- or 60-sec delay period, the rat was allowed to choose between two goal-boxes, one of which was identical to the box used at the beginning of the trial, the other of which was novel (to that session). Hippocampal damage had no effect on performance at either delay. Of interest also is the fact that a subsequent experiment, using the same animals, found that the hippocampal rats were severely impaired on a spatial DNMTS task in a T-maze, using a minimal delay. Aggleton and colleagues' 1986 report, then, is one that did find disruption of a spatial DNMTS task but nevertheless did not find disruption of a nonspatial DNMTS task using much longer delays. This pattern of outcomes is clearly extremely troublesome to any theory that supposes that the hippocampus is necessary for efficient short-term retention of all types of information.

Subsequent studies using similar designs have reinforced the findings of the Aggleton, Hunt, and Rawlins (1986) report. Rothblat and Kromer (1991), for example, tested fornicotomized rats in a DNMTS task with trial-unique objects and found no deficit at delays of up to 30 sec. Sutherland and McDonald (1990) used a design that differed slightly from that used by Aggleton and his colleagues in that only three different boxes were used, and rats were required to match to sample rather than to select the non-matching box: rats with neurotoxic hippocampal damage showed no impairment either in acquiring MTS or in responding appropriately after delays of up to 2 min.

An unusual type of DNMTS was investigated by Rasmussen, Barnes, and McNaughton (1989). In the sample phase of each trial, rats were given a forced run to one side of a Y-maze. In the choice phase, they were allowed to choose between two arms of the Y-maze, and the correct response was a body turn in the direction opposite to that experienced in the forced run. The location of the start arm was selected at random from trial to trial, so that the correct arm was sometimes the arm visited in the sample phase, and sometimes not. In other words, the problem could not be solved spatially by avoiding the place visited in the sample phase, but only by learning to turn (left or right) in the direction opposite to that of the forced-run turn (right or left). Rats with entorhinal lesions performed as efficiently as normals, even when delays of up to 60 sec were imposed between the forced run and the choice.

There are, then, examples of experiments on rats with hippocampal damage that have found no disruption in nonspatial DMTS and DNMTS designs. It should be added that the deficit seen in the Raffaelle and Olton (1988) report may not in any case have been due to the imposition in that experiment of a delay between the sample and the choice phases. Jagielo et al. (1990) found that rats with hippocampal lesions could not master a simultaneous nonspatial MTS task in which rats had to learn simply to select the arm (of a T-maze) that matched the start arm (which could be either black or white); since this task involved no delay, it appears that in some circumstances hippocampal rats cannot master MTS tasks. The deficit is clearly not general, as is shown by the successful performance of hippocampal rats in the DMTS and DNMTS tasks described above; but the Jagielo et al. result suggests that the deficit in DMTS observed by Raffaelle and Olton (1988) may have been due, not to a memory deficit, but to some demand imposed by the MTS requirement itself. The important question why rats sometimes do and sometimes do not show deficits in MTS and NMTS designs is one about which it is probably not helpful to speculate at present. What should be emphasized, however, is that when *spatial* DNMTS designs have been used, a hippocampal deficit is consistently observed in both rats (e.g., Rasmussen, Barnes, and McNaughton 1989) and monkeys (e.g., Murray et al. 1989). It appears that the evidence from MTS and NMTS procedures is therefore better accommodated by the spatial mapping theory than by the working memory theory.

Working Memory in Human Amnesics

A final difficulty for the working memory theory is posed by findings on human hippocampal amnesics: although these individuals do have serious difficulty in storing new information, they do not in general show any difficulty in retaining information for short periods of a few seconds or so, or, indeed, for as long as rehearsal is allowed (e.g., Sidman, Stoddard, and Mohr 1968). The conclusion generally drawn is that working memory in human amnesics is not defective. Just as human amnesics do not seem to have lost access to internalized spatial maps, so they do not seem to have lost working memory capacity.

Although there may of course be a major difference between the functions of the human and the nonhuman hippocampus, a theory that could reconcile the human and the nonhuman data is surely much to be preferred. A family of such theories will be introduced shortly. But two topics remain to be discussed before leaving the physiological analysis of short-term memory. The first concerns anatomical localization; the second, the proposal that hippocampal damage disrupts consolidation, a process at one time believed to be involved in the transfer of information from short-term to long-term memory.

Problems of Anatomical Localization

We discussed in chapter 7 the potential involvement in spatial learning of extrahippocampal components of the various anatomical systems to which the hippocampus belongs. Reference was made there to work by Jarrard and his associates on the contrasting effects of different methods of damaging the hippocampus, and now that the working memory hypothesis of hippocampal function has been introduced, that work may be considered in rather more detail.

Aspiration Versus Radiofrequency Lesions

Jarrard's experiments have explored the effects of hippocampal damage on radial-maze tasks designed to allow measurement of reference memory and working memory errors. The procedures that he used incorporated features of the procedures used by Olton and Papas (1979) and Olton and Feustle (1981), and were designed to allow assessment of working memory versus reference memory deficits, and of spatial versus nonspatial deficits. Surgical procedures were carried out after extensive pretraining on each of two 8-arm radial-maze tasks. In each task, only four of the eight arms were baited, so that errors could be categorized as either reference memory errors (entries into arms that were never baited) or working memory errors (reentries into baited arms that had already been visited). In one version of the task—the place task—the baited arms remained in the same place throughout-(as in the Olton and Papas study). In another version—the cue task—the arms were differentiated by the presence of different textured floor inserts, and the correct arms were moved from one place to another between trials; this procedure was similar to that used by Olton and Feustle (1981), except that the positions of the arms were not altered within a trial.

Total aspiration of the hippocampus severely affected performance in the place, but not the cue, tasks; the hippocampectomized rats showed elevation of both reference memory and working memory errors in the place task (Jarrard 1985). This pattern of results therefore supported the spatial map theory as opposed to the working memory theory of hippocampal function. However, when the hippocampus was extensively damaged by radiofrequency lesions, both place and cue tasks were disrupted, the latter primarily as a result of an increase in working memory errors (Jarrard 1985). This outcome, of course, did support the working memory as opposed to the spatial map theory.

Neurotoxic Lesions

Both aspiration and radiofrequency lesions disrupt fibers of passage through the hippocampus, and their effects could therefore be the result of disruption of normal activity in regions at some distance from the hippocampus. Neurotoxic lesions have the advantage that they destroy cell bodies in the vicinity of their injection sites, but do not damage fibers; Jarrard has therefore used neurotoxic lesions in an effort to pinpoint which zones within the hippocampal formation are important in the effects seen following total hippocampal removal. The results have been quite unexpected.

In one experiment (Jarrard 1983), kainic acid was used to lesion the CA3 region of the hippocampus. The lesioned rats showed no deficits on the cue task, and a minor, transient deficit in the reference memory component of the place task; a subsequent experiment (Jarrard et al. 1984) found a precisely similar pattern of results following extensive damage of the dentate gyrus by injection of the neurotoxin colchicine. Finally, Jarrard (1985) used ibotenic acid to destroy the great majority of cells in the hippocampus (regions CA1, CA3, and the dentate gyrus): the outcome was again the same—no effect on the cue task and a transient impairment of the reference memory component of the place task. Figure 8.4 summarizes the results of this series of experiments.

Jarrard has very reasonably concluded that "our results clearly indicate that the hippocampus (CA1–CA3 cell fields and dentate gyrus) is not necessary for correct performance of the complex place and cue tasks" (Jarrard 1986:112).

The work that led to Jarrard's surprising (and not particularly welcome) conclusion involved exploration of the effects of hippocampal damage on rats that had extensive training prior to their operations. Subsequent work that has focused on postoperative acquisition may serve to restore faith in the importance of the hippocampus in maze learning.

Bouffard and Jarrard (1988) used only the place task described above and introduced the modification that the set of four baited arms was altered after every eleven trials. The rats were required to learn (postoperatively) eight versions (problems) in all, on each of which they were tested for eleven trials. Three groups were run: one group had extensive ibotenic lesions of the entire hippocampus (comparable to those of Jarrard's 1985 report); a second group had extensive ibotenate lesions of both the entorhinal cortex and the subiculum (start and endpoints of the hippocampal trisynaptic pathway); the third group consisted of operated and unoperated controls. The animals with the hippocampal lesions showed, compared to controls, a severe and lasting impairment of the eight problems, and anal-

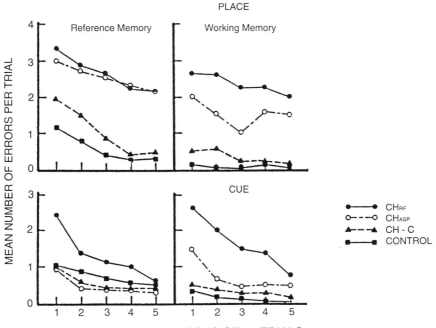

FIGURE 8.4. Effects of different types of hippocampal damage on memory in the radial maze. The graphs show the mean number of reference and working memory errors on the place (top) and cue (bottom) versions of the radial maze (see text for further details). CH$_{RF}$ = complete hippocampal, radiofrequency lesion; CH$_{ASP}$ = complete hippocampal, aspiration lesion; CH-C = complete hippocampal, ibotenic acid lesion; CONTROL = operated and unoperated controls. (*From* Jarrard 1985)

ysis of error patterns showed that this was due to increased numbers of both reference memory and working memory errors. Table 8.1 shows, however, that the animals with the combined entorhinal and subicular lesions showed no disruption of acquisition.

The absence of effect of the combined lesions contrasts with the disruptive effect of kainate subicular lesions reported by Jarrard (1983) on the preoperatively acquired place task: but Jarrard (1983) himself noted that those kainate injections had obtained damage at sites distant from the hippocampal formation, and Jarrard (1986) found that ibotenate lesions of the subiculum had only a minor transient effect of the (preoperatively acquired) place task (and no effect on the cue task).

TABLE 8.1

Comparison of Effects of Hippocampal and Subiculum/Entorhinal Lesions
on Memory in the Radial Maze

Lesion Group	Errors		
	WM	RM	Total
Hippocampus	1.86 (+/− 0.26)	4.43 (+/− 0.23)	6.26 (+/− 0.46)
Subiculum/entorhinal	0.38 (+/− 0.05)	2.72 (+/− 0.12)	3.11 (+/− 0.15)
Control	0.48 (+/− 0.05)	2.48 (+/− 0.09)	2.96 (+/− 0.11)

NOTE: Mean (+/− standard error of the mean) errors per trial for working memory (WM), reference memory (RM), and total errors for the three groups in the Bouffard and Jarrard (1988) study.

Conclusion

It is difficult to know what conclusions should be drawn from the attempts to localize the effects of hippocampal damage. Jarrard's work suggests that hippocampal damage (either total, or of hippocampal components) has remarkably little effect on preoperatively acquired radial-maze performance. But even this conclusion may be unsafe. Tilson et al. (1988) found that colchicine-induced lesions of the dentate gyrus did have a severe and lasting effect on preoperatively acquired performance in a conventional radial maze (in which all eight arms were baited at the start of each daily trial). Because asymptotic performance in this type of maze is attained more rapidly than in the complex place and cue tasks of Jarrard's experiments, the animals were given less preoperative training (fifteen as opposed to sixty trials). But whether that factor, or some other difference in the behavioral task used, or some aspect of the lesion technique is responsible for the difference between the Tilson group's 1988 result and the negative results obtained following apparently similar lesions by Jarrard et al. (1984), we simply do not know.

It may, then, be the case that rats that have received extensive preoperative training in mazes are relatively immune to hippocampal damage. That finding is surprising enough and would clearly require major modification of both the spatial mapping and working memory theories of hippocampal function. But the absence of effect of combined entorhinal-subicular damage on postoperative maze acquisition is equally unsettling: for this suggests that whatever role the hippocampus does play in maze learning is dependent upon neither its input to nor its output from neocortex—that, in other words, the trisynaptic pathway is irrelevant to that function.

Perhaps the best that can be done at present is to express the pious hope that further exploration of the effects of localized neurotoxic lesions will help uncover the proper interpretation of those effects and allow some understanding of the potential relevance of the known intrinsic physiology of the hippocampus to spatial and other forms of memory.

The Hippocampus and Consolidation

Consolidation Theory

The human amnesic deficit appears to be confined to long-term retention. The selective disruption of long-term and not short-term retention has been used to support the claim that there is a real distinction between stores serving short-term and long-term memory (Baddeley and Warrington 1970; Squire 1987), and this is a proposal to which we shall return. The fact that amnesics can recall events that occurred prior to the occurrence of hippocampal damage has been used to support the notion that amnesics can retrieve information from long-term memory and that what they can not do is to transfer information from short- to long-term memory. We shall discuss here what was at one time a common corollary of this notion—namely, the idea (e.g., Milner 1970) that transfer from short-term memory to long-term memory was mediated by a process of consolidation, that the longer an item survived in short-term memory the more it became consolidated and was thus retained as long-term memory. This notion in turn gained support from experimental work on the induction of retrograde amnesia in animals by electroconvulsive shock. Such work showed a temporal gradient so that recent but not old memories were forgotten following electroconvulsive shock: memories were susceptible to disruption for a relatively brief period—up to a few seconds (e.g., Chorover and Schiller 1965)—a period that seemed to be in general agreement with the decay times proposed by cognitive psychologists for items in short-term memory. The notion was, then, that items consolidated while in short-term memory, so that any event (such as electroconvulsive shock) that disrupted consolidation would disrupt retention of recent events, the memories for which were not yet fully consolidated into long-term memory. Less recent events would no longer be in short-term memory; their consolidation would have been completed, so that they would no longer be susceptible to electroconvulsive shock.

Time Course of Consolidation

A major difficulty facing consolidation theory was the fact that different experimental procedures obtained findings that led to different estimates of the temporal gradient of retrograde amnesia, some showing retrograde amnesia extending back to memories established several hours before delivery of electroconvulsive shock. It has now become clear that the amnesic effect of electroconvulsive shock is not an all-or-none but a graded effect that varies with such factors as the strength, duration, and number of electroconvulsive shock deliveries, and with the sensitivity of the behavioral technique used to assess retrograde amnesia (e.g., Schneider et al. 1969). It has also become clear that electroconvulsive shock may disrupt memory for events that occurred (in mice: Squire and Spanis 1984) up to three weeks previously or (in humans: Squire and Cohen 1979) up to three years previously; these times far exceed, of course, any notion of the decay time of items in short-term memory.

Relationship Between Anterograde and Retrograde Amnesia

Although it is not now possible to equate consolidation with persistence in short-term memory, the longer time constant of consolidation prompted an interesting hypothesis (Squire, Cohen, and Nadel 1984), which will be discussed after the presentation of some data pertinent to the relationship between anterograde and retrograde amnesia. One important generalization is that human anterograde amnesia is invariably accompanied by some degree of retrograde amnesia. This is true of humans whose anterograde amnesia is attributable to circumscribed brain damage, of humans who have experienced traumatic head injuries, and of patients suffering from Korsakoff's Syndrome (a syndrome associated with alcohol abuse; Korsakoff patients may show pathology in a number of areas, including the dorsomedial thalamus, the mammillary bodies, and the frontal cortex); it is also the case that humans who have been subjected to a course of electroconvulsive shock therapy show not only retrograde amnesia but also anterograde amnesia (Cohen and Squire 1981).

In some cases, retrograde amnesia shows no clear sign of a temporal gradient and extends to remote memory—memory for events that may have occurred decades before the onset of amnesia. This applies in particular to Korsakoff patients and may reflect a more general cognitive deficit that manifests itself in tasks that do not directly tax memory (Shimamura and Squire 1986). But in other cases, retrograde amnesia is clearly limited to events that occurred within a relatively short time (up to a few years) before the onset of amnesia. H.M., for example, showed a degree of amnesia for events that occurred eleven years or less prior to his operation (Corkin 1984). His amnesia was not total for those years: he showed normal recall in a test that showed faces which had been famous at various times over the two decades prior to his operation (but very poor recognition of faces that had become famous over the two decades following his operation) (Marslen-Wilson and Teuber 1975).

The invariable co-occurrence of retrograde amnesia and anterograde amnesia led to the hypothesis (Squire, Cohen, and Nadel 1984) that both reflect the same cause—namely, disruption of consolidation, a process now envisaged as continuing over a number of years in humans. A prediction that can be derived from this proposal is that the severity of anterograde amnesia should correlate with the extent of retrograde amnesia, and there is positive evidence on this score for patients with traumatic head injuries (Russell and Nathan 1946; Squire and Cohen 1984). There is, however, not yet supportive evidence from patients with circumscribed brain damage, and not, in particular, from patients with medial temporal lobe damage. This may, of course, reflect the paucity of such patients and the difficulty of providing precise estimates of the duration of retrograde amnesia and the severity of anterograde amnesia.

The nonhuman literature has so far contributed little to this debate, since until recently a temporally limited retrograde amnesia following hippocampal damage had not been reported in animals. Two recent reports do, however, suggest a potential role for the hippocampus in some consolidation-like process. Winocur (1990) conducted two experiments in which rats acquired a preference for a food with a particular flavor as a consequence of a single brief (15- or 30-min) interaction with another rat that had eaten food of that flavor. One group of operated rats had dorsal hippocampal lesions; another, dorsomedial thalamic lesions (that destroyed the entire dorsomedial nucleus). Animals were trained postoperatively, and retention tests were administered either immediately or after a one-, two-, four- or eight-day interval. Sham-operated control and dorsomedial thalamic rats showed a gradual forgetting of the socially acquired preference. Hippocampal rats' performance was normal when tested immediately or one day after training; the strength of their preference was, however, much weaker than that of the other two groups when tested after intervals of two days or more. In other words, hippocampal rats showed more rapid forgetting of information that was acquired normally—an instance of anterograde amnesia.

Winocur's second experiment explored retention of preferences acquired preoperatively. Surgery followed training either immediately or after a two-, five-, or ten-day interval, and testing took place ten days after surgery. Sham-operated controls showed forgetting—there was an inverse monotonic relationship between strength of preference and the age of the memory on which that preference was based. Hippocampal rats showed a quite different pattern. Their retention of old memories (established five or ten days prior to surgery) was normal, but they showed very poor retention of recent memories (established either immediately prior or two days prior to surgery). Preferences based on recent memories in hippocampal rats were significantly weaker than those based on older memories, precisely the opposite relationship to that seen in control animals, and an instance of temporally graded retrograde amnesia. The dorsomedial thalamic rats also showed a temporally graded retrograde amnesia, but it was less severe than that seen in the hippocampal rats, and observed only when surgery immediately followed training. This latter finding provides some (admittedly weak) support for the Squire, Cohen, and Nadel (1984) hypothesis, since dorsomedial rats showed no anterograde amnesia and weak retrograde amnesia, whereas hippocampal rats showed both anterograde amnesia and a stronger retrograde amnesia.

A report by Zola-Morgan and Squire (1990) agrees with the Winocur (1990) study in finding a temporally graded retrograde amnesia following hippocampal lesions in cynomolgus monkeys. Their study concerned object discriminations that were acquired at intervals of from two to sixteen weeks prior to surgery; testing took place two weeks after surgery. Hippocampal monkeys showed, compared to unoperated controls, retrograde amnesia for recent discriminations (discriminations established two or four weeks prior to surgery) but not for older discriminations (discriminations established eight, twelve, or sixteen weeks prior to surgery). And whereas normal monkeys showed better performance for recently acquired discriminations, the hippocampal monkeys showed a trend in the opposite direction.

There is evidence from both these reports that recent memories are more susceptible than old memories to disruption by hippocampal damage (although the time courses seem to be very different in rats and monkeys), and evidence also that hippocampal animals show better absolute levels of recall for older memories than for recent memories—and this, despite the fact that older memories are in normals weaker than more recent memories. Zola-Morgan and Squire (1990) argue that the superiority of older memories following hippocampal damage may be explained by supposing that information is gradually transferred (consolidated) from a temporary (hippocampus-dependent) store to a more permanent store, independent of the hippocampus and probably in the neocortex. Normals have access to both stores, and their performance reflects output from both the temporary and the permanent store. Hippocampal animals have access only to the more permanent store, a store that gradually acquires information from the temporary store, that process of acquisition being halted by hippocampal damage.

Both human and nonhuman data point to the conclusion that memories gradually become more resistant to a variety of types of disruption and that this process of strengthening, or consolidation, persists over long periods. The paucity of relevant data means, however, that the question whether the hippocampus is involved in that process remains at present an open question.

Some Long-Term Memories Are Preserved in Human Amnesia

The realization that consolidation is a process that long outlives the time for which items remain in short-term memory does not, of course, weaken the argument that the selective disruption of long-term and not short-term memory tasks implies a real distinction between short- and long-term memory stores. There are, however, problems facing the proposal that the amnesic deficit lies solely in a failure to transfer information from short- to long-term memory—one major difficulty being the fact that human hippocampal amnesics clearly are able to learn and retain over long periods certain types of new information. It is on the reasons for the immunity of some kinds of information to amnesia that much current theorizing about human amnesia focuses. A similar concern has arisen in studies of memory following hippocampal damage in nonhumans, and it is to that subject that we now return.

"Cognitive" Theories of Hippocampal Memory Function

Our consideration of theories of hippocampal function will end by discussing a family of theories, each of which supposes that there are (at least) two types of memory—one a cognitive system with (at least in humans) access to conscious processing, the other a more automatic system that may have limited access to higher-level cognitive processing.

A defect of these theories is that so far it has proved difficult to specify exactly which learning tasks engage "cognitive" processes and which do not, therefore making it problematic to generate predictions concerning lesion effects on hitherto untested tasks. What this may reflect, of course, is our currently incomplete understanding of learning processes. It may well be that by finding out which tasks are disrupted and which are not, we may gain insights into the precise domains of cognitive and noncognitive processing. Thus, a cognitive theory of hippocampal function may usefully point to tasks that are critical to understanding hippocampal function; and the pattern of deficits that emerges may contribute to refining the hypothesis.

Although the theories to be discussed have been characterized here as "cognitive," this is intended as no more than a convenient shorthand, since they are in effect a subclass of cognitive theories: *all* the major theories of hippocampal function appeal to concepts (selective attention and working memory, for example) that are derived from cognitive psychology. The "cognitive" theories have much in common with the spatial mapping theory (which also points to a contrast between a high-level and a lower-level system), but the concepts appealed to by cognitive theories are taken explicitly from human cognitive psychology. And although working memory is also a concept derived from human cognitive psychology, Olton's theory of hippocampal function differs importantly from the theories characterized here as cognitive in that his theory does not appeal to a distinction between a cognitive and a less cognitive system. One advantage of the "cognitive" theories is that they show much better promise of providing a unitary account of human and nonhuman data.

Hippocampus and Recognition Memory

The first thoroughgoing cognitive theory of hippocampal function in nonhumans was advanced by Gaffan (e.g., 1972, 1974). His theory posited disruption by hippocampal damage of one cognitive process, that of recognition. My discussions of the mapping and working memory theories of hippocampal function concluded with references to work on human hippocampal amnesics, work that suggested that both spatial mapping and working memory were unaffected. One of the attractions of the recognition memory theory of hippocampal function in animals is that it was originally formulated in the light of deficits observed in humans. One widely reported characteristic of human amnesics is their failure to recognize, whether assessed formally in laboratory experiments (e.g., Huppert and Piercy 1977) or, more strikingly, informally assessed: H.M., for example, "still fails to recognize people who are close neighbors or family friends but who got to know him only after the operation" (Milner, Corkin, and Teuber 1968:216).

Experimental Support for the Recognition Hypothesis

The clear deficits in recognition in human amnesics led Gaffan to propose his theory, and so to design experiments specifically to tap the process of recognition in nonhumans. We shall consider two of those experiments here.

Novelty and Exploration

The first report (Gaffan 1972) used a simple design, originally introduced by Dember (1956). Rats were allowed to explore for five minutes a T-maze having one black and one white arm (for some rats, the left arm was black; for others, white). The rats were then removed from the maze, and one arm was changed so that both arms were identical (for some rats, both black; for some, both white). Following this manipulation, then, one arm had changed, from black to white or vice-versa. The rats were replaced in the start-box and allowed to choose between the two arms: whereas all the control rats now selected the changed arm, the fornicotomized rats chose at random, showing no preference between the arms.

Gaffan's report should be considered along with the findings on exploration in hippocampal animals, discussed in chapter 3. It will be recalled that, although hippocampal animals showed no disruption of habituation of phasic orienting responses, they did show prolongation of active investigatory and exploratory behavior. It was argued there that the pattern of findings supported the view that hippocampals simply fail to recognize stimuli and therefore explore them despite previous exposure. A similar argument was brought to bear in chapter 7 when considering the disruptive effects of hippocampectomy on latent inhibition: it appeared that hippocampal subjects responded to previously exposed stimuli as though they were novel. A similar interpretation may apply to Gaffan's result: because hippocampal rats suffered from a failure to recognize, both the changed and the unchanged arm of the maze appeared novel and attracted investigation. The hippocampal rats, therefore, unlike the controls, showed no preference for the changed arm.

Recognition Versus Associative Learning

A second report (Gaffan 1974) concerned the performance of rhesus monkeys and began with an investigation of the effects of fornicotomy on a DMTS task that differed from previous conventional designs in that a large pool of junk objects was used. In Gaffan's study, 300 objects were used, so that each object was used only once a week. Response to an object shown in the sample phase was rewarded. After a delay of 10 sec, that object, along with another object (novel that week), was shown; choice of the previously presented (and rewarded) object was rewarded. The fornicotomized animals acquired efficient performance on this task as rapidly as normals: however, as can be seen from figure 8.5, when the delay was increased from 10 to 70 or 130 sec, their performance was dramatically disrupted (in contrast to controls, whose performance showed little effect of the increase in delay).

Two further experiments suggested that the deficit seen in fornicotomized animals at the longer delays was due to a specific disruption of recognition memory rather than to a general disruption of some temporary memory store. One experiment explored associative memory. In the first phase of each trial, monkeys were shown ten objects covering a central food well, one after the other with a 20-sec interval between objects. Half of the objects concealed a reward (obtained by the monkey), half did not. In the second phase, the same ten objects were presented again, but now each object was placed over the right food well, and there was, over the left food well, a brass disk. Objects rewarded in the first phase were re-

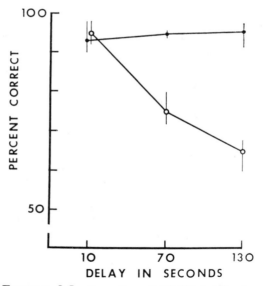

FIGURE 8.5. disruption of DMTS by fornicotomy. The graph shows mean performance
(and range) of fornicotomized and control monkeys at three retention intervals. *Open circles:*
fornicotomized monkeys; *filled circles:* controls.
(*From* Gaffan 1974)

warded in the second phase; objects that had been without reward again did not conceal reward, but on trials in which a nonrewarded object was present, the brass disk concealed a reward. The monkeys had therefore to reselect objects that had concealed a reward, and to select the brass disk in preference to objects that had not concealed reward. Figure 8.6 summarizes the results of the experiment and shows that fornicotomy did not impair performance despite the fact that information concerning reward and nonreward had to be retained for 200 sec.

The third experiment was identical to the second, except that in the first phase of each trial only five objects were presented, with a 40-sec interval between objects, and each of the objects was rewarded. The monkeys had therefore to learn to select in the choice phase an object previously seen and rewarded in preference to the brass disk, and to select the brass disk

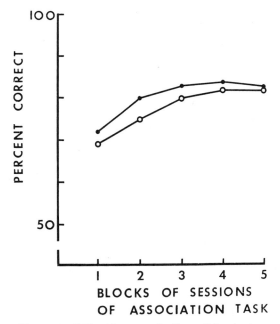

FIGURE 8.6. Absence of effect of fornicotomy on the 1-trial association task used by Gaffan (1974). The graph shows mean performance on successive 5-day blocks (there were three trials, each involving ten objects, each day). *Open circles:* fornicotomized monkeys; *filled* circles: controls. (*From* Gaffan 1974)

in preference to a novel object, not previously seen that week. Figure 8.7
shows that fornicotomized animals were, as in the first experiment, severely disrupted.

A recognition account of hippocampal function can readily accommodate the pattern of deficits obtained. The use of a large pool of objects (a
technique now very widely adopted in studies of hippocampal function)
ensured that the objects that had not been presented as samples in the first
and third experiments should have been markedly different in familiarity
from those that had been presented; this would enable controls readily to
perform successfully according to the relative familiarity of the objects
presented in the choice phase. Inability to discriminate familiar from un-

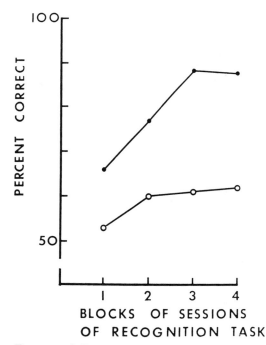

FIGURE 8.7. Disruption by fornicotomy of
performance on an analogue of a yes/no recognition task used by Gaffan (1974). The graph shows
mean performance on successive 5-day blocks
(there were two trials, each involving five rewarded objects, each day). *Open circles:* fornicotomized monkeys; *filled circles:* controls.
(*From* Gaffan 1974)

familiar objects—a consequence of the loss of recognition memory—
would clearly disrupt that performance. The second experiment, however,
required animals to discriminate between objects that had all been recently
presented and so were equated for familiarity; discrimination in that experiment could be based only on the associations formed in the first phase
between objects and reward or nonreward.

Role of Size of Stimulus Pool

Since Gaffan's original (1974) report there have been a number of studies
of the effects of hippocampal damage on monkey recognition memory in
experiments using a large pool of stimuli, and the great majority of the
reports agree in finding disruption by the lesions in both DMTS (e.g.,
Gaffan 1974; Gaffan and Weiskrantz 1980) and DNMTS designs (e.g.,
Mishkin 1978; Owen and Butler 1981, 1984; Mahut, Zola-Morgan, and
Moss 1982).

One question raised by these reports is whether in fact the use of a large
pool of stimuli is critical to obtaining a deficit in hippocampal animals. A
study by Owen and Butler (1981) suggests that it is. Normal and fornix-
lesioned monkeys were tested in two versions of DNMTS tasks. In one
version, only two objects were used throughout testing; in the other version, objects were drawn from a large pool so that each object was used
only once each week. The fornix-lesioned animals showed a disruption in
the latter (large-pool) task, a disruption that became more marked as the
delay was increased from 10 to 130 sec. But when only two objects were
used, fornix-lesioned animals showed no disruption at any delay—and
this, despite the fact that the task was more difficult than the large-pool
task (see Mishkin and Delacour 1975).

The results obtained by Owen and Butler (1981) support the recognition memory theory of hippocampal function. In the large-pool version of
DNMTS, an object recently presented as a sample would differ markedly
in familiarity from an object not seen for some seven days; in the two-
object version, both objects would be familiar and seen repeatedly each
day, so that the familiarity dimension would be of little value in performing the task. The results do, however, raise a problem: how is the two-
object task solved, if not by relying upon the relative familiarity of the
objects? Owen and Butler suggest that successful performance depends
upon visual short-term memory—that, in other words, a trace or representation of the sample stimulus is maintained in short-term memory, a store
that shows rapid decay. The rapid fall in accuracy (in both fornix-lesioned
and control animals) as the delay was increased (performance fell to little

better than chance at the 130-sec delay) supports such an account. Their proposal shows, moreover, good agreement with a theoretical account of MTS advanced by Roberts and Grant (e.g., 1976), an account based solely on behavioral data obtained in experiments on pigeons in which a small number of stimuli were used repeatedly within sessions. It is therefore plausible to suppose that visual short-term memory is involved in DMTS when few stimuli are used, and the proposal may also account for the fact that most studies have found little if any effect of hippocampal damage on large-pool DMTS or DNMTS tasks at short delays. If it is assumed that presentation of a sample obtains both a representation of the sample in short-term visual memory (a multipurpose store that may be used for both recognition and association formation) and a long-term representation of the sample, stored in parallel in recognition memory, then access to recognition memory would not be essential for efficient short-term recognition but would be essential when long retention intervals are used.

Summary

A number of lines of evidence do, then, suggest that hippocampal damage may disrupt the process of recognition. We have seen direct evidence for that proposition in humans; and seen also that hippocampal damage in nonhumans prolongs active investigatory behavior, and obtains a pattern of response to preexposed stimuli that parallels that shown to novel stimuli; moreover, in monkeys hippocampal damage disrupts choice performance based on the relative familiarity of stimuli.

Failure of recognition memory could also account for at least some of the deficits obtained in tasks that do not seem overtly to concern recognition. Novelty elicits approach and investigation: thus an animal in a maze with arms that it does not recognize will tend to explore those arms, despite the opposing pull of associations of some arms with reward, and some with nonreward. It may be that much of the susceptibility of learning about places to hippocampal damage can be accounted for by supposing that the tendency to explore (apparently) unfamiliar places overcomes the tendency to approach (equally unfamiliar) places associated with reward, and results in random progress through mazes.

Difficulties for the Recognition Memory Hypothesis

Although it is important to see that a deficit in recognition could by itself result in a range of other deficits, it hardly seems likely that it could explain all the deficits obtained following hippocampal damage: consider, for example, the susceptibility to hippocampal damage of performance in the rabbit eyelid-conditioning paradigm when nonoptimal interstimulus intervals are used; or the disruption of reversal but not of acquisition or extinction in the same paradigm. And although Gaffan (1974) reported results that supported the view that associative memory was intact, he has since reported other findings that have caused him to revise that view and, indeed, to abandon the recognition memory hypothesis.

Hippocampal Damage May Disrupt Associative Learning

One example of disruption of associative memory by hippocampal damage was provided by an experiment (Gaffan et al. 1984) that resembled one of those reported by Gaffan (1974) but had a very different outcome. In Gaffan's 1974 report, monkeys were shown a series of objects, half of which were rewarded, half not rewarded; the monkeys had then to select objects that had been rewarded and to avoid objects that had not been rewarded. Fornix lesions did not disrupt performance, a finding that suggested that the lesions had not disrupted associative memory. The Gaffan et al. (1984) report described a similar experiment but one in which monkeys had to choose objects that had not been rewarded in preference to objects that had been rewarded. They had, in other words, to make a choice that opposed the associative strengths that had just been built up. Since there was (as in the Gaffan 1974 study) no systematic difference in relative familiarity between the correct and the incorrect objects, performance should have been dependent upon associative memory. But monkeys with fornix lesions were severely impaired on this task.

It appears, then, that hippocampal damage may in some circumstances disrupt performance in tasks in which the relative familiarity of the stimuli is not an important cue. Further problems are posed by reports of hippocampal damage that fails to disrupt performance in tasks in which relative familiarity of the stimuli is the relevant cue.

Hippocampal Damage Does Not Invariably Disrupt Recognition

Although most reports agree that hippocampal damage does lead to a disruption of recognition performance in experiments using large stimulus pools in DMTS and DNMTS designs, some studies (e.g., Mishkin 1978) have found that the disruption is mild, and in at least two studies (Aggleton, Hunt, and Rawlins 1986; Murray and Mishkin 1984) no reliable dis-

ruption was seen with delays of 60 sec and more. Attempts have been
made (e.g., Bachevalier, Saunders, and Mishkin 1985; Ringo 1988) to
explain the differences between the studies using monkeys that find mild
impairments (e.g., Mishkin 1978) and those (e.g., Gaffan 1974; Zola-
Morgan and Squire 1986) that find severe impairments. It is not yet clear
that the differences between studies are fully understood, although it
seems to be the case that in studies in which animals are given extensive
preoperative training (as in most of the reports from Mishkin's laboratory)
the effects of hippocampal damage on recognition performance are mild.
Rather than going here into detailed examination of potential explanations
of the differences, it will be appropriate to note the important fact that
monkeys and rats with hippocampal damage are under at least some circumstances capable of relatively efficient recognition performance.

An Animal Model of Global Amnesia

The preceding discussion has highlighted two difficulties facing Gaffan's
original recognition memory theory of hippocampal function: there are
instances of performance that is disrupted in tasks in which recognition
does not seem to play an important role, and there are circumstances in
which hippocampal damage does not seriously disrupt recognition performance. Problems such as these have prompted two major modifications
to the recognition theory. One modification seeks to broaden the set of
cognitive processes disrupted so as to include not only recognition; the
other modification suggests that extrahippocampal damage may be necessary to obtain consistent effects on memory. Between them, the modifications promise to provide a convincing animal model of human global amnesia. We shall consider here the latter proposal first.

The contrast between the severe memory deficits observed in human
amnesics and the apparently milder deficits obtained in monkeys with hippocampal damage prompted Mishkin (e.g., 1978) to suggest that severe
anterograde amnesia in humans may not be due simply to hippocampal
damage but to damage to both the hippocampus and the amygdala. Detailed pathological data are not available for the great majority of human
amnesics, although we do, of course, have information on the intended
location of surgically inflicted damage for those whose amnesia was a
consequence of surgery. The most famous of these cases is H.M., and in
his case the surgery involved removal of the hippocampus, the amygdala,
and adjacent cortical areas. Scoville and Milner (1957), after reviewing
the series of patients given temporal lobe surgery, concluded that amnesia

depended upon the extent of hippocampal damage, but Mishkin et al. (1982) argued that their case was far from conclusive, and Zola-Morgan and colleagues pointed out in 1982 that "a clear case of human amnesia with lesions restricted to the hippocampal formation has not been reported" (Zola-Morgan, Squire, and Mishkin 1982:1339).

The amygdala has been introduced previously as a component of the limbic system, but little has been said of its anatomy or function. Some background in those areas is necessary for evaluation of Mishkin's proposal.

Amygdala: Anatomy

The amygdala consists of a complex of nuclei that forms a compact group in the anterior temporal lobe; the name itself derives from the Greek for "almond" and reflects its ovoid shape in primates. The amygdala lies immediately rostral to the tip of the horn of the lateral ventricle, underneath primary olfactory cortex, with which one of the amygdaloid nuclei fuses. The nuclear complex has been subdivided into constituent nuclei in different ways in different species, and in different ways by different anatomists in the same species. One major distinction that is widely drawn is between the basolateral and corticomedial divisions of the amygdala. However, as our major interest in this area will concern the effects of lesions in primates, and as attempts to distinguish between the effects of lesions of different regions of the primate amygdala have met with limited success (e.g., Aggleton and Passingham 1981), we shall not delve here into the confusing area of amygdalar subdivisions or of their different connectivities (for a recent survey of amygdalar neuroanatomy, see Amaral 1987, on which much of what follows is based).

Connections

The amygdala shows connections, most of which are reciprocal, with a large number of subcortical and cortical regions; we shall consider subcortical connections first.

There are reciprocal connections (carried by both the stria terminalis and the ventral amygdalofugal pathway) with the hypothalamus, and connections also with a variety of brainstem nuclei concerned with visceral and autonomic activity. The amygdala projects also to those regions of the basal forebrain (the basal nucleus of Meynert and the nucleus of the diagonal band of Broca) that contain magnocellular cells that provide extensive cholinergic input to the neocortex and the hippocampus.

The amygdala projects to (but does not receive projections from) the striatum (the caudate nucleus and putamen, pivotal structures of the extrapyramidal motor system) and the dorsomedial nucleus of the thalamus (a major source of input to prefrontal cortex).

There are extensive reciprocal connections between the amygdala and the hippocampal formation, most of which involve the subicular complex and the entorhinal cortex; there are, however, also direct amygdalar projections to the hippocampus proper (regions CA1 and CA3).

The amygdala receives, via the cortex, input from all the senses. There are projections from unimodal visual- and auditory-association cortex, a direct projection from primary olfactory cortex, and projections from multimodal association areas in orbitofrontal cortex and temporal polar cortex. Just as was the case with the hippocampus, the only projection from primary sensory cortex is that from olfactory cortex. However, unlike the hippocampus, the amygdala does receive projections from unimodal association cortex. A further contrast with hippocampal cortical connections lies in the fact that the amygdala projects very extensively throughout the neocortex, and projects to areas that do not project directly to it. There are, for example, no direct projections to the amygdala from either parietal or occipital cortex—but the amygdala sends projections to sites within those regions as well as to most of the regions (including prefrontal cortex) from which it receives projections.

Conclusions

The amygdala is well suited to monitor highly processed information from the senses, and, through its widespread projections to cortical zones, perhaps to modulate that input. The strong connections with the hypothalamus suggest a potential role in motivation and those with the striatum and brainstem, a potential role in skeletal and autonomic responding. The connections with the hippocampal formation and with prefrontal cortex suggest also that the amygdala may form part of a system concerned with high-level analysis and integration of sensory information. But, of course, the anatomical data can only suggest possibilities, likely roles. To gain more specific information about amygdalar function, lesion studies must be introduced.

Effects of Amygdalar Damage

Reduction of Fear

The most striking effect of bilateral amygdalectomy in a wide range of mammals, including primates, is a dramatic taming of the animal. Amygdalectomized monkeys show much reduced levels of fearful and aggressive responses to such normally alarming stimuli as humans and toy snakes (Aggleton and Passingham 1981). They show changes also in the items that they will examine and put into their mouths, and will indeed eat substances normally rejected, such as meat and feces (Weiskrantz 1956). Amygdalectomy may also lead to hypersexuality, which may manifest itself in attempts to copulate with partners of the same sex or of different species (Kling 1968; Schreiner and Kling 1953). These abnormalities constitute the principal features of the Kluver-Bucy syndrome, although the lesions used by Kluver and Bucy (1937) involved structures outside the amygdala, including hippocampus and temporal cortex.

It may be that most of the phenomena described above are due to a common cause, the reduction of fear. Ingestion of unusual substances may be due to a reduction in neophobia (Aggleton and Passingham 1982), and hypersexuality may be due to a reduced reluctance to approach other animals (Valenstein 1973).

In the light of the observations of reduced emotionality toward aversive stimuli, it is not surprising that there have been many reports of impaired fear conditioning following amygdalectomy, involving both behavioral (e.g., conditioned suppression: Weiskrantz 1956) and autonomic indices (e.g., Kapp et al. 1979). These effects could in turn be due to one of two causes—to loss of the motivational system of fear (or, what amounts to the same thing, to loss of the capacity to express fear), or to loss of the system or systems that identify stimuli as aversive.

Support for the latter of the two possibilities derives from experiments that have explored the effects of unilateral disconnection of the amygdala from visual input. Downer (1961) destroyed the amygdala of one hemisphere and cut the forebrain commissures (this prevented interhemispheric transfer of output from the intact amygdala but allowed bilateral access of tactile and visual stimulation to the intact amygdala). The monkeys showed normal affective responses to stimuli perceived with either eye. Downer then sectioned the optic chiasma, so that the intact amygdala could receive input from the ipsilateral eye only. The monkeys now showed emotional responses only to stimuli seen with the eye ipsilateral to the intact amygdala; they showed no fear of stimuli seen with the other eye. These monkeys possessed, then, a motivational fear system and were capable of expressing fear: but visual stimuli that were cut off from the amygdala were not classified as fear-inducing.

A similar point was made in an experiment by Gaffan and Harrison (1987) using, again, monkeys with unilateral amygdalectomy and forebrain commissurotomy. When visual association cortex (including all inferotemporal cortex and part of the prestriate cortex) was removed from the hemisphere ipsilateral to the intact amygdala, the monkeys showed no fear of visual stimuli (seen with both eyes), while still reacting emotively to tactile stimulation. Visual and tactile input to the amygdala is funneled through association cortex, thus removal of visual (but not of tactile) association cortex ipsilateral to the only intact amygdala prevented classification of visual (but not of tactile) stimuli as fear-inducing.

Disruption of Stimulus-Reinforcer Association Formation

Amygdalectomy also disrupts performance motivated by appetitive reinforcers in ways that do not seem simply to be attributable to reduced fear. The effects of amygdalectomy on acquisition of object discriminations in monkeys are inconsistent, but there is very wide agreement that discrimination reversal learning is disrupted by'amygdalar damage (Squire and Zola-Morgan 1983; Gaffan and Harrison 1987).

In an attempt to characterize the deficit in reversal learning, Jones and Mishkin (1972) analyzed patterns of responding within reversals. For this purpose, reversal sessions (each of which consisted of thirty trials) were classified into one of three stages: Stage 1 consisted of sessions in which 21 or more errors occurred; Stage 2 consisted of sessions in which the animals scored between 10 and 20 correct; and Stage 3 consisted of sessions in which animals scored between 21 and 27 correct choices. In this final stage, then, animals were performing at better than chance level, but had not yet achieved the criterion (28 correct trials).

Four groups of monkeys were run on both object and place reversals: one group had lesions of orbitofrontal cortex; a second group, of the hippocampus and hippocampal gyrus; a third group, of the amygdala and temporal pole (including temporal polar cortex); and unoperated controls made up the fourth group. The results are shown on figures 8.8 and 8.9 and may be summarized briefly. Orbitofrontal and amygdalar lesions disrupted both place and object reversals, whereas hippocampal lesions disrupted place reversals only. The disruptions seen in the hippocampal and orbitofrontal animals in the place-reversal task were qualitatively similar: both groups showed marked prolongation of Stage 1 responding—they showed, that is, an exaggerated perseveration of choice of the formerly positive stimulus. The orbitofrontal animals showed a similar perseverative pattern in object reversals also. The amygdalar animals, however, showed only a small increase in Stage 1 responding, but a large increase in duration of Stages 2 and 3.

Since the amygdalar animals showed relatively little difficulty in aban-

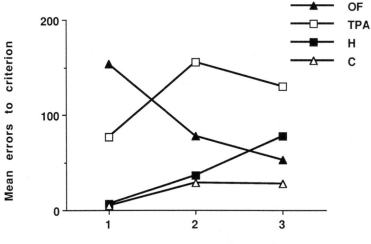

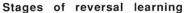

Stages of reversal learning

FIGURE 8.8. Performance on object-reversal learning of the four groups in the Jones and Mishkin (1972) study. The graph shows mean errors to criterion, divided into three stages (for further details, see text). OF = orbitofrontal lesions; TPA = lesions of temporal pole and amygdala; H = lesions of hippocampus and hippocampal gyrus; C = unoperated controls. (*Data from* Jones and Mishkin 1972)

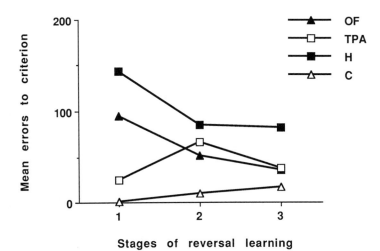

Stages of reversal learning

FIGURE 8.9. Performance on place-reversal learning of the four groups in the Jones and Mishkin (1972) study. The graph shows mean errors to criterion, divided into three stages (for further details, see text). OF = orbitofrontal lesions; TPA = lesions of temporal pole and amygdala; H = lesions of hippocampus and hippocampal gyrus; C: = unoperated controls. (*Data from* Jones and Mishkin 1972)

doning the former positive stimulus (and were markedly more efficient at this stage than were the orbitofrontal animals), Jones and Mishkin (1972) argued that the nature of the amygdalar deficit suggested a role for the amygdala in the formation of new stimulus-reinforcer associations. They also acknowledged, however, that the relatively minor and inconsistent effects of amygdalar lesions on original acquisition of new discriminations argued that other associative systems must be available, their relative inefficiency becoming apparent only when associative-learning demands were high, as might be expected to be the case in reversal learning.

The notion that amygdalar animals suffer from a peculiar deficit in establishing stimulus-reinforcer associations receives further support from a study (Spiegler and Mishkin 1981), which found marked disruption by amygdalar lesions of performance in a 1-trial object-reward task similar to that reported by Gaffan (1974). Spiegler and Mishkin tested monkeys in a version of the task in which two objects from a large pool were first shown singly, with one rewarded, the other not. Each object was then re-presented along with a gray card. An object that had been rewarded in the first phase was rewarded in the choice phase; when an object that had not been rewarded was presented in the choice phase, selection of the gray card was rewarded. Although, in contrast to Gaffan's (1974) finding of no effect of fornix damage, hippocampal lesions did lead to a deficit in post-operative reacquisition of the task, that effect was mild in comparison with the deficit seen following amygdalar lesions.

It should be emphasized at this point that Jones and Mishkin (1972) did not propose a *general* deficit in association formation following amygdalar damage, but a *specific* deficit in associations involving reinforcers, so that stimuli less readily acquire motivational or affective strength as a consequence of being paired with reinforcers. Two reports from Gaffan's laboratory serve to reinforce the point.

Gaffan and Harrison (1987) trained monkeys on a series of visual discriminations in which correct choices were rewarded by a distinctive auditory stimulus that had previously been established as a signal for food reward and so served as a secondary reinforcer; incorrect choices obtained an auditory stimulus that had previously accompanied nondelivery of food. Split-brain monkeys with unilateral amygdalectomy showed normal acquisition of this visual discrimination when contralateral visual association areas were removed (the procedure which, as we saw above, obtained tameness toward visual stimuli). But when auditory association cortex was removed (and visual association areas remained intact), the monkeys showed severely disrupted acquisition of the discriminations. A subsequent experiment (Gaffan, Gaffan, and Harrison 1988) confirmed that when unilateral amygdalectomy was accompanied by contralateral removal of visual association cortex, there was disruption of acquisition of visual discriminations in which correct choices gave immediate access to food.

Thus disconnection of the amygdala and visual association cortex did not disrupt acquisition of visual discriminations reinforced by an auditory secondary reinforcer, but did disrupt visual discriminations directly reinforced by a primary food reinforcer. The implication appears to be that the amygdala is involved in acquisition and maintenance of associations involving primary reinforcers: thus disconnection of the amygdala and auditory association areas disrupts the association between an auditory stimulus and food, and prevents that stimulus from acting effectively as a secondary reward. Associations that do not involve primary reinforcers are, however, immune to amygdalar/association-area disconnection.

Appetitive Versus Aversive Reinforcers

The notion that the amygdala is involved in associations between stimuli and primary reinforcers goes some way to providing a unitary account of the effects of amygdalectomy on both aversive and appetitively motivated behavior. There may, however, be important differences. It seems that amygdalectomy disrupts response not only to conditioned aversive stimuli—stimuli that have been associated with primary reinforcers—but to the primary aversive reinforcers themselves: thus, amygdalectomized animals do not appear to find *any* stimuli fear-inducing, even stimuli whose fear-inducing properties appear to be unlearned and common to all the members of a species. It hardly seems likely, for example, that the monkeys in the Aggleton and Passingham (1981) report had *learned* to fear toy snakes; and Kemble et al. (1984) have shown that amygdalectomized wild rats show markedly reduced fear to both humans and strange conspecifics—stimuli that require no prior training to arouse fear in intact wild rats.

By way of contrast with their reactions to primary aversive reinforcers, amygdalectomized monkeys do seem to react to and to discriminate between conventional foods normally. Aggleton and Passingham (1982) assessed preferences between three types of food (peanuts, raisins, and carrots). In one test, monkeys were allowed to choose between two of the foods, presented simultaneously; amygdalectomy had no effect of relative preferences between the foods. In a second test, animals were trained to work on progressive ratio schedules for the various foods. A progressive ratio gradually increases the number of responses required for a reinforcer until the animal abandons responding. The number of responses that a normal animal is prepared to produce for given food rewards varies with both palatability and amount of food, and with deprivation state, and so presumably provides a good index of the incentive value of a given food (Hodos 1961; Hodos and Kalman 1963). Amygdalectomy had no effect on performance for the three foods in the Aggleton and Passingham (1982) report: absolute rates of response were similar to those shown by normals and, like normals, amygdalectomized subjects worked harder for both raisins and peanuts than for carrots, worked harder for one peanut than for half a peanut, and worked harder for a raisin when they had not recently been fed than when they had recently been fed. Thus the motivational impact of primary food reinforcers does not diminish as a consequence of amygdalectomy, and this is a finding that contrasts with the effects of amygdalectomy on response to primary aversive reinforcers.

There have been relatively few studies of amygdalar function in monkeys, and studies using nonprimate mammals present a somewhat confusing picture due partly to conflict between the studies in locus of lesions (e.g., Sarter and Markowitsch 1985). For present purposes, we should note the evidence for the notion that the amygdala may play a central role in the association of neutral stimuli with primary reinforcers. In the context of Mishkin's proposal that the amygdala plays as important a role as the hippocampus in 1-trial recognition tasks, it should be noted that amygdalectomy alone, although it has a marked effect on 1-trial object-reward association, has little or no effect on other tasks involving brief delays, such as delayed response, DMTS or DNMTS, or the gap-trial procedure (Squire and Zola-Morgan 1983; Olton, Meck, and Church 1987). Moreover, in an experiment having a somewhat complicated design that required monkeys to remember in which of three possible locations an object had been shown in the sample phase, amygdalectomized monkeys showed only a mild and transient impairment of preoperatively established performance; hippocampectomized monkeys showed in the same 1-trial place-learning task a substantial and lasting impairment (Parkinson, Murray, and Mishkin 1988).

Effects of Combined Hippocampal/Amygdalar Lesions

The proposal (e.g., Mishkin 1978) that combined lesions of both the hippocampus and the amygdala are necessary (and sufficient) to obtain amnesic effects derived positive support from a series of experiments on recognition memory in which the effects of combined hippocampal/amygdalar lesions were compared to the effects of hippocampal or amygdalar damage alone. It should be noted here (and will turn out later to be of central importance) that the techniques used with monkeys for making the lesions involved in these experiments invariably also invaded cortical regions that adjoined the target (hippocampal, amygdalar, or both) areas.

The first relevant report was that of Mishkin (1978), who tested groups of normal controls and of animals having hippocampal removal, amygdalar removal, or combined amygdalar and hippocampal removal. The animals were trained preoperatively on a DNMTS task using trial-unique objects. The sample object was baited, and there was in preoperative training a 10-sec delay. Postoperatively, animals were retrained to criterion (90 correct choices in 100 trials), and then the effects of increasing delays were explored. Table 8.2 summarizes the results and shows that amygdalectomized and hippocampectomized animals showed a degree of retrograde amnesia for the task, and that the combined-lesion animals were profoundly impaired on reacquisition. It should be noted, however, that two of the three monkeys having combined lesions were able postoperatively to achieve criterion when a 10-sec delay was used (the third monkey had received damage not only to the hippocampus and amygdala but to visual association cortex also). When longer delays were introduced, both single-lesion groups showed a mild impairment whereas the combined group showed severe disruption.

In a subsequent report Overman, Ormsby, and Mishkin (1990) trained monkeys on a similar DNMTS task, using two-dimensional pictures as stimuli. Their procedure allowed the use of shorter delays than are pos-

TABLE 8.2

Effects of Removal of Amygdala and Hippocampus on Recognition Memory in Monkeys

Lesion Group	Preoperative		Postoperative		Delays (% correct)		
	Trials	Errors	Trials	Errors	30 sec	60 sec	120 sec
Unoperated controls	73	24	0	0	98	99	98
Amygdalar	100	33	140	39	94	93	94
Hippocampal	93	25	73	19	94	94	91
Hippocampal/amygdalar	130	32	987	270	68	57	60

SOURCE: Mishkin 1978.

NOTE: Scores in preoperative and postoperative columns are the mean numbers of trials and errors preceding criterion. Scores in delays columns are mean percentage correct in 100 trials at each of the three longer delays, tested in succession at the rate of 20 trials per day, except for the longest delay (120 sec), which was tested for 10 trials per day.

sible using the WGTA. Overman and colleagues found that monkeys with combined hippocampal/amygdalar lesions showed no postoperative deficits in performance at either a 1- or a 5-sec delay; significant deficits were observed only at delays of 10 sec and more. These reports therefore strongly support the conclusion that short-term recognition (with delays of up to approximately 10 sec) may be mediated by a system other than that which mediates long-term recognition; it will be recalled that in the course of the discussion of Gaffan's recognition memory hypothesis it was suggested (in agreement with Owen and Butler's 1981 proposal) that this system may be visual short-term memory.

There is evidence from rats also for an effect of combined hippocampal/amygdalar lesions that exceeds the summed effect of either amygdalar or hippocampal damage alone. Aggleton, Blindt, and Rawlins (1989) tested rats having either amygdalar or combined hippocampal/amygdalar lesions on the same nonspatial DNMTS task used in the Aggleton, Hunt, and Rawlins (1986) report (that found, it will be recalled, no effect of hippocampal damage on performance). Aggleton and colleagues (1989) found that although amygdalar damage itself had no significant disruptive effect on DNMTS tasks using delays of up to 60 sec, combined hippocampal/amygdalar damage had a disruptive effect on DNMTS when either a 20- or 60-sec delay was used; in agreement with the monkey work, no disruptive effect of combined lesions was seen at the 0-sec delay.

Effects of Combined Lesions of Structures Associated with the Hippocampus and Amygdala

A series of reports using the same DNMTS procedure showed that deficits could be obtained by damage to structures outside the amygdala and the hippocampus but connected with them; these reports agreed that in order to obtain what Aggleton and Mishkin (1983b) have called a "full-blown anterograde amnesia" it was necessary to damage structures associated with both the hippocampus and the amygdala.

Bachevalier, Parkinson, and Mishkin (1985) found that neither lesions of the fornix alone, nor lesions of the pathways (the stria terminalis and the ventral amygdalofugal pathway) that carry the output of the amygdala, had more than a mild effect on recognition: but combined lesions of those pathways had a major effect. Aggleton and Mishkin (1983a, 1983b) reported that damage centered on thalamic regions that show strong connections with either the hippocampus or the amygdala (with, respectively, the medial anterior thalamic nucleus and the magnocellular part of the dorsomedial nucleus) had only mild effects on recognition when either was carried out as a single lesion, but a marked effect when combined. The anterior thalamic nuclei and the magnocellular part of the dorsomedial nucleus in turn project to two subdivisions of cortex—orbitofrontal cortex and the cingulate gyrus. An extensive lesion of ventromedial prefrontal cortex that involved damage to both those regions had a severe effect on DNMTS whereas damage to the dorsolateral frontal cortex (target of the parvocellular part of the dorsomedial nucleus) did not disrupt performance (Bachevalier and Mishkin 1986). Similarly, Murray and Mishkin (1986) found that when lesions of rhinal cortex (which include areas such as the entorhinal cortex, which feed into the hippocampus) were combined with hippocampal lesions, performance was little worse than following hippocampal lesions alone; but when rhinal lesions were combined with amygdalar damage, a large deficit was seen. Finally, a study by Aggleton and Mishkin (1985) explored the effects of destruction of the mammillary bodies on DNMTS. The mammillary bodies are the primary target of the fornix but do not show strong connections with the amygdala. In accordance with the notion that damage to both hippocampal and amygdalar circuits is necessary for severe amnesic effects, damage to the mammillary bodies had only a mild effect on DNMTS performance.

Mishkin's conclusion was, then, that there are two anatomical systems, both of which must be damaged in order to obtain severe deficits in recognition: one consists of the hippocampus and structures associated with it; the other, of the amygdala and its associated structures. It should be emphasized in this context that the effects of the combined lesions are not modality specific: although Murray and Mishkin (1984) found that hippocampal lesions had no effect on their tactile version of DNMTS, and that amygdalar lesions had a mild effect, the effect of the combined lesion was again very marked.

It is clear, then, that consistent striking deficits in recognition memory may be obtained through the use of combined lesions. We turn now to the question of what processes other than recognition are disrupted by such damage and will preface that discussion by returning once again to human data, data that have inspired a theory that now finds application to nonhuman studies.

Skill Learning by Amnesics

Although human amnesics show a global anterograde amnesia in the sense that they do not show any ability to retain for more than a few seconds events that have happened since hippocampal damage occurred, they do show an ability to learn and to retain over long periods certain types of skilled performance. H.M. has shown overnight retention of a number of visuo-motor skills: figure 8.10 shows, for example, his performance on a mirror-drawing task in which he had to trace between two lines of a drawn star while watching his hand in a mirror. What is of particular interest is that H.M.—like other amnesics tested in skill-learning tasks—showed the improvement while at the same time denying any previous experience of the apparatus or of the task demands.

There have been reports that amnesics can learn not only motor skills but at least some cognitive skills. The most striking example concerns the "Tower of Hanoi" problem. Five circular disks of different sizes are arranged on the leftmost of three pegs, arranged according to size with the smallest disk at the top and the largest disk at the bottom. The task is to transfer the disks, one at a time, so that they end up on the rightmost disk with the smallest at the top and the largest at the bottom: at no point may a disk be placed upon a disk that is smaller than itself. The minimum number of moves necessary to solve this problem is 31, and only one sequence of moves can achieve this minimum number. Cohen (1984) tested a number of amnesics, including H.M., on this problem, asking

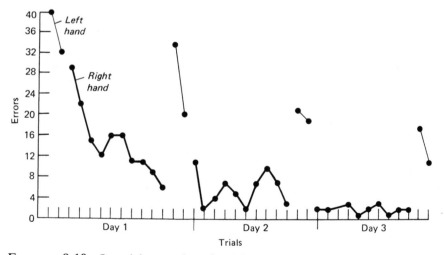

FIGURE 8.10. Overnight retention of a skill by patient, HM. The graph shows HM's performance over three days in a mirror-drawing test on a total of 31 trials using the right hand, and 8 trials using the left hand. (*From* Carlson 1977; *adapted from* Milner 1965)

them to complete it four times a day; table 8.3 summarizes their performance and that of control subjects over four days of testing, and shows that both groups had comparable rates of improvement across days. In this study the amnesics nevertheless showed little or no recollection of having had any previous experience of the problem. H.M.'s performance over eight days of testing and over a further four days testing carried out twelve months later is shown on table 8.4. It is clear that H.M.'s improved performance survived the 12-month interval relatively intact.

Declarative Versus Procedural Knowledge

The dissociation observed between the retention of skilled performance of a task and recognition of the task has led to a variety of proposals concerning the critical distinction between information that can be retained by amnesics and that which cannot. All the proposals have in common the notion that the information that is retained is implicit rather than explicit knowledge. One current proposal is that there is in human long-term memory a distinction between declarative and procedural knowledge, between "knowing that" and "knowing how." "Declarative knowledge is available to conscious awareness and includes the facts, lists, and data of conventional memory experiments. Procedural knowledge is implicit and available only by engaging the specific operations in which the knowledge is embedded. Declarative knowledge is created by adding new data structures. Procedural knowledge is created by modifying, biasing, or combining preexisting representations" (Squire, Shimamura, and Graf 1985:38). Squire and his colleagues suggest, then, that procedural memory is intact in human amnesics and that declarative memory is disrupted. To reiterate a point frequently made, if analysis of amnesics confirms the dissociation

TABLE 8.3

Overnight Retention by Amnesics of a Cognitive Skill

Group		Session Number			
		1	2	3	4
Amnesics ($N = 12$)	Mean	46.6	41.6	37.7	33.4
	Range	33–100	31–63	31–55	31–51
Controls ($N = 8$)	Mean	48.4	41.6	39.3	34.1
	Range	31–88	31–69	31–69	31–45

SOURCE: Cohen 1984.

NOTE: Number of moves to solution by amnesics and normal controls of the "Tower of Hanoi" problem (minimum number of moves = 31) on 4 daily sessions (4 trials per day).

TABLE   8.4

Long-term Retention by Patient H.M. of a Cognitive Skill

	Session Number			
	1	2	3	4
Mean	46.3	41.8	37.3	40.0
Range	39–53	34–46	31–42	35–51
	5	6	7	8
Mean	34.5	35.5	33.0	32.0
Range	31–39	35–37	31–35	31–35
	9	10	11	12
Mean	37.5	33.3	32.5	32.0
Range	31–47	31–37	31–35	31–35

SOURCE: Cohen 1984.

NOTE: Number of moves to solution by H.M. of the "Tower of Hanoi" problem (minimum number of moves = 31) on his first 8 daily sessions (4 trials per day), and on 4 further daily sessions carried out one year later.

between retention of procedural memories and loss of declarative memories, the case for there being in normals a real distinction between the processing of two different types of memories will be much strengthened.

Application to Nonhumans with Combined
Hippocampal/Amygdalar Lesions

It is clearly difficult to transfer directly to nonhumans the procedural/declarative distinction, since nonhumans can neither make declarative statements concerning their knowledge of events nor indicate what information is available to their consciousness. But we have already seen that a satisfactory analogue for nonhumans of recognition (a process of declarative memory) has been found, and ingenious proposals have been made concerning other types of learning in nonhumans that could be regarded as declarative as opposed to procedural. Those proposals may best be introduced in the context of further effects of combined hippocampal/amygdalar lesions, effects that conform to a pattern that shows striking parallels with the characteristics of human global amnesia.

Retrograde Amnesia for Object Discriminations But Not for Skills. First, it will be recalled that human amnesics show a (variable) degree of retrograde amnesia for events that occurred prior to the onset of amnesia. And given that conventional hippocampal lesions obtain retrograde amnesia in monkeys (Zola-Morgan and Squire 1990), it is not sur-

prising that combined hippocampal/amygdalar lesions also obtain retrograde amnesia. Salmon, Zola-Morgan, and Squire (1987) had monkeys
learn a large number of object discriminations at various intervals from
eight months to two weeks prior to combined hippocampal/amygdalar surgery. Figure 8.11 shows the results of a retention test carried out three
weeks after surgery. The lesioned animals showed a clear retrograde amnesia although, unlike the typical human finding, showing no sign of a
temporal gradient favoring older as opposed to younger memories—indeed, if anything, the opposite was found (it will, however, be recalled

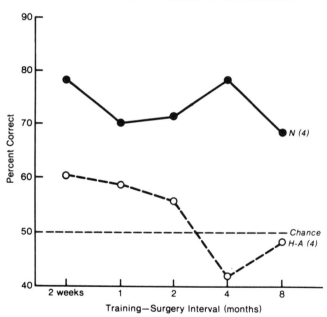

RETENTION TEST 3 WEEKS AFTER SURGERY

FIGURE 8.11. Retrograde amnesia for object discriminations following combined hippocampal/amygdalar damage in
monkeys. The graph shows performance on retention tests for
5 different sets of 20 object pairs, learned at five different intervals prior to surgery, and assessed three weeks after surgery.
Retention of all 100 object pairs was assessed by presenting
each pair for a single trial. N = normal monkeys; H-A =
monkeys with bilateral removal of the hippocampus and amygdala. Numbers in parentheses show the number of monkeys in
each group. (*From* Salmon, Zola-Morgan, and Squire 1987).

that Zola-Morgan and Squire [1990] did report a temporally graded retrograde amnesia following conventional hippocampal lesions).

Although human amnesics show retrograde amnesia for declarative
memories, they do not show retrograde amnesia for procedural memories
such as motor skills. Salmon, Zola-Morgan, and Squire (1987) accordingly taught monkeys not only object discriminations but also, some three
weeks before surgery, a motor skill. The apparatus consisted of a fixed
horizontal rod with a right-angle bend. At the beginning of each trial, a
circular candy with a hole in it (a Lifesaver) was placed at the fixed end
of the rod. In order to obtain the candy, the monkey had to manipulate it
along the rod and round the bend within 30 sec. Figure 8.12 shows the
rate of preoperative acquisition of this skill and postoperative retention
performance (tested some four to eight weeks after surgery). It is clearly
quite a difficult task for the monkey, but retention was not significantly
affected by the combined lesion.

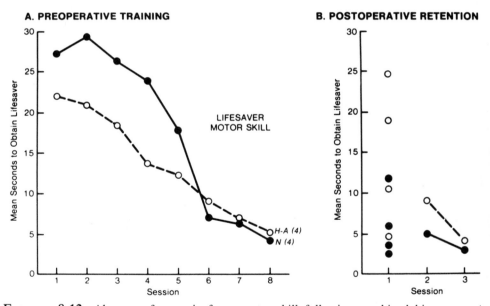

FIGURE 8.12. Absence of amnesia for a motor skill following combined hippocampo/
amygdalar lesions in monkeys. Fig. 8.12A shows performance on eight daily preoperative
sessions (six trials per session), and fig. 8.12B shows retention of the skill on three 6-trial
sessions. The first retention session was carried out four weeks after surgery; the second and
third sessions, eight weeks after surgery. N = normal monkeys; H-A = monkeys with bilateral removal of the hippocampus and amygdala. Numbers in parentheses show the number
of monkeys in each group. (*From* Salmon, Zola-Morgan, and Squire 1987)

Disrupted Acquisition of Object Discriminations But Not of Skills. If the parallel with human findings is to be maintained it will clearly have to be assumed that, because retention of object-discrimination learning is disrupted by hippocampal/amygdalar lesions, object-discrimination learning must be a declarative procedure. It should therefore be predicted that combined hippocampal/amygdalar lesions should disrupt postoperative acquisition and retention of object-discrimination learning. Before discussing the nature of object-discrimination learning, it may be best to see whether the prediction is confirmed.

Zola-Morgan and Squire (1984) examined postoperative acquisition of object discriminations in normal and hippocampal/amygdalar monkeys and found a substantial deficit in acquisition; a similar result was obtained by Salmon, Zola-Morgan, and Squire (1987). Moreover, there is evidence that once hippocampal/amygdalar subjects have achieved criterion on object discriminations, they show deficits in retention when tested 24 hours or five days later (Mahut, Moss, and Zola-Morgan 1981; Salmon, Zola-Morgan, and Squire 1987). By way of contrast, hippocampal/amygdalar–lesioned monkeys show no deficits in either postoperative acquisition or subsequent retention of motor skills (Zola-Morgan and Squire 1984; Salmon, Zola-Morgan, and Squire 1987).

Given the disruptive effects of hippocampal/amygdalar lesions on acquisition of conventional object discriminations, it is not surprising to find that lesioned animals also show severe impairments on the Spiegler and Mishkin (1981) 1-trial object-reward task. As we saw in a previous section concerned with the effects of amygdalectomy, hippocampal lesions had little effect on this task, and although amygdalar lesions did disrupt performance, figure 8.13 shows that when subsequently amygdalar lesions were added to the hippocampal lesions, and hippocampal lesions to the amygdalar lesions, the effect was greater than that of either single lesion (Mishkin et al. 1982).

Combined hippocampal/amygdalar lesions do, then, have dramatic effects on 1-trial recognition memory, 1-trial associative memory, and on the acquisition and retention of conventional object discriminations. They do not, however, affect either the acquisition or retention of motor skills. Can a case be made for the notion that the tasks that are disrupted involve declarative learning? Squire and Zola-Morgan believe that it can and base their argument partly upon the results of experiments that have studied the effects of hippocampal/amygdalar lesions on other types of discriminations.

Easy But Not Difficult Discriminations Are Disrupted. Although, as we

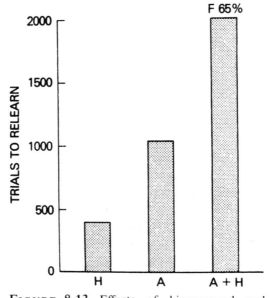

FIGURE 8.13. Effects of hippocampal and amygdalar damage on retention of the 1-trial object-reward association task used by Spiegler and Mishkin (1981) (for procedural details, see text). The graph shows mean trials to reattain criterion (90 correct trials in 100) on the task. A: bilateral amygdalectomy (N = 3); H: bilateral hippocampectomy (N = 3); A + H: second stage, combined ablation produced by superimposing A on preexisting H, and H on preexisting A (N = 5); F: failed to relearn within the limit of 2,000 trials (followed by average performance in final 100 trials). (*From* Mishkin et al. 1982)

have seen, hippocampal/amygdalar lesions disrupt object discriminations, a number of earlier reports involving hippocampal/amygdalar lesions found either no impairment in discrimination learning or relatively minor effects (for a review see Squire and Zola-Morgan 1983). And more recent studies have confirmed that conventional visual discriminations in which two-dimensional stimuli are used show little disruption following combined hippocampal/amygdalar lesions. Zola-Morgan and Squire (1984), for example, found no significant difference between normal and hippocampal/amygdalar–lesioned monkeys in trials to criterion in acquisition of two discriminations (between a square and a cross, and between N and W, the patterns consisting of white tape on a blue background). What is interesting about this finding is the fact that two-dimensional pattern discriminations are considerably more difficult for monkeys than are object discriminations. Whereas normal monkeys took on average 310 trials to master the two pattern discriminations, object discriminations, on which hippocampal/amygdalar animals show so marked a deficit, are typically solved by normals in a single session of some thirty to forty trials (e.g., Zola-Morgan and Squire 1984; Salmon, Zola-Morgan, and Squire 1987). Squire and Zola-Morgan (1983) reviewed forty-six previous reports of the effects of medial temporal damage (either hippocampal or combined hippocampal/amygdalar) on discrimination learning and found a significant tendency for disruptive lesion effects to be found on easy, but not on difficult, discriminations.

Selective Attention: A Skill Involved in Difficult Discriminations? Why should difficult discriminations tap procedural memory (and so, be immune to hippocampal/amygdalar damage), while easy tasks tap declarative knowledge (and so are disrupted by hippocampal/amygdalar damage)? Squire and Zola-Morgan (1983) adopt the notion (e.g., Sutherland and Mackintosh 1971) that discrimination learning involves two processes: first, the animal has to "tune in" to the appropriate dimension along which the stimuli are differentiated (e.g., pattern, brightness); second, the animal has to learn which of the two different outputs is rewarded. The former procedure may, according to Squire and Zola-Morgan, be an instance of skill learning whereas the latter involves declarative memory. Difficult discriminations are difficult precisely because it takes a long time for animals to tune in to the appropriate dimension, so that the skill-like component of learning occupies most of the solution period. Easy discriminations are those in which the relevant features are salient and attract attention, so that the dominant component in learning them is the declarative process of learning that one or the other stimulus is rewarded. Squire and Zola-Morgan's proposal that selective attention is skill-like and not disrupted by hippocampal damage inevitably brings to mind the proposal (Solomon 1977, discussed in chapter 6) that the hippocampus is critically concerned with selective attention. But it will be recalled that the discussion of Solomon's proposal, which concerned the analysis of work carried out on rabbits and rats, concluded that it currently gained little support from the somewhat contradictory literature available. There is, then, no difficulty in accepting that aspect of the Squire and Zola-Morgan proposal.

If discrimination learning invariably involves both procedural and declarative components, then difficult discriminations, although dominated by the procedural process, might nevertheless be expected to show at least a minor impairment (related to the declarative process). This in fact does appear to be the case. Although Zola-Morgan and Squire (1984) found no deficit in pattern-discrimination learning in terms of trials to criterion, there was a significant deficit when an errors-to-criterion measure was used to assess performance. The deficit was not large (mean errors for normals was 99, and 110 for hippocampal/amygdalar monkeys), and subsequent analysis revealed that the deficit was almost entirely due to the fact that hippocampal/amygdalar subjects made more errors than normals over the first five trials of each day. Zola-Morgan and Squire (1984) suggest that this may be due to a deficit in overnight retention of declarative (but not of procedural) information.

Classical Conditioning as Procedural Learning. The proposal that the process of learning which of two alternatives is rewarded is a declarative process (and so, susceptible to hippocampal damage) might appear to conflict with the fact that standard classical delay conditioning in the rabbit eyelid-conditioning preparation is not disrupted by hippocampal lesions. It is, however, clear that eyelid conditioning emerges slowly to an asymptote achieved only after a long series of trials (see, for example, figure 5.5). It is, in other words, a gradual incremental process and not one to which memories for specific trial outcomes appear relevant. Squire (1987) therefore suggests that classical conditioning is a procedural process. In this case it is reasonable to expect that information relevant to selection between two alternatives in a discrimination could accrue through the use of both the declarative and the procedural memory systems, so that disruption of the declarative system need not have a catastrophic effect on those choices. There will, in other words, be many associative tasks that are likely to engage both the procedural and the declarative systems in parallel; those tasks that are solved in relatively few trials may be assumed to be relying primarily upon declarative memory processes, and so to be liable to disruption by hippocampal damage; that disruption may, however, be mild, depending upon the relative rates of solution of the particular tasks achieved using the two systems independently.

Performance of Human Amnesics in Tasks Devised for Nonhumans. The findings reviewed in the preceding section have made out a good case for the parallel between the global amnesia seen in humans with limbic damage and the amnesic effects of combined hippocampal/amygdalar lesions in nonhuman primates. Although the distinction between procedural and declarative knowledge is not easily made in nonhumans, the speculations of Squire and Zola-Morgan concerning the skill-like aspects of attentional processes may provide a valuable way in which to begin the analysis of different learning tasks.

The case for a parallel between the animal model for amnesia and the human original is strengthened by evidence that human amnesics do indeed perform poorly when tested on the very tasks on which monkeys with hippocampal/amygdalar lesions perform poorly. Squire, Zola-Morgan, and Chen (1988), using a large pool of objects as stimuli, found poor performance by human amnesics on DNMTS tasks, on 1-trial associative learning, and on acquisition of simple object discriminations. Similarly, Aggleton et al. (1988), who projected slides of abstract paintings (not easily described verbally) found severe disruption of DMTS in amnesics.

Difficulties for the Animal Model of Global Amnesia

As was perhaps inevitable, work inspired by the hippocampal/amygdalar model of amnesia has thrown up findings that constitute serious challenges to the model, and we shall consider here two major problems. The first is a result that appears to challenge the basic notion that the animal data may be accounted for in terms of the procedural/declarative dichotomy; the second concerns what may be a less fundamental issue—namely, whether either the hippocampus or the amygdala is critically involved in global amnesia.

Discordant Lesion Effects

Concurrent Discriminations with a 24-Hour Intertrial Interval

An experiment by Malamut, Saunders, and Mishkin (1984) is important both because it emphasizes the remarkably specific nature of the deficit obtained by hippocampal/amygdalar lesions and because it appears to present serious problems for the interpretation of hippocampal/amygdalar lesions in terms of the procedural/declarative dichotomy. In the experiment, monkeys were trained on a set of twenty concurrent discriminations. The animals saw each day twenty pairs of objects; choice of one object was consistently rewarded, choice of the other object was never rewarded. The different pairs of objects were shown in the same order each day, but the position (left versus right) of the two objects in a pair varied irregularly from day to day. Once the animals reached criterion (90 percent correct choices on five consecutive days), another set of forty objects (twenty pairs) was introduced, and the same procedure was carried out. Since a given pair of objects was seen only once each day, the intertrial interval for each pair was 24 hours.

Two groups of animals were trained following bilateral hippocampal/amygdalar damage. These animals showed essentially normal acquisition of both discriminations except in cases in which histological examination revealed damage that extended to the rostral inferotemporal cortex (a visual association area). A third experimental group received combined lesions following acquisition of the two sets of concurrent discriminations. These animals (unlike controls) showed no retention for either of the preoperatively acquired sets and instead relearned them at the same rate as preoperatively. However, when tested on a third new set of twenty discriminations, their rate of acquisition was the same as that of controls. Subsequent testing in a conventional DMTS task with a large pool of objects showed, as anticipated, a substantial deficit in the animals with combined hippocampal/amygdalar lesions.

The results of the Malamut, Saunders, and Mishkin (1984) experiment may be summarized as follows: monkeys with combined hippocampal/amygdalar lesions showed normal acquisition of concurrent discriminations in which a 24-hour intertrial interval was used; they showed total retrograde amnesia for preoperatively acquired concurrent discriminations; and they showed severe disruption of short-term recognition. In view of the importance of the finding, it is worth noting that a dissociation between efficient acquisition of concurrent discriminations using a 24-hour intertrial interval and severe disruption of DNMTS has been obtained in two subsequent studies. Overman, Ormsby, and Mishkin (1990), found, as has already been noted, disruption by combined hippocampal/amygdalar lesions of DNMTS tasks using picture stimuli; but those same monkeys showed no deficit in acquisition of twenty concurrent picture discriminations, each pair of pictures being presented only once every 24 hours. Bachevalier and Mishkin (1986) tested monkeys with extensive lesions of ventromedial frontal cortex (an area that shows connections with both the hippocampal and the amygdalar systems). Their animals, it will be recalled, showed a severe deficit in DNMTS using objects; but they showed no deficit in acquisition of three sets of 20-pair object discriminations, with a 24-hour intertrial interval between presentations of the objects.

The observation (Malamut, Saunders, and Mishkin 1984) of retrograde amnesia for a task that showed no deficit in acquisition clearly poses a problem for any theory that supposes that the source of the retrograde amnesia is the same as that of anterograde amnesia, and, in particular, for the procedural/declarative interpretation of amnesia: if the concurrent task is procedural, then retrograde amnesia should not have been observed; if it is declarative, then no acquisition deficit should have been obtained.

Role of Intertrial Interval in Discrimination Learning

A further problem is posed for the procedural/declarative hypothesis by the fact that acquisition of the concurrent discriminations was not impaired in the Malamut, Saunders, and Mishkin (1984) report. These were, after all, simple object discriminations, and unoperated animals made less than 60 errors before attaining criterion—about three errors per discrimination. We have seen that, in conventional simple object discriminations, monkeys with combined lesions show deficits in acquisition; there is evidence too that monkeys with hippocampal/amygdalar lesions show deficits on concurrent object discriminations when five trials are given on each of eight discriminations each day (e.g., Zola-Morgan and Squire 1985).

Phillips et al. (1988) suggest that the distinction between the two types of concurrent discrimination lies in the effective intertrial interval. In the studies that have run concurrent discriminations with several presentations per day (e.g., Zola-Morgan and Squire 1985), the interval between re-presentations of each pair has typically been about 1–2 min. Phillips et al. suggest that in these circumstances normal animals make use of their cognitive memory system "by remembering object-reward associations from one trial to the next, an ability that earlier studies have shown is dependent on the limbic system" (Phillips et al. 1988:105, referring to Spiegler and Mishkin's 1981 study). This is a notion that could clearly be tested simply by increasing the intertrial interval between re-presentation of pairs in a concurrent-discrimination task until it exceeded the interval across which normals can retain object-reward associations formed in a single trial. Unfortunately, experiments have not yet been reported to show what that interval is, nor even to show (as is assumed in the Phillips et al. hypothesis) that it is in fact less than 24 hours. Given the somewhat surprising immunity of the 24-hour intertrial interval concurrent-discrimination tasks to hippocampal/amygdalar lesions in monkeys, it is interesting to note that human amnesics show disruption both on concurrent discriminations in which several trials of each discrimination occur each day and on concurrent discriminations in which each pair is shown only once each day (Aggleton et al. 1988; Squire, Zola-Morgan, and Chen 1988).

Memory Versus Habits

Although the reasons for the absence of effect of combined lesions on the concurrent-discrimination tasks of the Malamut, Saunders, and Mishkin (1984), Bachevalier and Mishkin (1986), and Overman, Ormsby, and Mishkin (1990) reports remain obscure, the findings do emphasize a dramatic contrast between two different methods of assessing memory. Since each pair was presented only once each day, some form of memory for the outcome of single trials must have persisted for at least 24 hours. But in the recognition task, the same animals apparently could not remember for more than a few seconds whether they had seen a given object or not.

Malamut, Saunders, and Mishkin discuss the contrast between the recognition task and the concurrent-discrimination task and suggest that the critical difference between them lies in the number of trials involved. They suggest that, where learning occurs in one trial, a cognitive memory system embracing processes of both recognition and association is involved, and that in multitrial learning a habit system is involved—a system that involves the formation of stimulus-response bonds very much in the way envisaged by Hull and his followers.

Mishkin rightly points out (e.g., Mishkin, Malamut, and Bachevalier 1984) that the proposed distinction between a cognitive memory system and an S-R habit system has profound implications for the analysis of learning in intact animals, and has implications also for both comparative and developmental psychology (e.g., Bachevalier and Mishkin 1984). The data are not yet available, however, that would allow us to choose between analyses in terms of the procedural/declarative dichotomy versus the memory/habit dichotomy. There is clearly a good measure of agreement between the proposals, each of which posits two learning systems, one of which is in some sense more cognitive than the other. It is clear too that although puzzles remain in the data on concurrent-discrimination learning, both Squire and Mishkin and their colleagues agree that tasks in which large numbers of learning trials are necessary tend to be immune to disruption by hippocampal/amygdalar lesions: there does seem to be some feature of tasks that are learned rapidly that engages a system that does not contribute to performance in tasks that are gradually acquired.

There is a parallel here too with one of the features of the mapping system envisaged by O'Keefe and Nadel (1978). Their theory supposes that the locale system, located in the hippocampus, is capable of rapid updating of information whereas the taxon system shows only incremental changes in habit strengths. These theories all agree, then, that limbic structures are critically involved in a system that is more flexible and more cognitive than some other system for learning that is independent of limbic structures and is concerned with the gradual formation and modification of habits or skills the nature of which are less accessible to conscious awareness.

Role of Cortex Adjoining the Hippocampus and the Amygdala

The experiments reviewed above have succeeded in providing the best parallel between nonhuman and human amnesic effects following limbic damage. It therefore seems clear that further work using lesioned animals should help clarify the nature and proper interpretation of that amnesia. But the techniques conventionally used for making both hippocampal and amygdalar lesions in monkeys have also resulted in the removal of parts of the cortex adjoining those areas; the cortical regions involved lie in or adjoin the rhinal sulcus and include perirhinal, entorhinal, periamygdaloid, and parahippocampal cortex. It is now clear that invasion of these cortical areas is responsible for the severe deficits obtained following combined hippocampal/amygdalar lesions. Studies on monkeys will now be discussed that show: first, that damage to the amygdala itself does not make any contribution to global amnesia; second, that cortical damage alone produces memory deficits comparable to those obtained following the conventional hippocampal/amygdalar lesion, deficits that are more severe than those obtained by damage confined to the hippocampal formation (and excluding adjoining cortex). Before discussing these findings, it may be well to caution that they concern only monkeys. The techniques used by Aggleton, Blindt, and Rawlins (1989) for making hippocampal and amygdalar lesions in rats caused minimal invasion of adjoining cortical regions: it will be recalled that the combined hippocampal/amygdalar lesions of that study obtained deficits in retention that were not seen following either lesion alone (deficits that did, however, seem less severe than those reported following conventional hippocampal/amygdalar lesions in monkeys).

Amygdalar Lesions That Avoid Cortical Damage Do Not Potentiate Memory Deficits

Zola-Morgan, Squire, and Amaral (1989) explored the effects of lesions that were confined to the amygdala and did not invade adjoining cortical regions. These lesions did influence the emotional reactivity of the monkeys but did not disrupt performance on a variety of memory tasks. The tasks included DNMTS (with trial-unique objects), retention of object discriminations, and concurrent discrimination learning (with five trials each day for each pair of objects). Conventional hippocampal lesions (lesions that included damage to adjoining cortical structures) did disrupt performance in those same tasks. When conventional amygdalar lesions (lesions that include additional cortical damage) are added to (conventional) hippocampal damage, performance is, as we have previously seen, worse than that seen following conventional hippocampal lesions. However, figure 8.14 shows that when amygdalar lesions that avoided cortical damage

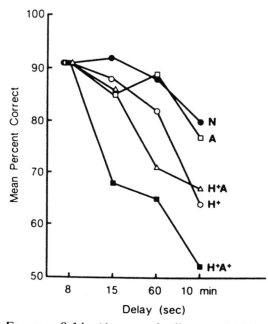

FIGURE 8.14. Absence of effect on DNMTS tasks of amygdalar lesions that spare adjacent cortical regions. N = normal (unoperated) monkeys; A = monkeys with amygdalar lesions that spared adjoining cortical regions; H$^+$ = monkeys with conventional lesions of the hippocampal formation; H$^+$A = monkeys with conventional hippocampal lesions combined with amygdalar lesions that spared adjoining cortical regions; H$^+$A$^+$ = monkeys with conventional lesions of the hippocampal formation combined with amygdalar lesions that invaded adjoining cortical regions. (*From* Zola-Morgan, Squire, and Amaral 1989b)

were added to conventional hippocampal lesions, no further deterioration was observed. These results show that damage to the amygdala proper does not disrupt memory processes and does not exacerbate the disruption obtained in memory tasks following hippocampal damage. The results show also that damage to cortical regions adjoining the amygdala does potentiate the disruption obtained by conventional hippocampal damage.

It should be emphasized here that although damage to cortical areas adjoining the amygdala is sufficient to reproduce the effects on memory tasks of conventional amygdalar damage, that cortical damage does not reproduce other effects that are obtained by conventional amygdalar damage; in particular, cortical damage alone does not result in the emotional changes that are seen following amygdalar damage. It seems likely, therefore, that the amygdala proper does indeed play a role in stimulus-reward associations but does not play a general role in recent memory.

Amnesia Following Lesions Confined to Cortical Regions

To complement the work showing an absence of effect of amygdalar lesions on memory, there is now evidence that hippocampal involvement is not necessary for severe memory impairment. Zola-Morgan et al. (1989) tested monkeys with damage to cortical regions (perirhinal and parahippocampal cortex) that are normally damaged when conventional combined hippocampal/amygdalar lesions are made; the lesions spared entorhinal cortex (which is also routinely damaged in the course of conventional hippocampal lesions), but transection of the white matter underlying the perirhinal cortex ensured that the entorhinal cortex was deprived of all cortical input. The monkeys were tested on three tasks (DNMTS, object discrimination, and concurrent discrimination with several presentations each day) known to be susceptible to disruption by conventional hippocampal/amygdalar lesions. The monkeys showed impairments on all three tasks, and the degree of impairment was comparable to that seen in monkeys with conventional hippocampal/amygdalar lesions. Hippocampal damage does not, then, in fact contribute to the memory impairments seen in monkeys following conventional hippocampal/amygdalar lesions; those impairments may all be accounted for by the effects of the cortical removals involved in those combined lesions.

Effects of Damage Restricted to the Hippocampus

There is, however, evidence that hippocampal damage alone does obtain memory deficits, albeit deficits that are less severe than those following removal of both perirhinal and parahippocampal cortex. We have already seen, for example, reports of memory deficits in both monkeys (e.g., Gaffan 1974) and rats (e.g., Olton and Papas 1979) following fornicotomy, a technique that avoids damage to cortex adjoining the hippocampus. Squire (1992) also reports more recent work, using techniques that confine damage to the hippocampal formation (the hippocampus proper, the dentate gyrus, and the subiculum) that finds a memory impairment (in a DNMTS task) equivalent to that seen following conventional hippocampal damage (but less severe, of course, than that seen following lesions that involve more extensive destruction of perirhinal and parahippocampal cortex).

Damage Restricted to the Hippocampus in a Human Amnesic (R.B.). Support for the involvement in memory of the hippocampus proper is available from a report by Zola-Morgan, Squire, and Amaral (1986), who were able to examine the brain of an amnesic patient (R.B.). R.B. had shown anterograde amnesia (with a restricted retrograde amnesia) following cerebral ischemia while recovering from a cardiac operation in 1978. He died from heart failure in 1983, and histological examination found a striking bilateral loss of cells in the CA1 region of the hippocampus. There was minor pathology in a few other areas that are not believed to be involved in global amnesia (in somatosensory cortex, in the globus pallidus, and in the cerebellum, for example); there was also some amygdalar damage, but of extremely limited extent (small foci of less than 1 mm^3). In general, all the subdivisions of the amygdala had a normal appearance. This report provides, then, good evidence that at least in humans hippocampal damage alone is sufficient to cause amnesia. It should be added that, although it is difficult to compare severity of amnesia across patients, it appears that R.B.'s amnesia, although severe, was not as profound as that seen in H.M. (in whom cortical regions adjoining the amygdala and hippocampus were removed); this report does not, therefore, run counter to the notion that damage to extrahippocampal structures plays a critical role in global amnesia in humans.

Behavioral Implications

The recent shift in focus from the hippocampus as a region necessarily involved in global amnesia poses difficulties for attempts to interpret memory function in terms of features specific to that structure (in terms, for example, of the detailed anatomical and physiological organization of the hippocampus). But no such problems are raised for behavioral psychologists, whose major interest lies in the nature of the behavioral breakdowns. The fact, for example, that the same monkey can learn concurrent discriminations with a very long intertrial interval but cannot master a DMTS task with a relatively short delay provides a behavioral dissociation that in itself points strongly to the existence of more than one memory system. The demonstration (Gaffan and Murray 1992) that this same dissociation may be obtained by rhinal cortical lesions that do not involve either the amygdala or the hippocampus has no direct bearing on the significance of the behavioral dissociation. It is true that the behavioral psychologist attempting to analyze and interpret a lesion-induced syndrome must be certain that the separate behavioral components of the syndrome could all be found (at least in principle) in the same animal. From this point of view, then, the behavioral psychologist does have an interest in locus and technique of lesions. But once it is established that one set of tasks is disrupted by the same lesion that does not affect another set of tasks, the psychologist is free to posit behavioral mechanisms that could account for the outcome and, at that point, the site of the lesion that produces the dissociation of interest is no longer relevant. In summary, it remains clear that certain types of learning task are immune to temporal limbic damage while others are profoundly affected. The question of major interest to psychologists—namely, whether the breakdowns point convincingly to a distinction between two types of memory system (between, for example, a declarative and a procedural domain of processing)—is not affected by shifts in our understanding concerning precisely which anatomical structures are necessarily involved in the breakdowns.

Current Status of Cognitive Theories of Hippocampal Function

We have seen in this and the preceding two chapters a bewildering array of facts and theories concerning the behavioral effects of hippocampal damage. It may be helpful to conclude this chapter with a brief résumé of the difficulties facing the various theories that have been discussed, followed by an assessment of the current status of "cognitive" theories of hippocampal function. This résumé will ignore questions of localization and will use "hippocampus" to refer rather freely to a variety of types of limbic damage, including combined (conventional) hippocampal/amygdalar damage.

Summary of Difficulties Facing Rival Theories

In chapter 6 we assessed the proposal that the hippocampus was involved in selective attention, and rejected that notion partly because some of the basic data in its support (the disruption of overshadowing and blocking by hippocampal damage) had been contradicted by subsequent reports, and partly because there are deficits (in, for example, maze learning and recognition memory tasks) that cannot be accounted for in terms of a deficit in selective attention.

Chapter 7 considered the notion that the hippocampus was concerned with contextual processing and with, in particular, the construction and use of a spatial map. That proposal was rejected partly because of data showing successful contextual processing in hippocampal animals, and partly, again, because there are hippocampal deficits (in reversal learning in the eyelid-conditioning preparation, for example) that seem resistant to explanation in terms of a contextual-processing deficit.

In the first part of this chapter we discussed the proposal that the hippocampus is critically involved in working memory, a proposal that was rejected partly because a number of tasks that should involve working memory (DNMTS with short delays, for example) are *not* disrupted by hippocampal damage, and partly because many tasks (such as the Morris water maze) that do not seem to require working memory *are* disrupted.

One negative feature of all those theories was the fact that they did not capture the central features of human hippocampal amnesia: hippocampal amnesic humans do not, for example, show any *special* difficulty in remembering spatial as opposed to nonspatial information, and generally show unimpaired performance on short-term memory tasks.

Cognitive Theories: Congruent with Basic Human Data

Recent work on human amnesics has emphasized that they can retain some information normally over long periods, while failing quite dramatically to retain other types of information. One of the best illustrations of this dissociation surely remains the report by Claparède (1911, cited by Weiskrantz and Warrington 1979). Claparède describes observations he made on a female patient with Korsakoff's Syndrome: "I tried the following experiment . . . to see if she would better retain an intense impression that set affectivity into play. I pricked her hand forcibly with a pin hidden between my fingers. This little pain was as quickly forgotten as indifferent perceptions and, shortly after the pricking, she remembered no more of it. However, when I moved my hand near hers again, she pulled back her hand in a reflex way and without knowing why. If, in fact, I demanded the reason for the withdrawal of her hand, she answered in a flurried way, 'Isn't it allowed to withdraw one's hand?.' . . . If I insisted, she would say to me, 'Perhaps there is a pin hidden in your hand.' To my question, 'What can make you suspect that I would like to prick you,' she would take up her refrain, 'It is an idea which came into my head,' or sometimes she would try to justify herself with 'Sometimes pins are hidden in hands.' But she never recognized this idea of pricking as a memory" (Weiskrantz and Warrington 1979:187). The latter part of this chapter has introduced cognitive theories of hippocampal function, theories that have had the virtue that they do capture the dissociation seen in Claparède's patient.

The first cognitive proposal discussed was due to Gaffan and was that hippocampal damage disrupted recognition memory while leaving associative memory intact. Gaffan's proposal received good support from experimental work on a range of tasks that might be supposed to involve recognition in nonhumans. It did appear, however, that the hypothesis was too narrow in the sense that some tasks that did not appear to require recognition (learning to select an object recently seen and not rewarded, for example) did show disruption following hippocampal damage; moreover, there were a number of reports showing relatively little disruption of recognition following hippocampal damage.

The final hypothesis constituted in effect an expansion of the recognition hypothesis, so that the failure of recognition was treated as one instance of disruption of a declarative memory system, a system now distinguished not from associative memory but from procedural memory. This proposal, which supposes that short-term memory remains intact following hippocampal damage, maintains the parallel with the human deficit and has resulted in an impressive series of demonstrations of comparable performance (in a variety of tasks) by human amnesics and limbic-damaged monkeys.

Can Basic Evidence for Rival Theories Be Accommodated Within the Procedural/Declarative Framework?

We have discussed one set of findings—on concurrent-discrimination learning with a 24-hour intertrial interval—that cannot easily be accommodated within the procedural/declarative framework. Are there substantial bodies of discordant data? It would be tedious here to go through all the experimental results that have been cited in previous chapters, to see whether or not they can be accommodated satisfactorily. But a consideration of some of the findings that have provided good support for other theories will help to set the current status of the theory in perspective.

The best evidence in support of the selective attention hypothesis was the disruption by hippocampal damage of latent inhibition; it has already been argued that this finding can readily be interpreted as a consequence of a failure of recognition memory, and so, as support for the procedural/declarative dichotomy.

The best evidence for the spatial mapping hypothesis derives from the severe disruption of maze learning by hippocampal damage, and it is frankly not easy at present to accommodate the maze learning data in terms of the procedural/declarative dichotomy. It was suggested in the discussion of Gaffan's recognition memory hypothesis that failure to recognize a piece of apparatus would result in exploration of that apparatus, and that exploration would conflict with approach to arms or regions associated with reward. Such an account might explain why hippocampal rats do not swim toward the site of a hidden platform in the Morris maze, but would find it difficult to explain why they do successfully swim toward a visible platform in the same apparatus, and difficult to explain why hippocampal rats can learn to avoid arms in a radial maze that are never rewarded.

Squire (1987) suggests that "Declarative memory includes memory for spatial location but is not limited to it" (Squire 1987:223), a proposal that in effect attempts to incorporate the spatial mapping theory into the procedural/declarative dichotomy. This proposal is surely too sweeping and faces some of the problems facing the spatial mapping hypothesis: hippocampal rats, for example, seem exceedingly reliant upon contextual information, rather than vice versa (Winocur and Olds 1978). And if spatial information is simply on a par with other information, why are spatial reversals more susceptible to disruption than nonspatial reversals (e.g., Mahut 1971)?

Olton's working memory theory of hippocampal function received good support from the demonstration that fornicotomized rats could learn to avoid arms of a radial maze that were never baited, but could not remember within a trial which baited arms had already been visited. Since learning to avoid unbaited arms is a gradual, incremental process, it may reasonably be regarded as an instance of procedural learning. This proposal does, however, face a serious difficulty: although the fornicotomized rats of the Olton and Papas (1979) study did learn to avoid unbaited arms, they showed no retention of preoperatively acquired memory for unbaited arms. Thus, as we saw in considering the Malamut, Saunders, and Mishkin (1984) experiment on 24-hour intertrial interval concurrent-discrimination learning, there appears to be postoperative amnesia for information that is best interpreted as procedural.

At first sight, the deficit shown by fornicotomized rats in the working memory component of the radial maze is problematic for a theory that supposes that short-term memory (regarded as equivalent in nonhumans to working memory) is intact following hippocampal damage. But there are peculiar behavioral features of working memory in the radial maze, and prominent amongst these is the fact that rats can remember over long intervals which arms have been entered within a trial: Beatty and Shavalia (1980) found that if a delay of 4 hours was imposed between the first four and the second four choices of a trial in an 8-arm maze, accuracy (selection of arms not previously entered) over the second four choices was better than 90 percent. This surprising result implies that in this task rats hold information about choices in a long-term store; Squire's proposal that hippocampal damage prevents access of declarative information to long-term memory can therefore accommodate this finding.

Evidence in support of Gaffan's recognition memory theory does, of course, also support the procedural/declarative dichotomy since recognition memory is a species of declarative memory. It is worth inquiring, however, whether the evidence that weakened Gaffan's theory can be accommodated any better within the procedural/declarative dichotomy. We shall consider two examples here. The first is the Gaffan et al. (1984) report that fornicotomized monkeys could learn to select an object that had recently been seen in association with reward but could not learn to select an object that had been seen in association with nonreward. The fact that Spiegler and Mishkin (1981) have shown that hippocampal damage may in fact obtain a mild disruption of learning to select an object associated with reward does not alter the basic question why learning to select objects not associated with reward should prove differentially susceptible to fornix damage.

The tasks in question are both 1-trial learning tasks and should therefore rely upon the declarative system. Learning to select an object associated with nonreward is clearly less "automatic" than learning to select one associated with reward; it could be argued that the less automatic a task is, the more its reliance upon declarative as opposed to procedural memory. But, applied to the current problem, this proposal would require us to suppose a considerable reliance upon procedural memory in the "automatic" version of the task, despite its being a 1-trial learning procedure. Given that we have already argued that procedural and declarative processes should occur in parallel in associative tasks, this may be an assumption that could be adopted. It would, however, mean that we could no longer use rate of learning as an indicator of the relative involvement of the declarative and procedural systems.

A second difficulty facing the recognition theory was the disruption in the rabbit eyelid-conditioning preparation of reversal learning, of trace conditioning, and of delay conditioning using nonoptimal interstimulus intervals. All these procedures show slow acquisition rates in comparison with the standard delay procedure, using an optimal interstimulus interval. If slow learning rate is an indicator of the involvement of the procedural system, then that system should have been engaged in the tasks that hippocampal lesions disrupted. But, again, the tasks that were disrupted were in a sense all less automatic than the standard task. Perhaps they should be seen as multitrial tasks that, because of their deviation from automaticity, nevertheless rely upon declarative memory.

Thus although the procedural/declarative dichotomy enjoys the advantage of providing an intuitively satisfying account of the basic features of human hippocampal amnesia and has led to valuable new insights into the nature of the dysfunction obtained by hippocampal damage in nonhumans, it does, like its rival theories, face many unsolved problems. It is not clear that it provides an account of spatial learning deficits, and there is as yet no unequivocal way of deciding the extent to which a given task relies upon declarative as opposed to procedural memory, a problem that leads to a danger of circular explanations: without an independent criterion of the extent to which particular tasks rely upon procedural versus declarative memory, there is a temptation to conclude too easily that those tasks that yield deficits following hippocampal damage involve declarative memory, and that those that do not, involve procedural memory.

Concluding Comments: Progress Toward Characterization of Cognitive Capacities

The clear conclusion of the discussions of this and the preceding two chapters is that all current theories of hippocampal function find difficulties in accommodating certain bodies of data. As has already been argued, it may be that hippocampal damage disrupts more than one system, so that not all the deficits are to be explained in the same way; it may be that none of the current theories has yet hit upon the basic nature of some pervasive source of disruption; and it may be that one of the current theories is substantially correct, but that we have not yet understood the proper behavioral analysis of some of the tasks. Finally, it may be that some confusion exists as a result of the use of different types of lesions and of different species of animals. We have considered in this survey results obtained from the use of a variety of techniques on rats, monkeys, and rabbits, and it may be the case that some of the deficits discussed would not occur together in any preparation.

The difficulties facing current theories should not be allowed to obscure the progress that has been made. Although the notion that the hippocampus is primarily concerned with working memory was rejected, we have appealed to the notion that short-term memory is *not* disrupted by hippocampal damage. This, for example, has seemed the best way of explaining the many reports of tasks (e.g., DNMTS using trial-unique objects) that are not disrupted by hippocampal damage when relatively short (10 sec or so) delays are used, but are disrupted when longer delays are used. To the extent that this proposal provides a convincing account of the data, the notion that there is a real dichotomy between short- and long-term memory gains support. The (lesion-based) case for that dichotomy is clearly not so strong in nonhumans as in humans, but this may reflect the fact that short-term memory in nonhumans has been less well explored behaviorally. Although controversy exists over the question whether there is in humans a distinction between mechanisms involved in short- and long-term memory, there is good general agreement among those cognitive psychologists who posit the existence of a discrete short-term memory store over a set of tasks that should be selectively sensitive to disruption of that store; thus Baddeley and Warrington were able to compare the performance of normal control and amnesic humans "using a range of standard laboratory memory tasks varying in the extent to which performance is assumed to depend on STM and LTM" (Baddeley and Warrington 1970:177). No such general agreement on the extent to which a set of tasks engage short- as opposed to long-term memory is currently to be found in the literature on nonhuman memory.

Work on nonhumans has, however, provided strong support for the claim that analysis of the disruptions induced by hippocampal damage has revealed a contrast between two systems of learning, one simpler and more automatic than the other, more cognitive, system. There currently exist a number of ways of characterizing the distinction between the two systems, and table 8.5 shows a listing prepared by Squire (1987) of terms used by proponents of various theories. It may not yet be possible to make a final decision in favor of a particular characterization, but that does not alter the fact that what has already been established carries important implications for behavioral psychologists.

The experimental work discussed in this chapter has been driven by hypotheses derived from cognitive psychology, and it is perhaps inevitable that the theoretical impetus for work in neuroscience should be provided by behavioral theories. We should note here that physiological findings themselves feed back into behavioral theory (modifications to which may result in turn in novel and testable physiological predictions). The work

TABLE 8.5

Alternative Characterizations of Two Memory Systems Uncovered by Hippocampal Damage

Fact memory	Skill memory
Declarative	Procedural
Memory	Habit
Explicit	Implicit
Knowing that	Knowing how
Cognitive mediation	Semantic
Conscious recollection	Skills
Elaboration	Integration
Memory with record	Memory without record
Autobiographical memory	Perceptual memory
Representational memory	Dispositional memory
Vertical association	Horizontal association
Locale	Taxon
Episodic	Semantic
Working	Reference

SOURCE: Squire 1987.

that has been introduced in this chapter has largely concerned studies on nonhumans, and the dichotomy of systems that is proposed has special relevance for theorists concerned with animal learning. Current theories of learning in animals deal primarily with laws governing the formation of associations. It seems likely that, to the extent that any of the proposed systems of laws is valid, those laws apply to the operation of only one of the learning systems identified by physiological work (and presumably, to the simpler of the systems). If our interpretation of the physiological data is valid, learning theories will be seriously incomplete until they produce a further set of laws that will successfully characterize the operations of the cognitive system. This argument highlights the interdependence of physiological and behavioral psychology. The fact that we cannot provide currently a fully satisfactory account of the behavioral effects of hippo-campal lesions was, in a sense, inevitable: given that these lesions affect a cognitive as opposed to some simpler system, and that, particularly for animals, we possess no complete formal account of the properties of the cognitive system, lesion effects are bound to be unpredictable. Further physiological work, informed (as before) by concepts drawn from behav-ioral theory, should help to clarify the range of tasks that are susceptible to hippocampal damage. The results of those investigations should aid the work of behavioral psychologists attempting to specify the properties of the more cognitive of the two systems for learning and memory.

9. Unexplored Avenues

Tripartite Organization of This Chapter

This final chapter will consider three areas that, despite their importance, have received little attention elsewhere in this book. Discussion of the first two areas will introduce two disciplines—comparative neurology and computational neuroscience—that may help unravel some of the problems thrown up in attempts to understand telencephalic function in mammalian learning. These disciplines have received relatively little attention not only in this book, but, until recently, in the neuroscience community in general. The third area is that of neocortical function, and in discussing that area one focus of interest will be upon the degree to which understanding of neocortical function has progressed since Lashley's day.

Two Outstanding Problems

The preceding chapters have shown many good reasons for the current interest in the hippocampus, and perhaps the most compelling reasons have been the discovery there of LTP (long-term potentiation) and the series of demonstrations of relatively specific cognitive deficits following hippocampal damage. But two clear difficulties have arisen in considering the available data: first, it has not so far proved possible to generate a theory of hippocampal function that accommodates satisfactorily the entire range of effects reported as consequences of hippocampal damage; second, we cannot yet see how to integrate the phenomenon of LTP—an associative process—into a general account of the hippocampus, a structure that does not appear to play a primary role in association formation. We shall consider now the possible value of two disciplines in helping overcome these difficulties.

A. COMPARATIVE VERTEBRATE NEUROLOGY

The first unexplored avenue may be briefly characterized as comparative vertebrate neurology, and it will be suggested here that work in this field might contribute to untangling the behavioral role of the hippocampus.

Importance of Dissociation

The vast majority of work on hippocampal function has used rats, rabbits, or monkeys as subjects. A bewildering array of behavioral deficits consequent upon hippocampal damage has been thrown up: deficits, for example, in latent inhibition, in reversal learning, in maze learning, in timing behavior, in recognition memory. Theories of hippocampal function have generally attempted to accommodate all these deficits within a single explanatory framework. But, as has been suggested in previous chapters, it may be the case that not all these deficits are due to disruption of a single system—some deficits may have one cause, some a quite different cause. It would, then, be interesting to know whether all these deficits invariably co-occur, or whether some of them might not in come circumstances be dissociable. Dissociable hippocampal deficits—deficits that may occur independently of one another—must be assumed to have different causes and could therefore not be accounted for by any single theory of hippocampal function.

Dissociation by Variation in Physiological Technique

How might dissociable deficits be teased apart? One method would be to use different types of physiological interference: if there is more than one type of behavioral system represented in the hippocampus, it might be that one of the systems was more susceptible to a given type of interference (e.g., to a lesion in a particular subregion or to depletion of a specific neurotransmitter) than some other system. There are two difficulties with this approach. First, the use of different types of interference has not as a matter of fact been particularly fruitful: as we have seen, variation in lesion type has not so much clarified hippocampal function as increased the confusion about function. Second, negative results are not helpful: even if more than one system is represented in the hippocampus, the systems might be widely represented throughout the hippocampus and so not independently susceptible to damage in different subregions; moreover, even if different systems did occupy different subregions, direct disruption of function of one region might nevertheless invariably indirectly disrupt normal function in adjacent regions (by, for example, altering local background field potentials). Thus a series of failures to establish dissociations within the hippocampus would not rule out the possibility of the existence there of fundamentally independent behavioral systems.

A Comparative Approach to Dissociation

A second method of seeking dissociable deficits is to explore the effects of hippocampal lesions in different species. Now although a number of mammalian species have been used, no convincing demonstration of a species difference amongst them in hippocampal function has been reported. This may be because there has been relatively little overlap between the types of procedure used with different species: work on rabbits, for example, has concentrated on classical conditioning of the eyelid response; work on rats, on maze learning; and work on monkeys, on various visual discrimination tasks, normally using objects as discriminanda. But the failure to demonstrate intramammalian species differences may reflect the fact that there are amongst mammals no differences in hippocampal function to be found. There are, after all, at least general similarities across mammalian species in hippocampal deficits: deficits in latent inhibition and in reversal learning are seen in both rabbits and rats; and deficits in spatial learning are reported in both rats and monkeys. It may, then, be that the behavioral systems represented in the hippocampus are essentially the same in all mammalian species. This possibility gains support from the fact that, despite differences in hippocampal size (differences that are closely correlated with differences in brain size), hippocampal organization is similar—at least in gross anatomy—throughout mammals. All mammals show the same pattern of two interlocked sets of cells—the hippocampus proper and the dentate gyrus—and the same orderly layered structure. But there is a group of vertebrates whose hippocampus appears very different from that of mammals, despite their being clearly homologous structures. That group is the class of birds.

Avian Telencephalic Organization

Mammals and birds have evolved independently since the appearance of the first reptiles, some 300 million years ago, and, as can be seen from figure 9.1, there are striking differences between the anatomical organization of the telencephalon of the two classes. There is no neocortex in birds, and the avian telencephalon is dominated by nuclear regions known as the paleostriatal, archistriatal, neostriatal, and hyperstriatal complexes. It is now generally agreed that the avian archistriatal complex corresponds to the mammalian amygdaloid complex; the paleostriatal complex, to the mammalian basal ganglia; and the neostriatal and hyperstriatal complexes, to the neocortex (for a discussion of the evidence for correspondence between these regions, and for a review of their involvement in learning, see Macphail 1982).

Avian Hippocampal Complex

It is also generally agreed that both the mammalian and the avian hippocampus developed from the reptilian dorsomedial cortex, but whereas the mammalian hippocampus has migrated laterally, the avian hippocampus remains in the original dorsomedial position. There are not only topological grounds on which to base the homology between the avian hippocampal formation (the hippocampus and the adjoining parahippocampal area) and the mammalian formation. General support is available from a number of sources, including embryological (Källén 1962) and neurochemical studies (e.g., Brauth et al. 1986; Dietl, Cortés, and Palacios 1988a; Krebs, Erichsen, and Bingman 1991; Reiner et al. 1984). More specific evidence of parallels between avian and mammalian hippocampus derives

---

FIGURE **9.1.** Transverse sections through the pigeon telencephalon. The figures at the side of each drawing indicate the location of the section (in millimeters anterior to the interaural zero), using the vertical plane of the Karten and Hodos (1967) atlas. Ad = archistriatum dorsale; APH = area parahippocampalis; Av = archistriatum ventrale; Cb = cerebellum; CDL = area corticoidea dorsolateralis; E = ectostriatum; HA = hyperstriatum accessorium; HD = hyperstriatum dorsale; Hp = hippocampus; HV = hyperstriatum ventrale; HVdv = hyperstriatum ventrale dorso-ventrale; HVvv = hyperstriatum ventrale ventroventrale; IHA = nucleus intercalatus hyperstriati accessorii; LPO = lobus parolfactorius; N = neostriatum; NB = nucleus basalis; NC = neostriatum caudale; PA = paleostriatum augmentatum; Pi = cortex piriformis; PP = paleostriatum primitivum; SL = nucleus septalis lateralis; Va = vallecula. (*After* Karten and Hodos 1967)

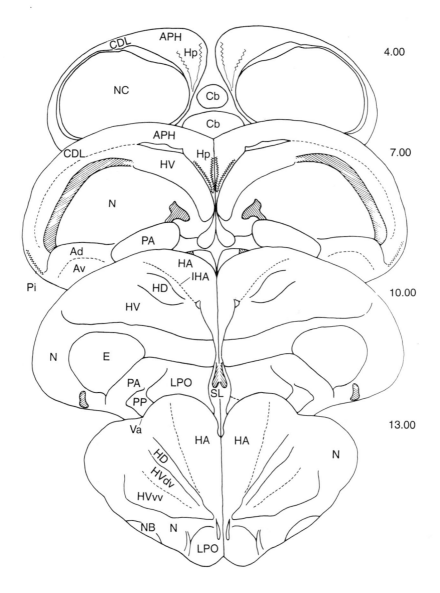

from studies of their respective afferent and efferent connectivities (Krayniak and Siegel 1978a, 1978b; Berk and Hawkin 1985; Casini, Bingman, and Bagnoli 1986; Kitt and Brauth 1986; Benowitz and Karten 1976).

The main body of the avian hippocampus consists of a V-shaped layer of densely packed cells that contains within and above the limbs of the V a dorsomedial zone having little obvious structure. Erichsen, Bingman, and Krebs (1991) have proposed, on the basis of immunocytochemical evidence, that the V-shaped structure (which does contain pyramidlike cells) may correspond to the hippocampus proper of mammals, and that the dorsomedial region (which contains some granule-like cells) may correspond to the mammalian dentate gyrus.

The parallels between the avian and mammalian hippocampus should not be exaggerated: although there is evidence for the existence of intrinsic connections within the avian hippocampal complex (Casini, Bingman, and Bagnoli 1986; Krebs, Erichsen, and Bingman 1991), there is no evidence currently of any system in birds equivalent to the mammalian hippocampal trisynaptic pathway (and Erichsen, Bingman, and Krebs [1991] have reported failures to identify a mossy-fiber system in birds using anatomical techniques that are successful in mammals). Similarly, although there is evidence for cholinergic projections to the avian hippocampus (Krebs, Erichsen, and Bingman 1991), a study of pigeon muscarinic cholinergic receptors (Dietl, Cortés, and Palacios 1988b) found that they occurred in very low densities in the hippocampal complex (whereas the rat hippocampus shows high densities of muscarinic receptors). And the parallels in connectivity, although striking, are far from complete. Although the avian hippocampus, for example, projects to the septal area, it does not receive any direct input from the medial septal nucleus (Krayniak and Siegel 1978b). The potential significance of this observation emerges when it is recalled (from chapter 6) that the mammalian theta rhythm is driven by pacemaker cells in the medial septal nucleus.

The avian parahippocampal area shows parallels, in terms of connectivity, with the mammalian subicular complex (Benowitz and Karten 1976; Krayniak and Siegel 1978a). But it is a region that shows very little structure and does not, unlike the regions within the mammalian subicular complex, show any clear layering. And we simply do not know enough of avian brain organization to answer questions about, for example, connections of the avian hippocampal complex with "association areas."

Conclusions

The evidence summarized above points to three uncontroversial conclusions. First, there are sufficient parallels between the avian and mammalian hippocampus to establish a homology between those regions; second, there are more differences between any avian hippocampus and any mammalian hippocampus than there are between the hippocampi of any two mammalian species; third, in terms of anatomical differentiation, the avian hippocampus is considerably simpler than the mammalian hippocampus. These conclusions in turn encourage the view that if more than one system is represented in the mammalian hippocampus, it is at least possible that some but not all of the same systems are represented in the avian hippocampus. With that notion in mind, we may turn now to consider studies of avian hippocampal function with a particular interest in potential involvement in spatial learning and in memory.

Avian Hippocampus and Spatial Learning

Homing by Pigeons After Hippocampal Damage

One of the most spectacular examples of spatial performance in the animal kingdom is surely the homing of pigeons: these birds return from wholly unfamiliar release sites at considerable distances from their home lofts, and the time taken for homing flights indicates that the route taken must be remarkably direct. There is general agreement that homing involves three components: a navigational system that allows the bird to calculate from any locus the bearing for home; a compass that allows the bird to fly on a given bearing; and a system for learning landmarks that comes into operation in the vicinity of home. The well-documented deficits in spatial learning following hippocampal damage in mammals lead naturally to an interest in the effects of similar damage on homing in pigeons, and a series of such studies has been reported by Bingman and his colleagues. The story that has emerged is not, as might have been anticipated, a simple one and is perhaps best approached chronologically.

Appropriate Orientation But Failure to Home

An early experiment (Bingman et al. 1984) found that hippocampal pigeons (pigeons having lesions of both the hippocampus and the parahippocampal area) failed to home from distant (more than 30 km from home) release sites, whether those sites were familiar or unfamiliar. But despite the failure to home successfully, the hippocampal birds did show efficient initial orientation on release: figure 9.2 shows that the direction in which most birds were flying when they vanished over the horizon was, like that of controls, very close to the true bearing for home. A second experiment from the same report found that, even when released within site of their

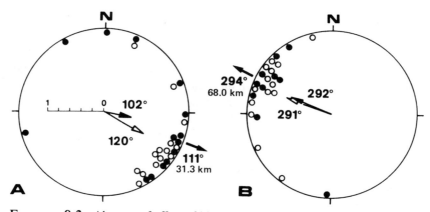

FIGURE 9.2. Absence of effect of hippocampal lesions on initial orientation of homing pigeons. Fig. 9.2A shows initial orientation in a release from a familiar site; fig. 9.2B shows initial orientation in a release from an unfamiliar site. Each dot on the periphery of the circles indicates the vanishing bearing of one bird. *Open dots:* unoperated controls; *filled dots:* hippocampal birds. The outer arrows indicate home, whose direction and distance are given. The inner arrows represent the mean vectors corresponding to open and filled dots; the length of the vectors can be read with the scale in fig. 9.2A. (*From* Bingman et al. 1984)

TABLE 9.1

Effect of Hippocampal Lesions on Entry into Visible Home Lofts

Lesion Group	Released	Landed Near Lofts	Entered	Entered Own Lofts	Entered Other Lofts	Disappeared
Sham-operated	6	6	6	5	1	0
Hippocampals	8	7	2	0	2	5
Operated controls	5	5	5	5	0	0

SOURCE: Bingman et al., 1984.

NOTE: Operated control birds had lesions of the hyperstriatal complex that invaded primarily hyperstriatum accessorium and hyperstriatum dorsale.

home lofts (some 800 m away), hippocampal birds failed to reenter their lofts. Observation of these birds found that hippocampal birds often approached and explored the loft area (where other pigeons were to be seen), but, as can be seen from table 9.1, that they generally did not enter the lofts and showed no tendency to explore their own as opposed to any other loft.

The combination of accurate initial orientation followed by failure to home from within site of the lofts encouraged the view that the deficit of hippocampal birds lay in "the recognition of the home loft and/or its immediate surroundings" (Bingman et al. 1984:105), a deficit that they regard as nonspatial (Bingman et al. 1987).

Successful Homing by Pigeons Given Postoperative Experience

Another early report (Bingman et al. 1985) found that postoperative experience was critical to the effects of hippocampal damage on homing. The pigeons in the 1984 report had only one or two days' postoperative experience of their home loft surroundings, and Bingman et al. (1985) found that when pigeons were given seven days' or so postoperative experience of their home lofts and allowed to see out (but not to fly) from them, hippocampal lesions no longer prevented homing from a release site 800 m from the home loft. Subsequent experiments (Bingman et al. 1987, 1988a) have shown that, given postoperative home-loft experience, hippocampal pigeons home successfully from distant sites (familiar and unfamiliar).

The remedial effects of postoperative home-loft experience imply that the recognition deficit applies only to preoperatively acquired cues—in other words, that hippocampal damage obtains retrograde amnesia for cues associated with the home loft. But this does not provide a complete explanation: Bingman et al. (1985) also reported that if pigeons were allowed seven days' postoperative experience of a novel loft, hippocampal pigeons did not then home successfully to that loft (nor to their preoperative home loft). Thus hippocampal birds that do home successfully cannot simply have learned the home-loft cues from scratch during their postoperative experience of them: some trace of their preoperative home-loft experience clearly remains.

Orientation of Anosmic Pigeons

Although our understanding of the pigeon's navigational system remains seriously incomplete, it appears that olfactory input plays an important role, since anosmic pigeons do not show appropriate initial orientation when released from unfamiliar sites (Benvenuti et al. 1973). Anosmic pigeons do, however, show appropriate orientation when released from familiar sites, and this finding is taken to show that the navigational system is redundant at familiar sites, where local landmarks may serve to allow efficient orientation. Hippocampal pigeons' ability to use landmarks at sites distant from the home loft can therefore be explored by looking at the performance of anosmic birds. The relevant experimental data indicate that, once again, postoperative experience is critical. Bingman et al. (1987, 1988b) reported the effects of anosmia on the initial orientation of hippocampal pigeons released at distant familiar sites (the pigeons had extensive postoperative experience of the home loft and could therefore be expected to recognize the home-loft cues). Anosmia was induced temporarily by injection of a local anesthetic into the nostrils (and the nostrils had been kept plugged during the journey to the release site). When the birds were released from sites with which they had had extensive preoperative (but no postoperative) experience, the initial orientation of hippocampal birds was (unlike that of controls) severely disrupted. But when the birds were released from sites with which they had become familiar postoperatively, anosmic hippocampal pigeons (like controls) showed efficient initial orientation.

Bingman et al. (1987) characterized the deficit of anosmic hippocampal pigeons as showing retrograde amnesia for spatial reference memories, and drew a parallel with the retrograde amnesia shown by fornicotomized rats in the radial maze for reference memory components of preoperatively established performance (e.g., Olton and Papas 1979; see chapter 8 above). The parallel is further supported by the fact that both hippocampal pigeons and fornicotomized rats show normal postoperative acquisition (or reacquisition) of spatial reference memory information (Bingman et al. 1988b; Olton and Papas 1979).

Hippocampal Pigeons Show Longer Flight Times

The results recounted this far point to a (retrograde) disruption of memory as opposed to a disruption of spatial mapping, since the latter proposal would anticipate no special difficulty associated with preoperatively as opposed to postoperatively acquired information. But there is one further finding which indicates that in fact processing of postoperatively acquired information is disrupted by hippocampal damage.

The measures of homing performance reported above have been accuracy of initial orientation and success or failure in returning to enter the home loft. Bingman has in his more recent studies also used another measure—the time taken to complete the flight home—and has found that hippocampal birds released from distant sites consistently take longer to fly home than do controls, whether the release sites are unfamiliar or familiar (due to either pre- or postoperative experience) (Bingman et al. 1987, 1988a, 1988b). In other words, although hippocampal pigeons given postoperative home-loft experience show efficient initial orientation and return home successfully from unfamiliar and familiar sites, they do not make that flight as efficiently as normals.

Since (given appropriate postoperative experience) initial orientation is efficient and hippocampal pigeons successfully approach home-loft cues, Bingman et al. (1988a) argue that the deficit in flight times must concern performance during the middle stage of the flight home. Bingman and his colleagues suggest that pigeons "use landmarks, not necessarily visual, to direct a course to their loft in a manner distinct from their navigational map" (Bingman et al. 1988a:562), and "offer as a working hypothesis impaired use of landmarks to locate the home loft" (p. 563) to explain the poor performance of hippocampal pigeons.

The flight-time deficit of hippocampal pigeons is compared by Bingman et al. (1988a) to the impaired performance of hippocampal rats in the Morris water maze. Hippocampal rats in the water maze show deficits in the use of distal cues (features of the experimental room) while being capable of successfully approaching proximal cues (a visible platform) (Morris et al. 1982; see chapter 7 above). Similarly, hippocampal pigeons show deficits in the use of distal cues (landmarks on the middle stage of the route home) but successfully approach home-loft cues. These parallels indicate "remarkable similarity in the nature of spatial performance deficits that follow hippocampal lesions in both rats and pigeons, and support the general hypothesis of hippocampal function in spatial navigation" (Bingman et al. 1988a:563). Bingman and his colleagues accept the prima facie case for supposing that accurate initial orientation by hippocampal pigeons might seem to imply an intact navigational system, but argue that O'Keefe and Nadel's (1978) spatial mapping interpretation of hippocampal function might nevertheless apply to pigeons. This they do on the grounds that "because of the complex nature of the pigeon navigational map, and its reliance on non-visual cues, it is not clear where it would fall into O'Keefe and Nadel's scheme" (Bingman et al. 1987:154–55).

Two Deficits: Is a Unitary Account Possible?

Bingman and his colleagues have identified two distinct deficits associated with hippocampal damage in pigeons: retrograde amnesia for preoperatively acquired information (both nonspatial and spatial), and a lasting postoperative deficit in use of distal cues. They have pointed to parallels between those deficits and deficits seen following hippocampal damage in rats, and have suggested that the deficit in use of distal cues reflects a disruption of spatial mapping. However, they do not suppose (e.g., Bingman et al. 1988b) that the retrograde amnesia deficits can be accommodated within a mapping hypothesis; so that in effect they propose that the two deficits have different underlying causes. If only for the sake of parsimony, a unitary account of hippocampal function is to be preferred, and it will be suggested here that one might be provided by appealing to the procedural/declarative dichotomy.

The most striking effect of hippocampal damage on homing is a retrograde amnesia for both proximal and distal cues. This deficit is reminiscent of the retrograde amnesia found in hippocampal monkeys for object discriminations (Salmon, Zola-Morgan and Squire 1987). Similarly, the disruption seen in hippocampal pigeons in postoperative use of landmarks on the route home finds a parallel in the disruption seen in monkeys in postoperative acquisition and retention of object discriminations (Zola-Morgan and Squire 1984). The effects of hippocampal damage on homing in pigeons do, then, seem close to those reported in hippocampal monkeys learning and remembering object discriminations.

The declarative processing account of hippocampal function (introduced in chapter 8) supposes that (easy) object discriminations are disrupted because discrimination between multidimensional stimuli relies primarily upon declarative processing and very little upon the procedural process of learning to attend to the relevant dimension. The parallel between avian and mammalian hippocampal function may, then, be extended a little further with the observation that, like objects, visual landmarks are multidimensional items with multiple redundant features. Thus, if hippocampal pigeons suffer from a deficit in declarative processing, they might be expected to show retrograde amnesia for preoperatively acquired information about landmarks, and a persistent postoperative impairment in learning to use landmarks. It cannot be pretended that this declarative account of pigeon hippocampal function can accommodate all the data on homing without strain. One obvious problem is that the current proposal would expect deficits in postoperative learning about those items (home-loft cues and release-site landmarks) for which retrograde amnesia is seen; but we have found no evidence for any such deficits, and this is a difficulty that can currently be overcome only by the unsatisfactory assumption that the measures used are simply less sensitive than the flight-time measure.

Conclusions

Whatever the interpretation put upon the deficits, it is clear that there are plausible parallels between the effects of hippocampal damage in pigeons on homing and certain effects seen following hippocampal damage in mammals. At the least, therefore, these data suggest that there may indeed be some processes in common to the functions of the avian and the mammalian hippocampus. This review of the effects of hippocampal lesions on homing by pigeons has favored an account in terms of dysfunction of a general memory process rather than in terms of a spatial mapping dysfunction. Problematic for a spatial mapping account were, first, that a retrograde amnesia (for both spatial and nonspatial information) has been found, and second, that the absence of any effect of hippocampal damage on the navigational system demonstrates that at least one mapping system is immune to hippocampal damage in pigeons. Nevertheless, we have also seen that an account of avian hippocampal function in terms of spatial mapping could account for postoperative deficits in flight times, and we shall find somewhat better support for a specifically spatial account in the following section, which explores the role of the hippocampus in another type of avian spatial memory.

Cache Recovery by Food-storing Birds

A second spectacular example of spatial performance in birds is provided by food-storing birds of the Paridae (tit or chickadee), Corvidae (crow), and Sittidae (nuthatch) families. These birds may, over the course of a season, hide thousands of seeds in caches, recovering them hours, days, even months later. Field observations and laboratory studies have combined to show that the birds use memory in recovering these caches (rather than, for example, caching in sites having some specific sensory characteristic and searching only in sites with that characteristic: Sherry 1984). There are now grounds for supposing that the hippocampus is involved in cache recovery by food-storing birds.

Food-Storing Species Possess an Enlarged Hippocampus

One type of relevant evidence has been provided by two recent reports concerning the size of the hippocampal complex (hippocampus and parahippocampal area) in storing and nonstoring birds. Krebs et al. (1989) examined the brains of 52 individuals, the birds coming from thirty-five species (or subspecies) of European passerines (songbirds) that belonged in turn to nine different families; nine of the species were food-storing birds (all of these were parids, corvids, or sittids). Sherry et al. (1989) examined the brains of 28 individuals, drawn from twenty-three species of North American passerines that belonged to thirteen families and subfamilies (three of the species were food-storing birds from the parid, corvid, and sittid families).

The main findings of both reports were identical. The largest single determinants of hippocampal size were, unsurprisingly, body weight and telencephalon size; but when those effects were parceled out (in a multiple regression analysis), there emerged a highly significant relationship between food storing and hippocampal volume. A striking example of the difference in hippocampal size between species may be found in comparing the data reported by Krebs et al. (1989) for two parid species—the marsh tit (*Parus palustris*) and the great tit (*P. major*). The marsh tit, a small food-storing bird, weighed 11 gm; the great tit, a nonstoring bird, weighed 20 gm. But the hippocampal volume of the marsh tit was some 30 percent larger than that of the great tit, and this despite the fact that the rest of the telencephalon of the great tit was some 20 percent larger than that of the marsh tit.

Both reports considered other potential factors and, in light of the data on homing after hippocampal damage, it is important to note that migrating species did not possess significantly larger hippocampal volume than nonmigrants; this negative finding may be compared with the absence of effect of hippocampal lesions on navigation in pigeons. The authors of the two reports suggest that food-storing birds have evolved a specialized memory capacity and that that specialized capacity is reflected in an enlarged hippocampal complex. Their data do not, however, address the question whether any such specialized capacity might be restricted to spatial locations or whether food-storing species may have developed a memory that is generally superior to that of nonfood-storers, whatever the type of information to be retained. Direct support for the possibility of hippocampal involvement in a spatial-memory system is provided by a study of the effects of hippocampal damage in food-storing birds.

Hippocampal Lesions Disrupt Cache Recovery

Sherry and Vaccarino (1989) trained nine black-capped chickadees (*P. atricapillus,* a North American food-storing parid species) in an aviary that contained six artificial "trees." The trees were in fact large branches held upright in metal containers, and each tree had drilled in it twelve holes (suitable for hiding seeds). In one experiment, hungry chickadees were allowed 10-min access to as many sunflower seeds as they wished, which they both ate and cached. They were then removed to their home cages, and three hours later they were allowed to reenter the aviary and to search for the cached seeds (all of which had in fact been removed in the interim).

Following preoperative experience in this caching task, three chickadees were subjected to hippocampal damage, three to control lesions of comparable size in the hyperstriatum accessorium (an adjoining telencephalic region), and three remained unoperated controls. The lesions were relatively small—a mean of only 38 percent of the hippocampus (excluding the parahippocampal area) was destroyed—but their effects were striking. Hippocampals stored as many seeds as controls, ate as many seeds at the time that they were freely available (for caching or eating), and made as many searches altogether; but whereas approximately 50 percent of all cache-recovery searches made by control birds (operated and unoperated) were of sites that had been used to cache seeds, less than 10 percent of postoperative searches by hippocampal birds were of cache sites, and their performance provided no evidence of any recall for those sites in the cache-recovery phase.

Retrograde Amnesia for Places but Not for Cues. A second experiment attempted to define further the nature of the lesion-induced deficit. The same trees were used, but caches were now made by the experimenters, who before each daily trial hid six seeds in holes in the trees. In one condition the same six holes were used on every trial, and the birds were given preoperative training until they had achieved a criterion of three visits to baited sites from the first six searches of each day for five consecutive days. In another condition, the locales of the six holes that contained a seed varied from day to day, but there was a large (5 x 5 cm) white (or, for some birds, black) card close to each of those six holes and black (or white) cards close to all the other holes; the birds in this condition were also trained to criterion preoperatively. Twelve birds were trained in the former (place) condition, and twelve in the latter (cue condition). Four of the birds in each condition were then given small hippocampal lesions; four birds, hyperstriatal lesions; and four remained unoperated.

Postoperative retention tests showed that, relative to unoperated and operated controls, hippocampal birds were unimpaired in the cue condition but severely impaired in the place condition. Whereas control subjects in the place condition scored postoperatively just under five searches of baited sites in their first six searches, hippocampals scored only two searches of baited sites. All groups in the cue condition showed just under four baited-site searches in their first six searches postoperatively; the cue condition was, then, for controls the more difficult task, but was the easier one for the hippocampal birds. These data indicate then a lesion-induced retrograde amnesia for spatial but not for cue information in hippocampal chickadees.

Interpretation in Terms of the Procedural/Declarative Dichotomy. The results of Sherry and Vaccarino's second (1989) experiment provide the best evidence of spatial specificity of hippocampal function in birds. But this finding too is amenable to an alternative account that draws attention once again to the potential significance of the availability of multiple redundant cues. Spatially defined cache sites (like landmarks and objects) possess many cues, all of which could serve to control appropriate behavior. In the cue version of this task, however, birds would have to learn (like monkeys performing visual discriminations) the feature that was relevant (brightness of the card) and to ignore those other features peculiar to the cache site that were not relevant. Perhaps, then, the spatial condition obtained disruption precisely because (like object discriminations for monkeys) it was easy and the cue condition did not because (like visual discriminations for monkeys), it was difficult. An account of this kind could, then, interpret the Sherry and Vaccarino (1989) data in terms of the distinction between procedural and declarative memory in precisely the same way as has been suggested by Squire and his colleagues (e.g., Squire and Zola-Morgan 1983; see chapter 8 above) in attempting to account for the susceptibility of easy, but not difficult, discriminations to hippocampal damage in monkeys.

Role of Avian Hippocampus in Conventional Memory Tasks

Given the indications for a role of the avian hippocampus in memory, there have been disappointingly few studies using more conventional laboratory tasks. Sahgal (1984) reported that hippocampal damage (which included extensive invasion of the parahippocampal area) disrupted performance of pigeons in a recognition-task lesion in the Konorski pair-comparison task. In this task each trial began with the illumination of a center key with red or green light (for 3 sec). After a delay, both side keys were lit with either red or green (each key with the same color); if that color was the same as that previously shown on the center key, responses to the left key were rewarded; if the side key color differed from the center key color, the right key was correct. Note that this is not a recognition task that can be compared to those used by, say, Gaffan (e.g., 1972) or Mishkin (e.g., 1978), since the animal has not to decide whether it has (ever) previously seen the color shown on the side keys but must remember, instead, which of two familiar color stimuli was exposed most recently on the center key.

Sahgal reported that although the hippocampal pigeons showed efficient performance in a simultaneous version of the task (in which the center key remained illuminated when the side keys were lit), their performance declined more rapidly than that of controls as delays of increasing duration were introduced. There was, however, a serious problem with that report: there was in fact no significant difference between the performance of the hippocampal and the control birds when overall performance in the delay conditions was assessed. But one hippocampal pigeon outperformed all the others (including the controls), and only when that bird was discarded as an outlier (a decision that received statistical support) did a significant difference emerge. Although the lesion reconstructions showed that the outlier had a smaller lesion than the other four hippocampal birds, this difference was not large, and the bird had suffered substantial bilateral invasion of the hippocampus. Experiments in our laboratory (Good, unpublished) have failed to replicate the Sahgal finding—which should, perhaps, be regarded with some caution.

Experiments in our laboratory have shown a number of consequences of hippocampal damage in pigeons that show parallels with those seen in mammals. These include: attenuation of the disruptive effect on acquisition of a discrimination of preexposure of the discriminanda, an effect analogous to the attenuation of latent inhibition (Good 1988); deficits in differential reinforcement of low rate (DRL) schedules—in which animals are rewarded for generating low response rates (Reilly and Good 1989); deficits in a spatial DNMTS task (Reilly and Good 1987), and in reversals of both color and position discriminations (Good 1988). But our experiments (Good and Macphail, in preparation) have failed to detect any effect of extensive hippocampal damage on either a conventional DMTS task (using red and green as sample stimuli) or a recognition task whose design (Macphail and Reilly 1989) may be compared to those used by Gaffan (e.g., 1974) and Mishkin (e.g., 1978): in this procedure, pigeons are rewarded for responding to slides (pictures of various scenes and objects) that they have never seen before, and not rewarded for responding to slides that they have seen before (once only, for 10 sec). We have, in summary, found no evidence of disruption of memory but have uncovered one effect (disruption of acquisition of spatial DNMTS) that could imply a spatial function for the pigeon hippocampus.

Avian Versus Mammalian Hippocampus: Some Speculations

The work carried out on avian hippocampal function to date has clearly only scratched the surface of a fascinating problem. It should be added here that in confining ourselves to a consideration of avian hippocampal function we have considered only a small fraction of comparative neurological work using birds (although it is true that very little work is currently being reported on the neurology of learning in nonmammals other than birds; see Macphail [1982] for a survey of that literature). Other workers have investigated avian telencephalic involvement in song-learning (e.g., Konishi 1985) and in imprinting (e.g., Horn 1985), and the impressive results of that work have been used to support the notion that there exists in birds a number of relatively independent specialized learning capacities (Sherry and Schacter 1987).

Neurological Differences Imply Behavioral Differences

Work on avian hippocampus was introduced here with the notion that the apparently simpler avian structure might find represented in it some, but not all, of the systems represented in the mammalian hippocampus. The results available to date, showing as they do effects that might be attributed either to specifically spatial disruption, or to more general memory disruption, encourage the view that at least some mammalian hippocampal systems find their counterparts in the avian hippocampus. But it may be instructive to consider the implications of some (hypothetical) major difference between birds and mammals in hippocampal function: suppose, for example, that evidence accumulates that convinces neuroscientists that whereas the mammalian hippocampus does contain a spatial map, the avian hippocampus does not—what would such a conclusion imply? A spatial map located in a nonhippocampal region would, presumably, be likely to possess very different properties from the mammalian, hippocampally located map. One major implication that would emerge is, therefore, that behavioral scientists should then seek (and expect to find) major differences between the organization of spatial behavior in birds and mammals. And, just as contrasts between the behavior of brain-damaged and normal individuals may throw light on the organization of behavior in intact animals, contrasts between the spatial behavior of birds and mammals might then contribute to the analysis of that behavior in both classes of animal (for a somewhat more detailed version of this argument, see Macphail 1982).

Behavioral Differences Imply Neurological Differences

The case made out above was that differences in hippocampal organization of behavioral functions should be reflected in differences in behavioral performance. One might, then, ask in turn whether there are to be found any differences in behavior between birds and mammals that might suggest differences in hippocampal function? It has proved remarkably difficult to find differences amongst vertebrate species in cognitive capacities (e.g., Macphail 1982, 1985b, 1987), and birds do seem to perform with great efficiency across a wide range of spatial and memory tasks: a variety of birds have, for example, been shown to perform at a high level of accuracy in various types of radial maze (e.g., Roberts and Van Veld-huizen 1985; Spetch and Edwards 1986; Krebs 1990; Hilton and Krebs 1990). Perhaps, then, it will not be surprising to find comparable telencephalic representation in birds and mammals of the systems that underlie such tasks. There is, however, a recent report of a behavioral difference between pigeons and rats that might reflect a difference in hippocampal organization, and this work concerns timing.

Timing in Rats and Pigeons

It will be recalled (from chapter 8) that rats show very accurate timing of the duration of stimuli when tested using the peak-trial procedure: when trained to anticipate food reward for the first response emitted after a given stimulus has persisted for a certain interval, rats show on trials in which reward is omitted maximal rates of response at the point during the stimulus when the trained interval has elapsed. A similar capacity is seen in pigeons (Roberts, Cheng, and Cohen 1989). It will also be recalled that when a gap is inserted into a timed stimulus, intact rats appear to remember over the gap the duration of the stimulus that had preceded it and to continue timing from that point when the gap terminates: fornix-lesioned rats, by contrast, reset their internal clocks when gaps occur (a finding that Olton, Meck, and Church [1987] interpreted as indicating failure of working memory). Roberts, Cheng, and Cohen (1989) found that, like hippocampal rats, intact pigeons reset their internal clocks when gaps occur in timed stimuli. Pigeons perform efficiently in a wide range of working memory tasks (e.g., radial maze: Roberts and Van Veldhuizen 1985); there seems, therefore, no reason why pigeons should not remember across a gap of a few seconds the duration of a signal that preceded the gap. Nevertheless, unlike normal rats, pigeons reset their internal clocks in the gap-trial procedure. The difference between the behavior of intact rats and pigeons suggests that timing in pigeons is organized differently than in rats; the fact that hippocampal damage has the consequence that rats now behave like (intact) pigeons suggests in turn that perhaps the pigeon hippocampus does not possess the system involved in timing in rats that is responsible for continuation of timing across gaps. An intriguing question that now arises is, then, whether hippocampal damage in pigeons will have the same effect on the peak-trial procedure that it does in rats; it will be recalled (from chapter 8) that such damage in rats appears to reduce the apparent duration of a signal. And if hippocampal damage in pigeons has no such effect, we might well conclude that the rat hippocampus contains a system not present in the avian hippocampus. And if other research continued to uncover parallels between birds and mammals

in effects of hippocampal damage on spatial and memory tasks, we might
further conclude that explanation of effects of hippocampal damage in rats
on spatial and memory performance should not endeavor to encompass
their effects on timing behavior.

Conclusions

Much of the foregoing discussion has been speculative, directed at illu-
minating potential rather than actual benefits of comparative neurology,
and we shall conclude this consideration of avian neurology with one final
speculation. Suppose that, despite all the anatomical contrasts between the
two structures, experimental work forces the conclusion that the avian and
the mammalian hippocampus play indistinguishable roles in behavior.
Would such an outcome deprive the work of any value? This surely would
not be so, if only because the very differences in anatomical structure
would indicate that it would not be fruitful to attempt to interpret hippocampal function in terms of anatomical features seen in one structure but
not in the other. A similar argument applies, of course, to physiological
properties of the structures: we do not yet know whether the avian hippocampus contains place or displace cells, nor whether a theta rhythm occurs
there. And although a form of long-term potentiation has been demonstrated in the avian hippocampus (Wieraszko and Ball 1991), we do not
yet know its physiological basis—whether or not, for example, it is dependent upon NMDA (N-methyl-D-aspartate) receptors; it is, however,
worth noting in this context that Bradley and his colleagues (Bradley, Delisle Burns, and Webb 1991; Bradley et al. 1991) have reported an NMDA
receptor-dependent LTP in the intermediate medial ventral hyperstriatum
of the chick brain, a region associated with both imprinting and passive
avoidance learning (Horn 1985; Patterson, Gilbert, and Rose 1990). The
absence of any one of those physiological phenomena—place cells, theta
rhythm, NMDA receptor-dependent LTP—in a structure whose function paralleled that of mammalian hippocampus would argue that the
absent phenomenon is not involved in the essentials of hippocampal processing.

It is, then, possible that comparative neurology may make a contribution not only to disentangling the function of the hippocampus, but also
to our second outstanding problem, the interpretation of the role of LTP
in behavior. But a second discipline may offer more promise of success in
tackling that problem, and it is to that we shall now turn.

B. COMPUTATIONAL NEUROSCIENCE

The second unexplored avenue may be characterized as computational neuroscience. Our particular interest will be to see whether any of the high-level phenomena associated with the hippocampus may be shown to be explicable in terms of interactions between neurons having relatively simple properties, properties that could reasonably be expected to obtain in the hippocampus, given our knowledge of its anatomy and physiology.

Parallel Distributed Processing

Interest in the emergent properties of networks of interconnected simple units has waxed and waned over recent decades and is currently enjoying a resurgence, with a focus on parallel distributed-processing models of cognition. These models concern the analysis of networks consisting of layers of units that show rich interconnections; the layers consist of an input layer and an output layer (usually along with one or more "hidden" layers). The computational capacities of the individual units within a network are generally similar or identical, and the activity of a given unit is determined by the input (which may be excitatory or inhibitory) reaching it via connections with other units. Given the homogeneity of the units, the differing emergent properties of various networks are determined by the differences in the pattern of connectivities. Most parallel distributed-processing networks assume that connectivities may be modified in an adaptive manner, but where such modifications occur they are assumed to be determined entirely by locally available information—by such factors, for example, as the current level of activity in two interconnected units; it is explicitly supposed that no global factor may intervene so as to modulate sets of connections in a network in the light of information not locally available at those connections.

Information processing in these connectionist models is carried out in parallel by the units in the network. There is not, as there is in conventional computers, a single highly complex central processing unit that operates in a serial fashion and oversees all processing. Any complex processing capacity possessed by a network is an emergent property determined solely by its pattern of connectivity. The rich interconnections between layers of parallel distributed-processing networks are designed so that a given input generates widespread activity across units of a succeeding layer—gives rise, in other words, to a distributed representation. Rather than particular "lines" or units being dedicated to input of a specific origin, a unit in one layer may be activated by any of a number of units in some lower layer. The identity of an input is preserved by the pattern of activity across a layer, not by the activity of any specific unit or subset of units.

Support from Biological Considerations

The original impetus for work on parallel distributed-processing models came from cognitive psychologists, and this is reflected in the subtitle "Explorations in the Microstructure of Cognition" of the standard survey of the field (Rumelhart, McLelland, and the PDP Research Group 1986). The input and output units of their models have generally been psychological constructs such as words, actions, percepts, and so on. But that work has from the outset gained support from biological considerations. The notion that cognitive processing is carried out in parallel is virtually dictated by the knowledge of slow rates of response at the neuronal level (slow relative to the speed of computation in modern digital computers). The notion that representations might be distributed is in agreement with Lashley's well-known conclusion that individual memories are not stored in specific cells of the brain (Lashley 1950). It is, moreover, a notion that seems demanded by basic psychological facts. "A salient feature of the memory system is its enormous capacity for forming associations between elements selected virtually at random from an unlimited array of possibilities. . . . This has led many theorists to assume that memories are represented in a distributed form . . . and that the representations are densely interconnected" (Lynch 1986:18).

Our interest here specifically concerns networks whose units are neurons. Many of the properties of neurons are well suited to their serving as units in models that can be subjected to the formal analyses of parallel distributed-processing theorists. Neurons typically either fire or do not fire as a result of the net effect of a number of excitatory and inhibitory inputs. Different synaptic inputs may have very different "weights"—for example, synapses at dendritic loci distal from the soma are likely to be less effective than synapses at more proximal sites. Moreover, we know from analysis of the phenomenon of LTP that long-lasting changes in synaptic weights can occur as a result of events local to a synapse.

Distributed Processing in Cortex?

Support for the notion that distributed processing may be a widespread feature of the functional organization of the brain (or, at least, of the cortex) has been sought from data on brain size and neuronal density. Neocortical volume increases linearly with brain volume in mammals (Elias and Schwartz 1969). As neocortical volume increases, so does the number of neocortical neurons; but there are data to show that the increase in number of cortical neurons does not keep pace with the increase in cortical volume, so that cortical neurons in mammals with a large neocortex are less densely packed than those in mammals with a small neocortex (Bok 1959; Rockel, Hiorns, and Powell 1980). What is more pertinent here is that Bok (1959) reported that the mean dendritic length of what he termed "homologous" neurons in the neocortex of four mammalian species increased as brain size increased (and so, as both neocortical size and number of cortical neurons increased). A number of authors (e.g., Jerison 1973; Lynch 1986) have made the not unreasonable assumption that increased dendritic length is accompanied by an increase in the number of synaptic connections per cell. Before discussing the potential significance of any such increase in connectivity, it is necessary to note that there is currently no direct evidence to show an increase in the number of synapses per cell as neocortical volume increases. Moreover, Winfield, Gatter, and Powell (1980) found fewer synapses on the somata of neocortical cells in rhesus monkeys than on those of (smaller-brained) cats and rats (and the difference in synapse numbers could not be attributed to differences in cell size); although these data do not rule out the possibility that monkey cortical dendrites possess more synapses than those of cats or rats, the assumption that larger brains show increases in cortical connectivity should clearly be treated with some caution.

If we take note of the caveat outlined above but nevertheless adopt the common interpretation of Bok's (1959) data—namely, that the addition of extra neocortical neurons has required an increase in the mean number of connections per cell—it becomes of interest to ask why this should be. Lynch (1986) has provided an elegant demonstration of the way in which a distributed-processing system would require precisely such an increase. Lynch contrasts two types of neuronal arrangement, illustrated in figure 9.3. Two input cells are showing forming connections with two target cells, and each input cell is assumed to form two synapses. In one arrangement (that Lynch describes as topographic), each input cell forms two synapses on one target cell; in the other arrangement (that Lynch describes as combinatorial but will be described here as distributed), each input cell makes one synapse on each of the two target cells. Consider the effect on each arrangement of adding a further input and a further output cell. In the topographic system, only two further synapses are required, so that there would now be six synapses in all for the six cells. But in a distributed system in which each input showed a connection with all the target cells, the total number of synapses (see figure 9.3) would rise to nine, representing an increase in the mean number of connections per cell.

More specific support for a distributed organization from input cells onto an array of target cells is provided by the anatomy of various types

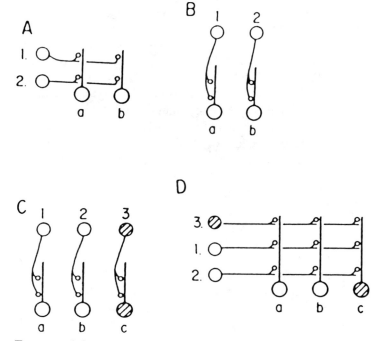

FIGURE 9.3. Comparison of a distributed with a topographic type of neuronal organization. Fig. 9.3A shows a distributed arrangement, in which the inputs (1 and 2) provide one contact for each of two target cells, a and b. Fig. 9.3B shows a topographic arrangement in which the two inputs are segregated so that input 1 provides two synapses for cell a and input 2 provides two synapses for cell b. Fig. 9.3C shows that an additional input—3—can be accommodated in the topographical arrangement by simply adding a third neuron to the target field, without any changes in the already present inputs and targets. Fig. 9.3D shows that a comparable accommodation of input 3 in the distributed arrangement would require not only an extra target neuron but also additional synapses that would involve the expansion of dendritic trees and axonal arborizations. (*After* Lynch 1986)

of cortex. We saw in chapter 4, for example, that in cerebellar cortex each of the incoming mossy fibers synapses onto several hundred granule cells, and that each granule cell projects (via parallel fibers) onto thousands of Purkinje cells. Similarly, the major output from entorhinal cortex cells (see chapter 6) is diffusely distributed via perforant path fibers to a considerably larger (about 20 percent larger, in monkeys: Rolls 1989) array of granule cells in the (archicortical) dentate gyrus.

Hebb-Marr Networks

Long before the current vogue for parallel distributed-processing models, Marr (1969, 1971) proposed formal models of ways in which the cerebellar and hippocampal cortices might function. Marr supposed in those models the existence of Hebbian synapses although at that time LTP, the phenomenon whose analysis has provided a mechanism for synaptic modification according to Hebb's principle, was still awaiting discovery. Modern work on connectionist models of hippocampal function owes a large debt to both Marr and Hebb, and McNaughton and Nadel (1989) have therefore suggested that current models should be known as "Hebb-Marr" networks. We shall now consider one of those models, with the object of determining to what extent it can provide a satisfactory account of high-level properties of hippocampal function in terms of known lower-level properties of hippocampal neurons and their interconnections.

The McNaughton and Morris Model

An Associational Array in the Dentate Gyrus?

McNaughton and Morris (1987) have provided an analysis of hippocampal organization in terms of the existence within the hippocampus of associative networks, and have argued that certain properties of these networks point to their involvement in spatial learning. In order to make clear the nature of the enterprise, I shall begin by discussing their model of the perforant path–dentate gyrus array in some detail. The account presented here will, first, point to the known features of hippocampal organization on which that model is based; second, list the basic structural assumptions of the model; third, list assumptions concerning relative synaptic strengths and the ways in which they change; fourth, show how the model operates and what properties emerge from its operation. Two major problems facing the model will be discussed after the remaining McNaughton and Morris proposals for hippocampal function have been outlined.

Features of the Perforant Pathway Incorporated in the Model

The McNaughton and Morris model of the perforant path–dentate gyrus array is based on the following anatomical and physiological features of the perforant pathway. The input to dentate gyrus cells (in rats, at least) derives from two distinct divisions of the perforant path (Wyss 1981): a medial pathway terminates in a restricted lamellar zone on synapses that are relatively close to the dentate gyrus cell bodies; a lateral pathway spreads somewhat more diffusely and terminates in dendritic regions distal to the dentate gyrus cell bodies, giving rise to weaker synapses than those of the medial pathway. Incoming perforant path fibers also distribute widely onto interneurons that inhibit the same granule cells that are excited by medial and lateral pathway fibers.

Assumptions Concerning Structural Organization

In order to allow the development of a formal model, McNaughton and Morris make a number of simplifying assumptions concerning hippocampal organization: (1) that the medial–dentate gyrus synapses are initially effective, and that the lateral–dentate gyrus synapses are initially ineffective (initially here means prior to any learning, and an effective synapse is one that obtains an impulse in the postsynaptic cell whenever an impulse occurs in the presynaptic cell); (2) that lateral fibers make synaptic contact with all dentate gyrus cells; and medial fibers, with only one dentate gyrus cell; (3) that initially ineffective lateral–dentate gyrus synapses are modified to become effective when a lateral input occurs simultaneously with a medial input (the mechanism of this modification is, of course, LTP, which is known to occur at the perforant path–dentate gyrus synaptic interface); (4) that the synapses onto inhibitory interneurons are initially effective and not modifiable.

Figure 9.4(i) is a schematic representation of an array that incorporates the assumptions outlined above, showing interconnections of six lateral fibers and six medial fibers with dendrites of six dentate gyrus cells, whose activity forms the output of the array.

Assumptions Concerning Synaptic Strengths

Before exploring the effects of various inputs on the output of the array shown in figure 9.4(i), assumptions must be made concerning the relative strengths of the synapses. In order for lateral activity to obtain any dentate

---

FIGURE **9.4.** Schematic representations of the various states of an associative array (for further details, see text)

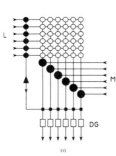

(i)

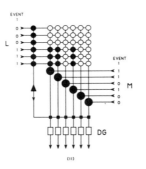

(ii)

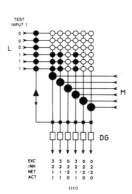

EXC	3	3	0	3	0	0
INH	2	2	2	2	2	2
NET	1	1	-2	1	-2	-2
ACT	1	1	0	1	0	0

(iii)

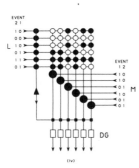

(iv)

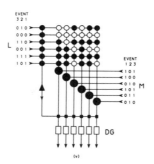

(v)

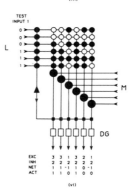

EXC	3	3	1	3	2	1
INH	2	2	2	2	2	2
NET	1	1	-1	1	1	0 -1
ACT	1	1	0	1	0	0

(vi)

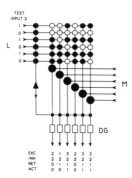

EXC	2	1	3	2	3	3
INH	2	2	2	2	2	2
NET	0	-1	1	0	1	1
ACT	0	0	1	0	1	1

(vii)

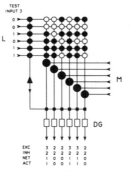

EXC	3	2	2	3	3	2
INH	2	2	2	2	2	2
NET	1	0	0	1	1	0
ACT	1	0	0	1	1	0

(viii)

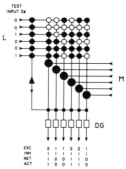

EXC	2	1	1	2	2	1
INH	1	1	1	1	1	1
NET	1	0	0	1	1	0
ACT	1	0	0	1	1	0

(ix)

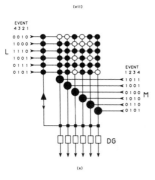

(x)

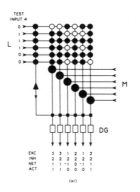

EXC	3	3	1	2	1	3
INH	2	2	2	2	2	2
NET	1	1	-1	0	-1	1
ACT	1	1	0	0	0	1

(xi)

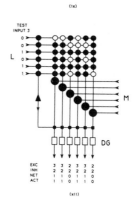

EXC	3	3	2	3	3	2
INH	2	2	2	2	2	2
NET	1	1	0	1	1	0
ACT	1	1	0	1	1	0

(xii)

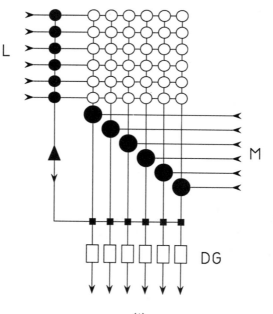

(i)

FIGURE 9.4(i). Input fibers from the lateral division of the perforant pathway (L) make effective excitatory synapses (*filled small circles*) onto interneurons (*filled inverted triangle*) that in turn make effective inhibitory synapses (*filled squares*) onto output cells (*open rectangles*) of the dentate gyrus (DG). Lateral fibers also make initially ineffective excitatory synapses (*open small circles*) onto all dentate gyrus cells. Each input fiber from the medial division of the perforant pathway (M) makes an initially effective "detonator" synapse (*filled large circles*) onto only one dentate gyrus cell.

gyrus output, the effectiveness of the inhibitory synapses must be less than that of excitatory synapses. For purposes of exposition, we will assume here: (1) that each effective lateral–dentate gyrus synapse contributes, in response to presynaptic activity, one unit of excitation to a dentate gyrus cell; (2) that there is a threshold in operation in the inhibitory pathway so that activation of one inhibitory synapse has no effect; that activation of two synapses contributes one unit of inhibition; that activation of three synapses (two units of inhibition, three synapses) contributes two units; and so on (this assumption is simpler than that adopted by McNaughton and Morris, who suppose that the inhibitory input performs the function of division. In the examples to be used here, the consequence of division is identical to that of the process assumed. For further details, and for a discussion of how a process of division might be realized in the nervous system, see McNaughton 1989); (3) that a dentate gyrus cell will fire when net excitatory strength (the algebraic sum of positive excitatory strength and negative inhibitory strength) is one or more; (4) that the medial–dentate gyrus synapses are sufficiently strong to overcome any lateral-generated inhibition, so that activity in a medial fiber invariably obtains activity in the dentate gyrus cell with which it makes synaptic contact (the invariable effectiveness of these synapses has led to their being termed "detonator" synapses).

Operation of the Model

Initially, activity in lateral fibers has no effect on dentate gyrus output; none of the lateral–dentate gyrus excitatory synapses is effective, and thus only inhibition may be generated (and then, only when two or more lateral fibers fire simultaneously). Firing of medial fibers does obtain dentate gyrus output, and since each medial fiber connects with a different single dentate gyrus cell, the pattern of that output reflects precisely the pattern of the input.

Association Formation. Consider now the effect on the array of events that obtain simultaneous activity in both medial and lateral fibers. Figure 9.4(ii) shows the state of the array after one such event; lateral synapses on the dendrites of the dentate gyrus cells that were simultaneously activated by the medial input have become effective. This array has the interesting property that if the same *lateral* input pattern recurs, the dentate gyrus output reflects the original *medial* input—see figure 9.4 (iii); the array performs, then, an associative function. Figures 9.4(iv) and 9.4(v) show the effects on the array of two more events involving both medial and lateral activity. What is considerably more interesting now is that when any one of the three original lateral inputs is tested, the dentate gyrus output reflects the pattern of medial activity that had originally co-occurred with the lateral input—figures 9.4(vi), 9.4(vii), and 9.4(viii). Two important features of this associative array should be noted: first, the information about the three events (co-occurrences of medial and lateral inputs) is distributed through the array, and six of the modified lateral–dentate gyrus synapses shown are "shared" in the sense that they were activated simultaneously with medial input in more than one of the three

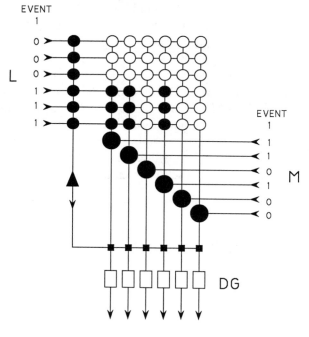

(ii)

FIGURE 9.4(ii). State of the array after Event 1, which consisted of the simultaneous activation of three of the lateral and three of the medial fibers. Nine of the 36 initially ineffective lateral–dentate synapses are now effective.

events; second, the inhibitory pathway, activity in which varies according to the total number of lateral fibers firing, plays a vital role.

Pattern Completion. The array shown in figure 9.4(v) has another valuable property—it is capable of a degree of "pattern completion" in that when given a lateral input that is an incomplete copy of one of the original inputs, it may nevertheless generate the output appropriate to the medial input that originally accompanied that input; this property is illustrated in figure 9.4(ix).

Saturation. Arrays of the kind discussed here allow the efficient storage of a number of associations concerning discrete events. But that efficiency is obtained precisely because it is a distributed system in which

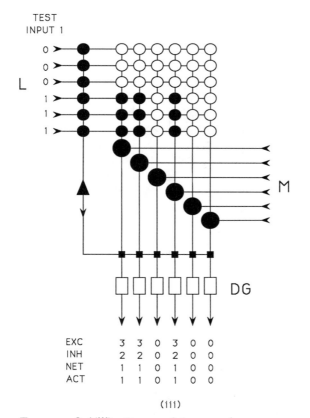

FIGURE **9.4(iii).** Output of the array in response
to a lateral-fiber test input that exactly duplicates the
lateral input component of Event 1. EXC = units of
excitation of dentate gyrus cells; INH = units of
inhibition of dentate gyrus cells; NET = net excitation (or inhibition) of dentate gyrus cells; ACT =
activity (1 = fire; 0 = no activity) of dentate gyrus
cells.

units are shared by different events. There is a price to pay for this efficiency: the system may become saturated if an attempt is made to store
too many events. Figure 9.4(x) shows the effect on the array of adding a
fourth event (again involving co-occurrence of medial and lateral inputs).
When the lateral input involved in the fourth event is subsequently presented alone—figure 9.4(xi)—the output once again accurately represents
the medial input of the fourth event; however, if the lateral input of the

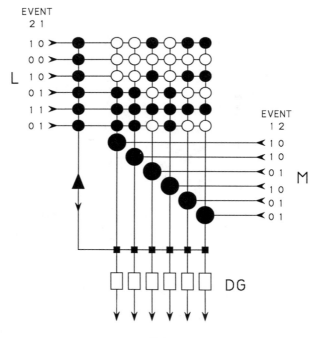

(iv)

FIGURE 9.4(iv). State of the array following a second event, which again consisted of the simultaneous activation of three of the lateral and three of the medial fibers. Eighteen of the 36 initially ineffective excitatory synapses of the lateral–dentate array are now effective.

third event is now tested again—figure 9.4(xii)—the output no longer faithfully represents the medial input of that event.

Formal Implementation in a Correlation Matrix. The McNaughton and Morris model of the perforant path–dentate gyrus array is, of course, a gross oversimplification. But the general principles involved may nevertheless be entirely valid, and the model has the important virtue that it allows us to see how rather precise information might be preserved in anatomically diffuse networks. The simplifying assumptions have also allowed the development of a model that is sufficiently formal for its properties to be analyzed mathematically. The array described is formally comparable to a correlation matrix (see McNaughton and Morris 1987), and the properties of any specific type of correlation matrix are readily established.

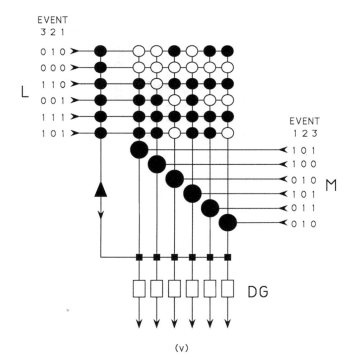

(v)

FIGURE **9.4(v)**. State of the array following a third event

Relevance to Spatial Learning

The McNaughton and Morris model proposes, then, that the dentate gyrus is an associative system: an initially ineffective stimulus, after being paired with a strong stimulus, acquires the capacity to obtain the output elicited by the strong stimulus. This is, of course, a description that applies equally well to simple conditioning: an initially ineffective CS obtains, after pairing with a UCS, a CR that typically closely resembles the UCR elicited by the UCS. An important feature of the system is that it allows pattern completion so that imperfect representations of the original weak stimulus may nevertheless elicit the learned output. This is a capacity that could be critical to the formation of associations involving the context (and so, to spatial learning). The complex pattern of cues available in a context on one occasion is not likely to be precisely reproduced on a subsequent occasion; moreover, we know that hippocampal place cells fire in a particular location despite substantial changes to salient environmental stimuli (see chapter 7). (For a more detailed account of how the types

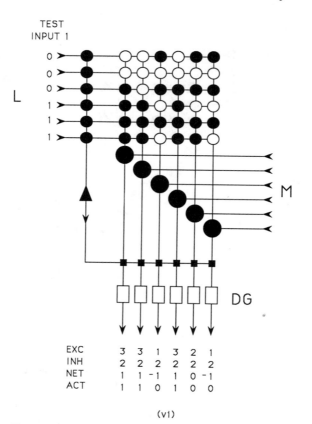

(vi)

FIGURE 9.4(vi), (vii), and (viii). Output of the array in response to lateral-fiber test inputs that exactly duplicate the lateral input component of Events 1, 2, and 3, respectively. Note that the output in each case reflects the medial component of the corresponding event.

of networks that McNaughton and Morris believe are to be found in the hippocampus might subserve spatial performance, see McNaughton 1989.)

Autocorrelative Arrays

The preceding section discussed the McNaughton and Morris model for the perforant path–dentate gyrus array in some detail so as to provide some flavor of the computational approach, and to show that formal anal-

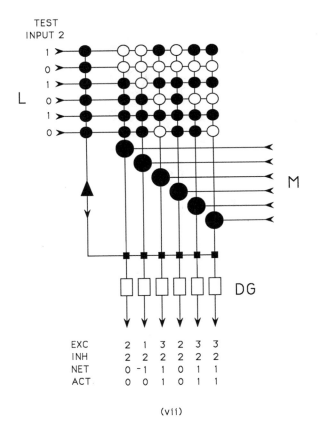

(vii)

yses can arrive at conclusions that are both intuitively surprising and theoretically useful. McNaughton and Morris (1987) discuss two further types
of array that may be instantiated in the hippocampal formation, and we
shall complete this account of their proposals by introducing those arrays
in considerably less detail.

The array that we have already discussed achieved heteroassociative
learning: two input patterns became associated, as a consequence of modification of synapses activated by only one of those patterns (the weak
input). Relatively minor alterations to the assumptions adopted can, not
surprisingly, lead to major changes in functional properties, and we shall
now consider two arrays that are capable of autoassociation. Such arrays
detect correlations within a given input pattern with the result that pattern
completion occurs and the output to imperfect versions of a familiar input
is the same as that to the complete version of that input. The notion that

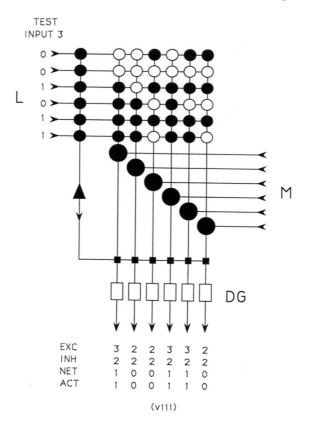

(viii)

pattern completion may be of particular importance in contextual learning should once again be borne in mind.

An Autocorrelative Array in the Dentate Gyrus?

A system that could perform autoassociation may exist, in parallel with the heteroassociative system, in the dentate gyrus. If, for example, the same (medial) perforant path fibers that make strong (detonator) synapses on single dentate gyrus cells also made weak (but modifiable) synapses onto many other dentate gyrus cells, an array having the properties of an autocorrelation matrix would be available (McNaughton and Morris 1987). There is evidence in fact that some of the synapses (about 3 percent) of the medial pathway are very much stronger (generating EPSPs—excitatory postsynaptic potentials—some ten to twenty times larger) than the others (McNaughton, Barnes, and Andersen 1981), and this leads

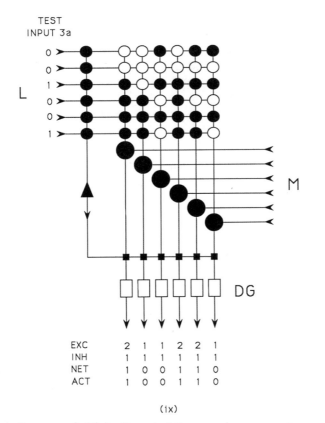

(ix)

FIGURE **9.4(ix).** Output of the array in response to a lateral-fiber test input that is an incomplete copy of the lateral input component of Event 3. Note that the output nevertheless accurately reflects the medial component of Event 3.

McNaughton and Morris to the suggestion that both auto- and heteroassociative arrays may coexist in the dentate gyrus.

An Autocorrelative Array in the CA3 Region?

McNaughton and Morris go on to discuss the potential properties of arrays in the CA3 region of the hippocampus. CA3 pyramidal cells receive input from the dentate gyrus granule cells (the output of the perforant path–dentate gyrus array). The projection is carried by the mossy-fiber system and forms part of the trisynaptic circuit. There are in mammals many more dentate gyrus cells than CA3 cells, but each mossy fiber makes very few

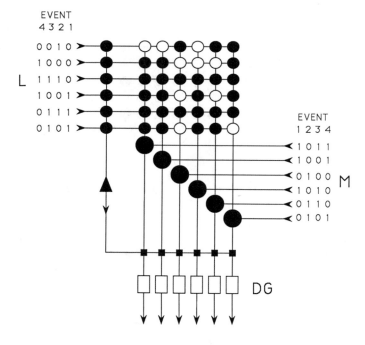

(x)

FIGURE 9.4(x). State of the array following a fourth event. Note that 26 of the 36 synapses in the lateral–dentate array are now effective.

contacts with CA3 cell dendrites. The net result is that the probability of a given CA3 cell receiving input from a specific dentate gyrus cell is very low (less than 1 in 10,000 in the rat: Rolls 1989). A given set of inputs from dentate gyrus cells is therefore unlikely to show any significant degree of overlap with any other set in CA3 cells with which synaptic contact is made; this array clearly is not suited to the type of heteroassociative function proposed for the dentate gyrus array. Another feature of CA3 suggests, however, a possible role. CA3 cells (see chapter 6) possess many longitudinal associational fibers that show diffuse synaptic connections across the CA3 dendritic field: CA3 cells, in other words, feed back excitation onto their own dendritic fields, and this is a feature that points to an autocorrelative function for the CA3 region. This analysis suggests, then, that the CA3 array may allow pattern completion. The McNaughton and Morris formalization of potential CA3 function emphasizes the notion that the autocorrelations will be between the current input and the "reentrant" (feedback) input to the array. Should there be a substantive delay

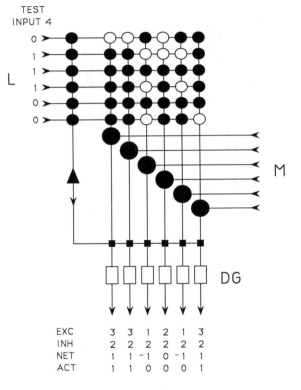

(xi)

FIGURE 9.4(xi). Output of the array in response to a lateral-fiber test input that duplicates the lateral input component of Event 4. The output accurately reflects the medial component of Event 4.

in the feedback circuit, so that the reentrant input occurred after the input that gave rise to that feedback had altered, a system would then be available that could form associations between inputs that succeeded each other, rather than between simultaneous inputs. A system of this kind could, then, on being given the first of a familiar series of events, reproduce the entire series.

Two Problems for the McNaughton and Morris Proposals

We may return now to the problem that led to the introduction of computational models and ask whether the proposals advanced by McNaughton and Morris (1987) have helped close the gap between "low-level" physi-

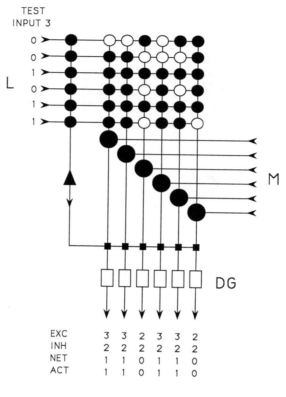

(xii)

FIGURE 9.4(xii). Output of the array in response
to a lateral-fiber test input that duplicates the lateral
input component of Event 3. Note that the output no
longer accurately reflects the medial component of
Event 3.

ological phenomena, such as LTP, and 'high-level' phenomena, such as
the disruption of maze learning by hippocampal damage.

We have seen the potential value of synapses of the Hebbian type in
both hetero- and autoassociative networks. We have seen also that the
anatomical organization of the hippocampus is compatible with the notion
that such networks are to be found there. Finally, we have seen that pattern
completion is a property of the networks outlined, and noted the argument
that pattern completion may be particularly relevant to spatial learning. It
is appropriate also to refer back to the discussion in chapter 6 of the potential role of LTP in learning: it will be recalled, for example, that there is

evidence that drugs that block LTP block spatial learning, and that induction of LTP prior to learning (a procedure that might produce saturation of hippocampal networks) has been found to disrupt acquisition of spatial (but to cause potentiation of nonspatial) learning.

The discussion thus far has emphasized the virtues of the associational arrays proposed by McNaughton and Morris (1987). There are, however, two major problems facing their proposals. The first is that predictions concerning the behavioral consequences of hippocampal damage are, at best, imprecise. There is very little in the networks discussed to show why hippocampal processing should be restricted to spatial learning: the occurrence of pattern completion could clearly be of value in many tasks that do not involve spatial information (generalization of learned responses to stimuli that are not identical to those used in training is, after all, a universal property of animal learning). The second problem is that our knowledge of the anatomy and physiology of the hippocampus would currently allow the postulation of alternative models incorporating different assumptions, assumptions that would not violate the known facts. Our detailed knowledge of the anatomy and physiology of the hippocampus is not sufficient to allow any degree of certainty concerning the validity of the assumptions incorporated in rival hypothetical networks; there is, moreover, much that is known that is not incorporated in current models. These two problems are not independent, given that, as has already been observed, small changes in assumptions may lead to large changes in function. To illustrate the general importance of the point, we shall introduce here an alternative account of hippocampal processing (Rolls 1989), an account whose assumptions differ from those made by McNaughton and Morris in one critical respect—namely, that no "detonator" synapses are proposed (and the question whether such synapses are to be found in, for example, the dentate gyrus, remains to be answered).

The Rolls Model

Categorization in the Dentate Gyrus?

Rolls assumes that the perforant path–dentate gyrus matrix has no detonator synapses, and incorporates both the feedforward inhibition of the McNaughton and Morris model (mediated by connections of perforant path fibers with inhibitory interneurons) and feedback inhibition (mediated by fibers from the granule cells themselves that synapse onto those same inhibitory interneurons). Rolls argues that such an arrangement is well suited to "categorize" incoming material. A categorizing array would detect and use the redundancy amongst input patterns to recode them efficiently into a relatively small number of output patterns. Rolls supports his analyses of this and the other stations of the hippocampal trisynaptic circuit with computer simulations that incorporate his assumptions and that do succeed in the various roles (e.g., in pattern separation) that are ascribed to the different components of his model.

Episodic Memory Formation in the CA3 Region?

Rolls agrees with McNaughton and Morris in assigning an autocorrelative role to the CA3 pyramidal cells, but argues that the rich interactions between the CA3 cells (mediated by the longitudinal associational fibers) serve to detect correlations between simultaneous events, the representations of which are to be found (as a consequence of the pattern separation achieved in the dentate gyrus) in quite different sets of CA3 cells. In other words, where McNaughton and Morris see one possible role of the CA3 autocorrelation process as completion of a familiar input pattern given only a part of that input, Rolls sees the input as a collection of independent input patterns, any one of which could serve to elicit the others. In effect, then, Rolls proposes that the CA3 region carries out the same pattern-associating role that McNaughton and Morris assign to the dentate gyrus. Rolls goes on to suggest that an associative function of the kind outlined constitutes in effect a system for episodic memory. "Each episode would be defined by a conjunction of a set of events, and each episodic memory would consist of the association of one set of events. An example of an episodic memory would be where, with whom, and what one ate at lunch on the preceding day" (Rolls 1989:294). Episodic memory is widely regarded as a type of declarative memory, and so this analysis is compatible with an analysis of hippocampal function (e.g., Squire 1987) in terms of the distinction between declarative and procedural memory.

Categorization in CA1?

Finally, Rolls argues that the overall organization of the CA1 region resembles that of the dentate gyrus region—it is, then, adapted to act as a categorizer. Rolls supposes that the role of the CA1 region is to produce an economical recoding of the episodic memory inputs received from the CA3 region (via the Schaffer collaterals, the final stage of the trisynaptic circuit). The output of the CA1 cells returns, via the subicular complex, to neocortex, and Rolls suggests that that output may be used to direct long-term storage (through, perhaps, some consolidation-like process) in the neocortex. Such a proposal could, then, account for the fact that humans with hippocampal amnesia cannot form new episodic memories but can recall pretraumatic episodic memories.

Current Status of the Computational Approach to Hippocampal Function

The discussion of a second computational model of hippocampal function (and there are others—see, for example, Lynch 1986; O'Keefe 1989) serves to emphasize the problems facing the McNaughton and Morris (1987) proposals. Like the McNaughton and Morris model, Rolls's (1989) model purports to account for a behavioral consequence of hippocampal damage (disruption of episodic memory, in this case). But, just as the link between the properties of the McNaughton and Morris matrix and spatial processing was, to say the least, tenuous, so is the link between the pattern-associating properties proposed by Rolls for the CA3 region and episodic memory formation. Thus despite the mathematical precision with which the properties of the arrays can be demonstrated, the behavioral role to be expected of arrays having these properties is far from clear. The contrasts between the two models further emphasize the fact that small changes in assumptions yield large changes in the functions proposed for the various hippocampal arrays; this is a serious problem, given that currently we have no way of deciding what set of assumptions best reflects the true low-level functional organization of the hippocampus. These difficulties point to the clear conclusion that computational considerations are not yet sufficiently stringent to allow us to choose between rival "high-level" accounts of hippocampal function. Connectionist models allow us to think in relatively concrete terms about ways in which the physiological and anatomical properties of the hippocampus might support specific modes of information processing. They show that current ways of thinking about hippocampal function (as, for example, a spatial mapping system or as a declarative memory system) can be made compatible with its lower-level features, but they do not help us to decide between current theories.

Two further points may be made here, each of which emphasizes the obvious fact that computational models of hippocampal function are incomplete and incorporate only a fraction of what is known of hippocampal physiology. The mossy fibers form large but relatively few synapses (the mosses) on their target cells (the CA3 pyramids), and both McNaughton and Morris (1987) and Rolls (1989) treat these synapses as strong synapses that are not modified. But we know that LTP does occur at the mossy-fiber CA3 pyramidal cell synapses (although we also know that this form of LTP is atypical in that, for example, NMDA receptors are not involved: Harris and Cotman 1986; Zalutsky and Nicoll 1990; see chapter 6 above). Similarly, both models assume that dentate gyrus provides a major source of input to the CA3 region (another source being provided by the direct perforant path projection from entorhinal cortex). But we know that selective damage to dentate gyrus cells does not affect the spatial selectivity of CA3 place cells (McNaughton et al. 1989; see chapter 7 above). If the dentate gyrus input to the CA3 region does play a critical role in CA3 processing, it is odd that one of the more striking higher-level phenomena observed in the CA3 region—the occurrence of place cells— is unaffected by removal of that input. It appears that, if we are to understand place cells, further attention must be paid to the ways in which the direct entorhinal cortex–CA3 projection is processed.

The general conclusion that emerges from this discussion is that the neuronal network approach represents promise currently unfulfilled. Computational neuroscience does allow us to see how neurons having known low-level properties could combine in networks to yield high-level properties of interest to behavioral psychologists. At present, however, it appears that many models may be compatible with known features of hippocampal anatomy and physiology; that no model incorporates all (or even most) of all that is already known of those low-level features; and that the behavioral implications of the models available are insufficiently precise to allow specific predictions (concerning, for example, the effects of hippocampal damage).

Computational neuroscience, then, shows how the gap between low-level and high-level phenomena could be bridged; but the gap still remains. It is of interest that the problems noted here find counterparts in criticisms directed by some cognitive psychologists at connectionist analyses of human cognitive activity (analyses that use psychological constructs rather than neurons as their basic units). Lachter and Bever, for example, argue that associationist models are simply not appropriate as accounts of the acquisition by humans of structural knowledge, that, in other words, "the structure of human behaviors such as language cannot be explained by associative networks" (Lachter and Bever 1988:243). It is their contention that, to the extent that connectionist models do succeed in modeling aspects of language competence in humans, they do so because they have covertly incorporated structural information. It may be that, in order to succeed, computational models of hippocampal function will require a considerably more structured organization than those assumed in current models. Hypotheses concerning the form such structures might take may develop in the light of advances in understanding of low-level features of hippocampal anatomy and physiology, or may develop as a consequence of attempts to understand what type of structures could give rise to the complex behavioral phenomena associated with hippocampal damage. But at present it does seem likely that, if computational models are to provide a convincing account of the behavioral function of the hippocampus, they will need to become considerably more complex than those currently proposed.

C. FUNCTIONS OF THE NEOCORTEX

Perceptual Processing in the Cortex

The potential role of the prefrontal cortex, the major multimodal cortical association area, was discussed in chapter 7, but little else has been said about the role of the remainder of the neocortex. There are two reasons for the lack of attention here to what certainly seemed to Lashley a critical structure for intelligence. The first is that it now appears that most of the (nonfrontal) neocortex, given over as it is to primary sensorimotor and unimodal association areas, is concerned with perceptual processing: the position taken here, as elsewhere (e.g., Macphail 1987) has been that perception should be treated as relatively independent of intelligence. The second reason is that the case for arguing a general role for neocortex in intelligence has in any case advanced surprisingly little since Lashley's day. In this section we shall consider data that confirm an important role for the neocortex in perceptual processing. The role of neocortex in general intelligence will be considered in the following, final, section.

Engram Storage

Neocortical involvement in perceptual processing may best be introduced by considering conclusions reached by Lashley, some four decades ago, on the localization of memory traces. Work on rats with lesions of a variety of neocortical sites convinced Lashley (1950) that for simple conditioning procedures "no part of the cerebral cortex is essential except the primary sensory area" (Lashley 1950:467). Lashley's experiments had shown, for example, that damage to motor cortex, to any primary nonvisual sensory cortex, or to any association area (visual or nonvisual) had no effect on the acquisition or retention of brightness discriminations. This conclusion led in turn to the notion that visual memories are stored in the very same cells that mediate the act of perception itself: "the same cells which bear the memory traces are also excited and play a part in every other visual reaction of the animal" (p. 477).

That same conclusion is also supported by a quite different type of evidence. Human hippocampal amnesics show retrograde amnesia but, as has been noted previously (see chapter 8), that retrograde amnesia is not total: old memories are likely to be immune to hippocampal damage. This observation has led to general acceptance of the notion that although the hippocampus plays a critical role in memory, it is not itself the site of memory storage (or at least, not of long-term memory storage). Mishkin, for example, argues from such considerations to the same conclusion that Lashley had reached: "The likeliest repository of memories . . . are the same areas of cortex where sensory impressions take shape" (Mishkin and Appenzeller 1987:67).

Role of Association Areas

Anatomy and Physiology of Inferotemporal Cortex

Recent work, particularly work using primates, does, however, require modification of Lashley's view that association areas played no role in discrimination learning. We noted in chapter 6 that the hippocampus receives (nonolfactory) sensory information from association areas rather than direct from primary cortical sensory areas. It was suggested there that the role of the association areas may be to extract relatively high-level and abstract properties from the raw primary input. This proposal will be supported here by describing work using monkeys on the unimodal belt of visual-association areas that run from the striate cortex (area OC in figure 9.5) to the temporal pole. Those areas may in fact be subdivided into a sizable number of anatomically and functionally discrete areas, but for our purposes it will be sufficient to allocate them to two zones: posterior inferotemporal cortex (PIT), which includes areas OA and OB of the prestriate cortex and area TEO of the inferotemporal cortex proper, and anterior inferotemporal cortex (AIT), which consists of area TE.

Projections from the primary visual cortex contribute to multiple representations of the visual field in PIT. Recordings from single cells in PIT show that cells in a given representation are sensitive to variations in one particular dimension—e.g., to color, direction of movement, orientation, etc. (Zeki 1978). It appears, therefore, that the function of each represen-

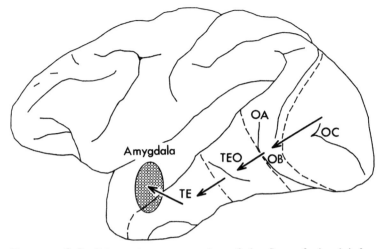

FIGURE 9.5. Schematic representation of the flow of visual information from the primary cortical visual area (OC) through the secondary areas (OB, OA, and TEO) that form the posterior inferotemporal cortex to the highest-order visual area (TE), which forms the anterior inferotemporal cortex. The figure shows that information from area TE projects directly into the medially located amygdaloid complex; there are also projections from area TE through multimodal association areas to the hippocampal formation. (*From* Amaral 1987)

tation is to analyze one of a number of visual dimensions. AIT receives projections from a variety of sites in PIT, and recordings in this region suggest that more abstract properties are now of interest. Receptive fields of AIT cells are large, and there is no retinotopic organization evident in AIT (Desimone and Gross 1976). The cells respond optimally not to simple stimuli such as spots or slits of light but to complex stimuli such as hands, faces, brushes, etc. (Gross, Rocha-Miranda, and Bender 1972); moreover, responses of AIT cells to visual stimuli in conscious animals may be modulated by such behavioral aspects of the test situation as whether a stimulus should be attended to or not (Richmond, Wurtz, and Sato 1983). These properties "suggest that inferotemporal neurons may be involved in spatially invariant visual processing such as recognition or classification of objects independent of their exact location in the visual field" (Gross, Bender, and Gerstein 1979:215). Similar but somewhat more specific conclusions have been reached by a number of workers in this field. Weiskrantz and Saunders have suggested that the function of AIT is the "storage of an object-centered prototype" (1984:1033); Mishkin (e.g., 1982) has argued that one of the central functions of the system that terminates in AIT is the synthesis of the various physical properties of a visual object into the unique configuration that identifies that particular unique object. The case for a function of this general kind can be made out by considering the outcomes of a number of experiments that contrast the effects of lesions at various sites in the cortical visual system.

Inferotemporal Lesions and Visual Discrimination Learning

Damage to inferotemporal cortex (AIT or PIT) does not cause scotomata in any part of the visual field and does not impair primary visual processing when assessed by psychophysical measures of thresholds for, for example, acuity, incremental brightness, or critical flicker-fusion (Dean 1976). Inferotemporal lesions do, however, cause deficits in a variety of types of visual discrimination (and do not cause deficits in nonvisual discriminations). First, consider the effects of cortical lesions on acquisition of a shape discrimination. Blake, Jarvis, and Mishkin (1977) studied acquisition by monkeys of a discrimination between two angles (in white, on a gray background); one angle was 90°, the other 10°. PIT lesions significantly impaired acquisition: monkeys with either AIT or lateral striate lesions (the latter being lesions that involved the foveal striate representation) showed an overall level of performance that was somewhat poorer than control performance, but with much overlap so that no significant deficit was found. PIT lesions had, then, a severe effect on shape discrimination, an effect more severe than that of either AIT or lateral striate lesions. This effect was not due to a gross visual sensory deficit: when monkeys were subsequently tested with the 90° stimulus as standard, using angles progressively closer to 90°, thresholds for discrimination between the angles were markedly impaired by lateral striate lesions, but not by either type of inferotemporal lesion.

Posterior Inferotemporal Cortex and Attention. Two subsequent experiments using the same animals pointed to the possibility that the PIT deficit might be attentional in nature. Acquisition of a second shape discrimination (an outline square versus a plus sign) was not disrupted in the PIT group (there were no significant group differences in this experiment). But in acquisition of a discrimination between two red cards, one of which was slightly less saturated (more pink) than the other, a PIT deficit once again emerged. One way of explaining these findings is to suggest that PIT animals show a deficit in identifying and attending to a relevant visual dimension—thus original acquisition of the (angle) shape discrimination was impaired. Having identified and learned to maintain attention to shape, however, PIT animals showed no deficit on the second (square versus plus) shape discrimination, but were impaired when a different visual dimension (hue saturation) was made relevant.

Anterior Inferotemporal Cortex and Object Identification. The severe effect of PIT lesions on shape and hue-saturation discriminations may be contrasted with the relative lack of effect of such lesions on a task for which object identification was necessary (Mishkin 1982). One such task is Mishkin's (e.g., 1978) DNMTS task, in which, it will be recalled, monkeys are required to recognize (and not to select) objects seen once only (10 sec previously). Figure 9.6 shows that monkeys with AIT lesions were severely impaired on the retention of this (preoperatively acquired) task, and that their impairment became more marked as the retention interval increased. It can also be seen from figure 9.6 that PIT lesions, like amygdalar or hippocampal lesions, caused little impairment; combined hippocampal/amygdalar lesions do, of course, cause severe impairment on this task, a degree of impairment that is similar to that seen following AIT lesions (Mishkin 1982).

The regions of rhinal cortex now believed to be responsible for the severe deficits in memory seen after conventional hippocampal/amygdalar lesions receive their visual input via the AIT, so that it is not, perhaps, surprising that tasks (such as object recognition) that are disrupted by hippocampal/amygdalar damage are also disrupted by AIT lesions. But AIT lesions also disrupt tasks that are not susceptible to disruption by hippocampal/amygdalar lesions. Malamut, Saunders, and Mishkin (1984), for example, found that combined hippocampal/amygdalar lesions did not disrupt the concurrent acquisition of twenty object discriminations, using a 24-hour intertrial interval; but Phillips et al. (1988) found that AIT damage did cause severe disruption of the acquisition of those same discriminations.

The implication of these findings is that wherever a task demands that a given object be discriminated from any of a large range of other objects—that, in other words, the configuration of cues that define a specific object must be learned—damage to AIT causes impairment. This impairment may be regarded as essentially perceptual in nature since it occurs irrespective of the nonvisual aspects of the task. It occurs, that is, both in what Mishkin would term habit-formation tasks (such as the concurrent task) and in genuine memory tasks (such as the DNMTS recognition task). Mishkin (e.g., 1982) proposes that memories for the configurations of

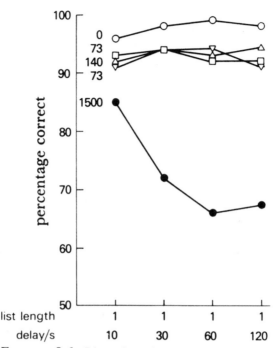

FIGURE 9.6. Disruption of DNMTS performance by lesions of area TE in monkeys. *Open circles:* un-operated controls; *upright triangles:* monkeys with amygdalar lesions; *inverted triangles:* monkeys with hippocampal lesions; *squares:* monkeys with lesions of area TEO; *filled circles:* monkeys with lesions of area TE. Numbers to the left of the curves indicate the average number of trials to relearn the basic task, which involved a delay of 10 sec. The first point on each curve is the average final score achieved on that condition, and animals were trained at the remaining three intervals for one week each (twenty trials per day). (*From* Mishkin 1982)

visual properties associated with individual objects are both formed and stored in AIT. Object memories are laid down automatically when the habit-forming system is engaged, but that process is slow and incremental. In contrast, when limbic memory mechanisms are activated (by, for example, the occurrence of a novel object), then rapid storage in AIT of the visual representation of objects is implemented, so enabling their recognition following only one presentation.

*Functions of Sensory Association Areas Outside the
Inferotemporal Cortex*

This discussion has focused on visual association areas in inferotemporal
cortex, largely because more is known about these areas than about any
other sensory association areas. There are other visual association areas,
and association areas serving other modalities. What is known of them
suggests that the scheme outlined by Mishkin may apply generally
throughout the unimodal sensory regions of the cortex. Another belt of
visual processing areas extends into the parietal cortex, and there is evidence that these regions are concerned with the analysis of location as
opposed to the sensory qualities of objects (Mishkin, Lewis, and Ungerleider 1982). And other primary cortices project, like the visual primary
cortex, into a series of mutually adjoining areas, and we have seen that
limbic damage affects memory for nonvisual information in just the same
way that it affects visual memory (Murray and Mishkin 1984).

Neocortex: A Mosaic of Modality-Specific Regions

We may, then, regard nonfrontal neocortex as a mosaic of regions that
analyze (to a greater or a lesser depth) sensory input and that (in the case
of motor cortical areas) organize the fine control of motor output. The
sensory areas not only analyze inputs but store representations that allow
the reidentification of those inputs on subsequent occasions; it is a reasonable surmise also that memories for fine motor skills are stored in motor
cortex. We know, moreover, that at least one region within the frontal
cortex is concerned with short-term retention of spatial information and
have seen the proposal (Goldman-Rakic 1987) that the frontal cortex may
be a mosaic of areas concerned with short-term retention of information
from different modalities.

The neocortex is heavily involved in memory—but what, it may well
be asked, is its role in intelligence? That question will form the basis of
the final discussion.

Epilogue: Neocortex and General Intelligence

The central focus of this final section of the book will be on the question
whether the neocortex contributes in a nonspecific manner to all tasks that
tap intelligence. But the opportunity will also be taken here to expand the
view so as to reflect very generally on the way in which the work reviewed
in the preceding chapters represents progress toward the three goals of

physiological psychology outlined in chapter 1. Those goals, it will be recalled, were: localization of function; identification of physiological substrates; and definition of cognitive functions. The third of these goals was identified in chapter 1 as being of the most interest to psychologists, and that bias will be maintained here through an emphasis on progress in our understanding of the nature of intelligence. To provide a yardstick against which to measure progress, our current conceptions will be contrasted with those held by Lashley.

The Definition of Intelligence

This book purports to survey the neuroscience of intelligence, but has so far provided no definition of that term. This is basically because although there is at least some measure of agreement about the fact that some tasks—complex problem-solving, for example—do tap intelligence, there is no such agreement over the boundaries of the set of tasks in which intelligence is involved. Lashley (1929) articulated precisely this problem, observing that neither the capacity to learn (anything) nor the capacity for insightful solutions to problems provided a satisfactory criterion of intelligence; the former criterion, in his view, would include too much, the latter limited the concept of intelligence too sharply. Lashley's (1929) conclusion was that there was little hope of finding a satisfactory definition of intelligence, and he argued that we should seek, in animals as in humans, constellations of activities correlating among themselves. Since that time, however, neither Lashley nor anyone else has in fact provided good behavioral evidence for correlations in levels of performance of animals across different tasks (see, for example, Macphail 1987). A behaviorally meaningful way of defining intelligence is, therefore, no more possible now than it was then.

Given that no formal definition of intelligence is possible, it seemed sensible to cast the net widely and to consider as potentially relevant data from both simple and complex tasks, and data on both acquisition and memory (Lashley also observed that although it is logically possible to distinguish between problem-solving and memory, it is experimentally difficult if not impossible to do so). It was sensible because, since we do not understand the nature of intelligence, any definition that restricted the topics to be considered would allow the possibility of exclusion from consideration of some topic that might in fact be relevant. Suppose, for example, that a definition was adopted that insisted that problem-solving was the prototypical function of intelligence; we might then exclude consideration of, say, habituation. But the mechanisms that are responsible for habituation may very well be involved in much more complex forms of learning (and might be best explored in a relatively simple behavioral paradigm): consider, for example, the role ascribed to habituation in the account of blocking provided by Hawkins and Kandel (1984; see chapter 4 above).

The Nature of Intelligence: Unitary or Mosaic?

In the preface to his 1929 monograph *Brain Mechanisms and Intelligence*, Lashley observed that the whole theory of learning and of intelligence was in confusion. The confusion derived partly from the problem of definition alluded to above, and partly from a deep division within the psychological community concerning the fundamental nature of intelligence. Psychologists who advanced theories of the nature of intelligence could be classified into two groups: one group believed that intelligence was a unitary capacity that determined, either on its own or in cooperation with task-specific capacities, the level of performance in all cognitive tasks; the other group believed that intelligence was the algebraic sum of diverse capacities. That dichotomy of psychological theories found a parallel in neurological theories of intelligence: one group of theorists held that intelligent activity was the outcome of the interaction of diverse and independent cortical areas; the other, that intelligence was a unitary cortical function that could add to the efficiency of specialized capacities. Some members of this latter group believed that intelligence could be located to some specific cortical region (the frontal lobes, for example); others believed that intelligence was a function of the whole cortex, acting as a unit.

Contemporary behavioral theories of intelligence still exhibit the same dichotomy to which Lashley referred. Few behavioral theorists now believe that intelligence is a unitary capacity that on its own can determine performance; there is, then, a general acceptance of the notion that intelligent performance of a given task will involve mechanisms that are relatively specific to that task. But the question whether there is or is not in addition some overriding factor that contributes to performance in all tasks that tap intelligence remains open, and we shall now consider the contribution made to the debate by physiological work.

Localization of Function and the Emergence of Structural Hypotheses

In chapter 1 the case was made out that physiological investigation might reveal the underlying structure of intellectual activity. The ensuing chapters have recounted a series of physiologically inspired hypotheses of a structural nature. These hypotheses have included proposals that have concerned: the distinction between habituation and sensitization; the role of sensitization in dishabituation and in classical conditioning; distinctions between short- and long-term storage mechanisms—for habituation, for sensitization, for spatial information, and for memories in general; a distinction between the processing of contextual information and of other types of information; distinctions between types of long-term memory (procedural versus declarative; recognition versus associative; habit versus memory). It can be argued that some of the dissociated processes (sensitization, for example) are simply not intelligent processes. But some of the dissociations involved (between, for example, declarative and procedural processing) do lie within the domain of what many psychologists would regard as intelligent activity: one implication of the higher-level dissociations is that intelligence is a far-from-unitary capacity, that intellectual activity involves the cooperation of a number of systems for learning and memory that are anatomically and functionally independent. There is as yet no universal consensus concerning the precise nature of the processes revealed in these higher-level dissociations. But most current theories posit a distinction between a cognitive, flexible system and a simpler, less flexible system. The notion that two such systems exist and operate in parallel constitutes an important example of progress toward the major goal of physiological psychology, the definition of cognitive functions.

The great majority of the work introduced in preceding chapters concerned mechanisms that were not located in neocortex. Lashley did agree with his contemporaries in believing that subcortical regions played little if any role in intelligence: his own experiments (Lashley 1929), for example, convinced him that the hippocampus played no role in maze learning. Thus to the extent that the mechanisms associated with these subcortical structures are properly regarded as mechanisms of intelligence, intelligence is not located solely in the neocortex (and this is a conclusion that reflects important advances in our understanding of localization of function since Lashley's day).

Physiological demonstrations of a structure to intelligence give further support to the widely held view that intellectual activity is indeed the outcome of the cooperation of a number of relatively independent devices. But they do not, of course, rule out the possibility that there is some other system that contributes to all intelligent activity. We shall now address that possibility by considering evidence that gives positive support to the view that something that could be regarded as "general intelligence" does play a role in certain tasks. Since the tasks in question are characterized as complex, this in turn may support the view of those (e.g., Maier and Schneirla 1935; Jolly 1987) who believe that intelligence is manifested only in complex tasks and not in such simple tasks as association formation. The basic evidence was provided by Lashley in the experiments, introduced briefly in chapter 1, that led to his concepts of mass action and equipotentiality.

Mass Action and Equipotentiality

In a series of experiments using rats in relatively complex mazes, Lashley found that acquisition and retention of maze habits could be disrupted by cortical lesions: the degree of disruption was related to the total extent of cortical damage but was independent of its locus within the cortex. Lashley (e.g., 1950) cited similar outcomes for experiments on other complex tasks using rats, and for tests of "higher-level functions" in monkeys. To accommodate these findings Lashley introduced the concepts of equipotentiality and mass action. All parts of the neocortex, he suggested, make an equal contribution to complex tasks (thus, locus of lesion is irrelevant); and the various parts of the cortex in some sense cooperate or mutually facilitate each other (thus, the greater the lesion size, the greater the disruption). It hardly needs to be added that Lashley was not proposing that all parts of the neocortex were equipotential for all tasks: we have already considered his conclusion that simple visual habits were served by the primary visual cortex alone.

The most powerful objection to Lashley's view has been (Hunter 1930) that the apparent equipotentiality of cortical regions in maze learning is an artifact of the progressive invasion by increasingly large lesions of specific sensory regions. Maze learning is a multisensory task that no doubt involves vision, touch, somesthesis, and even hearing. The more extensive the cortical damage, the more likely it is that serious disruption to one or more of those senses will occur. Thus, the argument goes, although lesions in different loci produce comparable increases in error scores, they do so for quite different reasons—the only common factor being sensory disruption.

Peripheral Versus Cortical Sensory Loss. Lashley (1950) countered Hunter's objection by citing experiments that showed, first, that occipital damage had more effect than blindness on maze learning in rats; second, that occipital damage disrupted maze learning in blind rats. Such results argue that the occipital cortex plays a role in maze learning over and above its specifically visual role. These experiments were in turn subject to crit-

icism on such grounds as, for example, that the lesions used were so large
that they extended beyond the primary visual area; and other experiments
with more restricted lesions (e.g., Pickett 1952) failed to substantiate
Lashley's claims (for further discussion see Zangwill 1961; Macphail
1982). Rather than review again that somewhat inconclusive material, we
shall describe here a recent study that highlights some of the problems
encountered in these studies.

Goodale and Dale (1981) trained rats in an 8-arm radial maze and then
subjected them either to peripheral blinding (enucleation) or to lesions of
primary visual cortex (area 17) and adjoining unimodal visual-association
cortex (areas 18 and 18a). Peripheral blinding obtained a small deficit,
whereas cortical damage had a very marked disruptive effect. This effect
was also seen in rats subjected to blinding and to cortical damage, and in
rats that had initially been blinded when they were subsequently subjected
to cortical damage. These data argue that neurons in the primary visual
cortex do indeed contribute to performance of complex nonvisual tasks.
But Goodale and Dale also reported a finding that is troublesome for Lashley's view: two rats had extensive posterior cortical lesions that were not
properly placed and, although as extensive as those of other lesioned animals, did not so extensively destroy visual cortical areas. These two rats
showed a considerably smaller deficit than the other lesioned animals.
This finding suggests that the locus of the lesion may be critical, and that
it is specifically the visual cortex that is critical for radial-maze performance, even in blind rats. Insofar as the Goodale and Dale (1981) data
confirm an involvement of visual cortical cells in nonvisual processing,
they provide support for Lashley's equipotentiality principle. But, as we
have seen, that support is qualified.

Physiological Substrates: The Synapse and Learning. Lashley observed that "we have today an almost universal acceptance of the theory
that learning consists of the modification of the resistance of specific synapses within definite conduction units of the nervous system" (Lashley
1929:125). Lashley's work on the effects of cortical damage on maze
learning had, however, made him extremely skeptical about this proposition. He had, for example, found that (postoperatively acquired) maze
performance was less well retained (over a period of forty days) by rats
with neocortical damage than by controls. The degree of impairment was
roughly proportional to the extent of cortical damage, and this suggested
to him that "the retention of the habit is conditioned by the total amount
of functional tissue in the cortex and not, primarily, by the inherent properties of the synapses themselves" (p. 126). Lashley, moreover, doubted

whether "the same neurons or synapses are involved even in two similar reactions to the same stimulus" (p. 173). He argued, therefore, that "it is not clear that the synapse is either essential or important for learning" (p. 127).

It hardly needs to be said that our general physiological understanding of the functioning of synapses has advanced dramatically since 1929, nor that there is by now a very much stronger case for supposing that modification of the efficacy of synaptic transmission does form the basis of learning and memory. We have (from the work reviewed in chapters 2 and 4) evidence to show directly involvement of specific synapses in learning in the invertebrate *Aplysia*. The work on LTP (reviewed in chapter 6) showed that vertebrate brain synapses can be modified as a consequence of brief physiological events, and there was evidence also that interference with at least that type of synaptic modification does indeed influence learning. Lashley's concern that modification of synapses as a learning mechanism would seem to imply that learning consisted in the modification of transmission along fixed lines of neurons may also be countered by the notion, introduced in this chapter, of parallel distributed processing in neuronal networks; that notion envisages learning as change in patterns of connectivity spread across populations of neurons. We shall return (briefly) to the relationship between mass action and parallel distributed processing after considering one final source of evidence concerning the neocortex and general intelligence.

Brain Damage and Intelligence in Humans. Whatever we do mean by intelligence, there is a widespread view that intellectual capacity reaches a peak in humans. It might therefore make most sense to explore the relationship between intelligence and the neocortex by considering human data. This book has attempted to keep the material considered within reasonable bounds by restricting its scope to nonhuman data. There have, of course, been numerous exceptions and, in particular, many references have been made to analyses of amnesia in humans. But an attempt to analyze neocortical involvement in intelligence in humans would in any case run into the difficulty referred to in chapter 8—namely, that language plays a major role in human intellectual processes. There is evidence (Teuber and Weinstein 1956) that cortical damage that causes aphasic symptoms is associated with poorer performance on an intelligence test that does not appear to be verbal in nature (in a visuo-spatial "hidden-figure" test); and evidence (Weinstein and Teuber 1957) that only left-hemisphere cortical damage (likely to be associated with aphasia) causes decrement in a standard intelligence test.

There is in fact surprisingly little evidence from humans that cortical damage causes decrements in intellectual performance over and above those in the comprehension and production of language. This may, of course, be because our language-dominated culture has developed language-dominated tests of intelligence, tests that are insensitive to variations in nonlinguistic intellectual skills.

Some relatively recent human work has attempted to overcome the problem of aphasia and has provided qualified support for Lashley's position. Kornhuber et al. (1985) examined the effect of cortical injuries on intelligence-test performance in children; recovery from aphasia following cortical injury is typically rapid in children. These workers found a significant correlation between lesion extent and intelligence test scores: lesion locus did not play a significant role, except that left-hemisphere lesions were associated with lower test scores than right-hemisphere lesions (despite the fact that none of the children showed clinical signs of aphasia). Although this report supports Lashley's proposal, that support must be qualified since the correlation emerged only in older (five years and more) children: children whose injuries occurred earlier in life showed no consistent relation between extent of damage and test performance.

Qualified support for the equipotentiality principle is also provided by a report on the effect of unilateral brain wounds on intelligence test scores of (right-handed) Vietnam veterans (Grafman et al. 1986). These authors found for each hemisphere a significant correlation between total brain volume loss and global intelligence test scores. But the brain damage was not restricted to cortex (although there was evidence that cortical damage was in fact critical), and the relationship between tissue loss and test score was much weaker than that between pre- and postinjury test performance.

Intelligence: A General Capacity of Neocortex

The available human and nonhuman data are far from conclusive, but they do suggest that it is perhaps not unreasonable to take seriously Lashley's proposal that all regions of the cortex contribute equally to all complex tasks: to adopt, however tentatively, his conclusion that the neocortex plays a very general role in problem-solving. And if that conclusion is adopted, then the implication for psychological theories of intelligence is that drawn by Lashley (1929)—namely, that there does exist a general capacity that enters into all intelligent activity.

Two observations may be made about this conclusion. The first is that the emergence of parallel distributed-processing models makes the notion readily digestible. What is being proposed, after all, is simply that complex multimodal information is processed in parallel throughout the neo-cortex by units whose individual computational capacities are similar. In a sense, mass action and equipotentiality are inevitable properties of parallel distributed-processing systems.

A second observation points to a paradox in Lashley's thinking. Lashley himself believed that relative brain size (brain size, that is, corrected by a factor that allows for differences in body weight) was "the only neurological character for which a correlation with behavioral capacity in different animals is supported by significant evidence" (Lashley 1949:33). Larger animals tend in general to have larger brains, and it is generally assumed that the increase in brain size with body weight reflects the operation of a somatic factor that requires more brain space for the processing of sensory and motor information as the body surface increases (e.g., Jerison 1973; Macphail 1982). But if all cortical cells—irrespective of their role in sensory or motor processing—contribute equally to complex tasks, then variations in absolute, not relative, cortical size should correlate with variations in general intelligence. Now although there are those (e.g., Jerison 1973) who agree with Lashley that intelligence is correlated with relative brain size (as well as those who do not—e.g., Macphail 1982), there is very little support for the belief that *absolute* brain size determines general intelligence. Thus acceptance of the notions of mass action and equipotentiality of cortical function in complex tasks should lead to acceptance of the notion that absolute brain size determines intelligence, but this is a counterintuitive notion that Lashley himself rejected.

A Fitting Conclusion

It is appropriate that this book should end with a discussion of Lashley, whose experiments and ideas provided so much of the early impetus for work on the physiological psychology of learning and memory. Appropriate, too, that it should end with a paradox. For all that we have learned since Lashley set us on our way is that there is much more that we have yet to understand. The eventual goal—an understanding of intelligent thought processes—poses problems more difficult than any that scientists (of any discipline) have solved heretofore. The progress made by neuroscience and the current pace of that progress give real grounds for optimism that our discipline will make substantial contributions to the unraveling of those problems.

Bibliography

Abrams, T. W. and E. R. Kandel. 1988. Is contiguity detection in classical conditioning a system or a cellular property? Learning in *Aplysia* suggests a possible molecular site. *Trends in Neurosciences* 11:128–135.

Abrams, T. W., L. Bernier, R. D. Hawkins, and E. R. Kandel. 1984. Possible roles of Ca^{++} and cAMP in activity-dependent facilitation, a mechanism for associative learning in *Aplysia*. *Society for Neuroscience Abstracts* 10:269.

Ackil, J. E., R. L. Mellgren, C. Halgren, and G. P. Frommer. 1969. Effects of CS pre-exposures on avoidance learning in rats with hippocampal lesions. *Journal of Comparative and Physiological Psychology* 69:739–747.

Acosta-Urquidi, J., D. L. Alkon, and J. T. Neary. 1984. Ca^{2+}-dependent protein kinase injection in a photoreceptor mimics biophysical effects of associative learning. *Science* 224:1254–1257.

Aggleton, J. P. and M. Mishkin. 1983a. Visual recognition impairment following medial thalamic lesions in monkeys. *Neuropsychologia* 21:189–197.

—— 1983b. Memory impairments following restricted medial thalamic lesions in monkeys. *Experimental Brain Research* 52:199–209.

—— 1985. Mammillary body lesions and visual recognition in monkeys. *Experimental Brain Research* 58:190–197.

Aggleton, J. P. and R. E. Passingham. 1981. The syndrome produced by lesions of the amygdala in monkeys (*Macaca mulatta*). *Journal of Comparative and Physiological Psychology* 95:961–977.

—— 1982. An assessment of the reinforcing properties of foods after amygdaloid lesions in rhesus monkeys. *Journal of Comparative and Physiological Psychology* 96:71–77.

Aggleton, J. P., H. S. Blindt, and J. N. P. Rawlins. 1989. Effects of amygdaloid and amygdaloid-hippocampal lesions on object recognition and spatial working memory in rats. *Behavioral Neuroscience* 103:962–974.

Aggleton, J. P., P. R. Hunt, and J. N. P. Rawlins. 1986. The effects of hippocampal lesions upon spatial and non-spatial tests of working memory. *Behavioural Brain Research* 19:133–146.

Aggleton, J. P., R. M. Nicol, A. E. Huston, and A. F. Fairbairn. 1988. The performance of amnesic subjects on tests of experimental amnesia in animals: Delayed matching-to-sample and concurrent learning. *Neuropsychologia* 26:265–272.

Akers, R. F., D. M. Lovinger, P. A. Colley, D. J. Linden, and A. Routtenberg. 1986. Translocation of protein kinase C activity may mediate hippocampal long-term potentiation. *Science* 231:587–589.

Alkon, D. L. 1974. Associative training of *Hermissenda*. *Journal of General Physiology* 64:70–84.

—— 1980. Membrane depolarization accumulates during acquisition of an associative behavioral change. *Science* 210:1375–1376.

—— 1983. Learning in a marine snail. *Scientific American* 249:64–74.

—— 1984. Calcium-mediated reduction of ionic currents: A biophysical memory trace. *Science* 226:1037–1045.

Alkon, D. L., J. Acosta-Urquidi, J. L. Olds, G. Kuzma, and J. T. Neary. 1983. Protein kinase injection reduces voltage-dependent potassium currents. *Science* 219:303–306.

Alkon, D. L., B. Bank, S. Naito, C. Chen, and J. Ram. 1987. Inhibition of protein synthesis prolongs Ca^{2+}-mediated reduction of K^+ currents in molluscan neurons. *Proceedings of the National Academy of Sciences* 84:6948–6952.

Alkon, D. L., M. Kubota, J. T. Neary, S. Naito, D. Coulter, and H. Rasmussen. 1986. C-kinase activation prolongs Ca^{2+}-dependent inactivation of K^+ currents. *Biochemical and Biophysical Research Communications* 134:1245–1253.

Alkon, D. L., H. Ikeno, J. Dworkin, D. L. McPhie, J. L. Olds, I. Lederhendler, L. Matzel, B. G. Schreurs, A. Kuzirian, C. Collin, and E. Yamoah. 1990. Contraction of neuronal branching volume: An anatomic correlate of Pavlovian conditioning. *Proceedings of the National Academy of Sciences* 87:1611–1614.

Altman, J., R. L. Brunner, and S. A. Bayer. 1973. The hippocampus and behavioral maturation. *Behavioral Biology* 8:557–596.

Amaral, D. G. 1987. Memory: Anatomical organization of candidate brain regions. In F. Plum, ed., *Handbook of Physiology*. Section 1, vol. 5, *Higher Functions of the Brain (Part 1)*, pp. 211–294. Bethesda, Md.: American Physiological Society.

Amaral, D. G. and M. P. Witter. 1989. The three-dimensional organization of the hippocampal formation: A review of anatomical data. *Neuroscience* 31:571–591.

Andersen, P. 1975. Organization of hippocampal neurons and their interconnections. In R. L. Isaacson and K. H. Pribram, eds., *The Hippocampus*. Vol. 1: *Structure and Development*, pp. 155–175. New York: Plenum Press.

Andersen, P., T. V. P. Bliss, and K. Skrede. 1971. Lamellar organization of hippocampal excitatory pathways. *Experimental Brain Research* 13:222–238.

Artola, A. and W. Singer. 1987. Long-term potentiation and NMDA receptors in rat visual cortex. *Nature* 330:649–652.

Bachevalier, J. and M. Mishkin. 1984. An early and a late developing system for learning and retention in infant monkeys. *Behavioral Neuroscience* 98:770–778.

—— 1986. Visual recognition impairment follows ventromedial but not dorsolateral prefrontal lesions in monkeys. *Behavioural Brain Research* 20:249–261.

Bachevalier, J., J. K. Parkinson, and M. Mishkin. 1985. Visual recognition in monkeys: Effects of separate vs. combined transection of fornix and amygdalofugal pathways. *Experimental Brain Research* 57:554–561.

Bachevalier, J., R. C. Saunders, and M. Mishkin. 1985. Visual recogni tion in monkeys: Effects of transection of fornix. *Experimental Brain Research* 57:547–553.

Baddeley, A. D. and G. J. Hitch. 1974. Working memory. In G. H. Bower, ed., *The Psychology of Learning and Motivation: Advances in Research and Theory*, 8:47–90. New York: Academic Press.

Baddeley, A. D. and E. W. Warrington. 1970. Amnesia and the distinction between long- and short-term memory. *Journal of Verbal Learning and Verbal Behavior* 9:176–189.

Bagshaw, M. H., D. P. Kimble, and K. H. Pribram. 1965. The GSR of monkeys during orienting and habituation and after ablation of the amygdala, hippocampus and inferotemporal cortex. *Neuropsychologia* 3:111–119.

Bailey, C. H. and M. Chen. 1983. Morphological basis of long-term habituation and sensitization in *Aplysia*. *Science* 220:91–93.

—— 1988a. Morphological basis of short-term habituation in *Aplysia*. *Journal of Neuroscience* 8:2452–2459.

—— 1988b. Long-term memory in *Aplysia* modulates the total number of varicosities of single identified sensory neurons. *Proceedings of the National Academy of Sciences* 85:2373–2377.

—— 1988c. Long-term sensitization in *Aplysia* increases the number of presynaptic contacts onto identified gill motor neuron L7. *Proceedings of the National Academy of Sciences* 85:9356–9359.

—— 1989. Time course of structural changes at identified sensory neuron synapses during long-term sensitization in *Aplysia*. *Journal of Neuroscience* 9:1774–1780.

Balsam, P. D. and A. Tomie, eds. 1985. *Context and Learning*. Hillsdale, N.J.: Lawrence Erlbaum.

Barnes, C. A. 1979. Memory deficits associated with senescence: A neurophysiological and behavioral study in the rat. *Journal of Comparative and Physiological Psychology* 93:74–104.

Barnes, C. A. and B. L. McNaughton. 1985. An age comparison of the rates of acquisition and forgetting of spatial information in relation to long-term enhancement of hippocampal synapses. *Behavioral Neuroscience* 99:1040–1048.

Barzilai, A., T. E. Kennedy, J. D. Sweatt, and E. R. Kandel. 1989. 5-HT modulates protein synthesis and the expression of specific proteins during long-term facilitation in *Aplysia* sensory neurons. *Neuron* 2:1577–1586.

Bear, M. F., L. N. Cooper, and F. F. Ebner. 1987. A physiological basis for a theory of synapse modification. *Science* 237:42–48.

Beatty, W. W. and D. A. Shavalia. 1980. Spatial memory in rats: Time course of working memory and effect of anesthetics. *Behavioral and Neural Biology* 28:454–462.

Becker, J. T., J. A. Walker, and D. S. Olton. 1980. Neuroanatomical bases of spatial memory. *Brain Research* 200:307–320.

Beggs, A. L., J. E. Steinmetz, and M. M. Patterson. 1985. Classical conditioning of a flexor nerve response in spinal cats: Effects of tibial nerve CS and a differential conditioning paradigm. *Behavioral Neuroscience* 99:496–508.

Beggs, A. L., J. E. Steinmetz, A. G. Romano, and M. M. Patterson. 1983. Extinction and retention of a classically conditioned flexor nerve response in acute spinal cat. *Behavioral Neuroscience* 97:530 –540.

Bekkers, J. M. and C. F. Stevens. 1990. Presynaptic mechanism for long-term potentiation in the hippocampus. *Nature* 346:724–729.

Benowitz, L. and H. J. Karten. 1976. The tractus infundibuli and other afferents to the parahippocampal region of the pigeon. *Brain Research* 102:174–180.

Benvenuti, F., V. Fiaschi, L. Fiore, and F. Papi. 1973. Homing performances of inexperienced and directionally trained pigeons subjected to olfactory nerve section. *Journal of Comparative Physiology* 83:81–92.

Béracochéa, D. J., F. Alaoui-Bouarraqui, and R. Jaffard. 1989. Impairment of memory in a delayed non-matching to place task following mamillary body lesions in mice. *Behavioural Brain Resaerch* 34:147–154.

Béracochéa, D. J., R. Jaffard, and L. E. Jarrard. 1989. Effects of anterior or dorsomedial thalamic ibotenic lesions on learning and memory in rats. *Behavioral and Neural Biology* 51:364–376.

Berger, T. W. 1984. Long-term potentiation of hippocampal synaptic transmission affects rate of behavioral learning. *Science* 224:627–630.

Berger, T. W. and W. B. Orr. 1983. Hippocampectomy selectively disrupts discrimination reversal conditioning of the rabbit nictitating membrane response. *Behavioural Brain Research* 8:49–68.

Berger, T. W. and R. F. Thompson. 1978. Neuronal plasticity in the limbic system during classical conditioning of the rabbit nictitating membrane response. I. The hippocampus. *Brain Research* 145:323–346.

Berger, T. W. and D. J. Weisz. 1987. Single unit analysis of hippocampal pyramidal and granule cells and their role in classical conditioning of the rabbit nictitating membrane response. In I. Gormezano, W. F. Prokasy, and R. F. Thompson, eds., *Classical Conditioning*, pp. 217–253. 3d ed. Hillsdale, N.J.: Lawrence Erlbaum.

Berger, T. W., B. Alger, and R. F. Thompson. 1976. Neuronal substrates of classical conditioning in the hippocampus. *Science* 8192:483–485.

Berger, T. W., S. D. Berry, and R. F. Thompson. 1986. Role of the hippocampus in classical conditioning of aversive and appetitive behaviors. In R. L. Isaacson and K. H. Pribram, eds., *The Hippocampus*, 4:203–239. New York: Plenum Press.

Berger, T. W., P. C. Rinaldi, D. J. Weisz, and R. F. Thompson. 1983. Single-unit analysis of different hippocampal cell types during classical conditioning of rabbit nictitating membrane response. *Journal of Neurophysiology* 50:1197–1219.

Bergold, P. J., J. D. Sweatt, I. Winicov, K. R. Weiss, E. R. Kandel, and J. H. Schwartz. 1990. Protein synthesis during acquisition of long-term facilitation is needed for the persistent loss of regulatory subunits of the *Aplysia* cyclic AMP dependent protein kinase. *Proceedings of the National Academy of Sciences* 87:3788–3791.

Berk, M. L. and R. F. Hawkin. 1985. Ascending projections of the mammillary region in the pigeon: Emphasis on telencephalic connections. *Journal of Comparative Neurology* 239:330–340.

Best, P. J. and J. B. Ranck. 1982. The reliability of the relationship between hippocampal unit activity and sensory-behavioral events in the rat. *Experimental Neurology* 75:652–664.

Bingman, V. P., P. Bagnoli, P. Ioalé, and G. Casini. 1984. Homing behavior of pigeons after telencephalic ablations. *Brain, Behavior, and Evolution* 24:94–108.

Bingman, V. P., P. Ioalé, G. Casini, and P. Bagnoli. 1985. Dorsomedial forebrain ablations and home-loft association behavior in homing pigeons. *Brain, Behavior, and Evolution* 26:1–9.

—— 1987. Impaired retention of preoperatively acquired spatial reference memory in homing pigeons following hippocampal ablation. *Behavioural Brain Research* 24:147–156.

—— 1988a. Hippocampal-ablated homing pigeons show a persistent impairment in the time taken to return home. *Journal of Comparative Physiology* A163:559–563.

—— 1988b. Unimpaired acquisition of spatial reference memory, but impaired homing performance in hippocampal-ablated pigeons. *Behavioural Brain Research* 27:179–187.

Black, A. H., L. Nadel, and J. O'Keefe. 1977. Hippocampal function in avoidance learning and punishment. *Psychological Bulletin* 84:1107–1129.

Blake, L., C. D. Jarvis, and M. Mishkin. 1977. Pattern discrimination thresholds after partial inferior temporal or lateral striate lesions in monkeys. *Brain Research* 120:209–220.

Bland, B. H. 1986. The physiology and pharmacology of hippocampal formation theta rhythms. *Progress in Neurobiology* 26:1–54.

Bliss, T. V. P. 1990. Maintenance is presynaptic. *Nature* 346:698–699.

Bliss, T. V. P. and A. R. Gardner-Medwin. 1973. Long-lasting potentiation of synaptic transmission in the dentate area of the unanaesthetized rabbit following stimulation of the perforant path. *Journal of Physiology* 232:357–374.

Bliss, T. V. P. and T. Lømo. 1973. Long-lasting potentiation of synaptic transmission in the dentate area of the anaesthetized rabbit following stimulation of the perforant path. *Journal of Physiology* 232:331–356.

Bliss, T. V. P., R. M. Douglas, M. L. Errington, and M. A. Lynch. 1986. Correlation between long-term potentiation and release of endogenous amino acids from dentate gyrus of anaesthetized rats. *Journal of Physiology* 377:391–408.

Blumberg, M. S. 1989. An allometric analysis of the frequency of hippocampal theta: The significance of brain metabolic rate. *Brain, Behavior, and Evolution* 34:351–356.

Bok, S. T. 1959. *Histonomy of the cerebral cortex*. Princeton, N.J.: Van Nostrand-Reinhold.

Borszcz, G. S., J. Cranney, and R. N. Leaton. 1989. Influence of long-term sensitization of the acoustic startle response in rats: Central gray lesions, preexposure, and extinction. *Journal of Experimental Psychology: Animal Behavior Processes* 15:54–64.

Bouffard, J.-P. and L. E. Jarrard. 1988. Acquisition of a complex place task in rats with selective ibotenate lesions of hippocampal formation: Combined lesions of subiculum and entorhinal cortex versus hippocampus. *Behavioral Neuroscience* 102:828–834.

Bradley, P. M., B. Delisle Burns, and A. C. Webb. 1991. Potentiation of synaptic responses in slices from the chick forebrain. *Proceedings of the Royal Society* B243:19–24.

Bradley, P. M., B. Delisle Burns, T. M. King, and A. C. Webb. 1991. Persistent potentiation of the locally evoked response recorded *in vitro* from the IHMV of the domestic chick. Paper presented at the Conference on Avian Learning and Plasticity, September 5–8, 1991, at the Open University, Milton Keynes, U.K.

Braha, O., N. Dale, B. Hochner, M. Klein, T. W. Abrams, and E. R. Kandel. 1990. Second messengers involved in the two processes of presynaptic facilitation that contribute to sensitization and dishabituation in *Aplysia* sensory neurons. *Proceedings of the National Academy of Sciences* 87:2040–2044.

Brauth, S. E., C. A. Kitt, A. Reiner, and R. Quirion. 1986. Neurotensin binding sites in the forebrain and midbrain of the pigeon. *Journal of Comparative Neurology* 253:358–373.

Breese, C. R., R. E. Hampson, and S. A. Deadwyler. 1989. Hippocampal place cells: Stereotypy and plasticity. *Journal of Neuroscience* 9:1097–1111.

Briggs, C. A., T. H. Brown, and D. A. McAfee. 1985. Neurophysiology and pharmacology of long-term potentiation in the rat sympathetic ganglion. *Journal of Physiology* 359:503–521.

Broadbent, D. E. 1958. *Perception and Communication.* London: Pergamon Press.

Brunelli, M., V. Castellucci, and E. R. Kandel. 1976. Synaptic facilitation and behavioral sensitization in *Aplysia:* Possible role of serotonin and cyclic AMP. *Science* 194:1178–1181.

Buchwald, J. S. and G. L. Humphrey. 1973. An analysis of habituation in the specific sensory system. In E. Stellar and J. M. Sprague, eds., *Progress in Physiological Psychology* 5: 1–75. New York: Academic Press.

Buonomano, D. V. and J. H. Byrne. 1990. Long-term synaptic changes produced by a cellular analog of classical conditioning in *Aplysia. Science* 249:420–423.

Butters, N. and D. N. Pandya. 1969. Retention of delayed-alternation: Effect of selective lesions of sulcus principalis. *Science* 165:1271–1273.

Byrne, J. H. 1987. Cellular analysis of associative learning. *Physiological Reviews* 67:329–439.

Carew, T. J. 1984. An introduction to cellular approaches used in the analysis of habituation and sensitization in *Aplysia.* In H. V. S. Peeke and L. Petrinovich, eds., *Habituation, Sensitization, and Behavior,* pp. 205–249. Orlando, Fla.: Academic Press.

Carew, T. J., V. Castellucci, and E. R. Kandel. 1971. An analysis of dishabituation and sensitization of the gill-withdrawal reflex in *Aplysia. International Journal of Neuroscience* 2:79–98.

—— 1979. Sensitization in *Aplysia:* Restoration of transmission in synapses inactivated by long-term habituation. *Science* 205:417–419.

Carew, T. J., R. D. Hawkins, and E. R. Kandel. 1983. Differential classical conditioning of a defensive withdrawal reflex in *Aplysia* californica. *Science* 219:397–400.

Carew, T. J., H. Pinsker, and E. R. Kandel. 1972. Long-term habituation of a defensive withdrawal reflex in *Aplysia. Science* 175:451–454.

Carew, T. J., E. T. Walters, and E. R. Kandel. 1981. Associative learning in *Aplysia:* Cellular correlates supporting a conditioned fear hypothesis. *Science* 211:501–504.

Carlson, N. R. 1977. *Physiology of Behavior.* Allyn and Bacon: Boston.

Casini, G., V. P. Bingman, and P. Bagnoli. 1986. Connections of the pigeon dorsomedial forebrain studied with WGA-HRP and 3H-Proline. *Journal of Comparative Neurology* 245:454–470.

Castellucci, V. F. and E. R. Kandel. 1974. A quantal analysis of the synaptic depression underlying habituation of the gill-withdrawal reflex in *Aplysia. Proceedings of the National Academy of Sciences (U.S.A.)* 71:5004–5008.

—— 1976. Presynaptic facilitation as a mechanism for behavioral sensitization in *Aplysia. Science* 194:1176–1178.

Castellucci, V. F., T. J. Carew, and E. R. Kandel. 1978. Cellular analysis of long-term habituation of the gill-withdrawal reflex of *Aplysia* californica. *Science* 202:1306–1308.

Castellucci, V. F., H. Pinsker, I. Kupfermann, and E. R. Kandel. 1970. Neuronal mechanisms of habituation and dishabituation of the gill-withdrawal reflex in *Aplysia. Science* 167:1745–1748.

Castellucci, V. F., S. Schacher, P. G. Montarolo, S. Mackey, D. L. Glanzman, R. D. Hawkins, T. W. Abrams, P. Goelet, and E. R. Kandel. 1986. Convergence of small molecule and peptide transmitters on a common molecular cascade. In T. Hökfelt, K. Fuxe, and B. Pernow, eds., *Co-Existence of Neuronal Messengers: A New Principle in Chemical Transmission,* pp. 83–102. Progress in Brain Research Series, vol. 68. Amsterdam: Elsevier.

Cegavske, C. F., T. A. Harrison, and Y. Torigoe. 1987. Identification of the substrates of the unconditioned response in the classically conditioned, rabbit, nictitating-membrane preparation. In I. Gormezano, W. F. Prokasy, and R. F. Thompson, eds., *Classical Conditioning,* pp. 65–91. 3d ed. Hillsdale, N.J.: Lawrence Erlbaum.

Chamizo, V. D. and N. J. Mackintosh. 1989. Latent learning and latent inhibition in maze discriminations. *Quarterly Journal of Experimental Psychology* 41B:21–31.

Chamizo, V. D., D. Sterio, and N. J. Mackintosh. 1985. Blocking and overshadowing between intra-maze and extra-maze cues: A test of the independence of locale and guidance learning. *Quarterly Journal of Experimental Psychology* 37B:235–253.

Chapman, P. F., J. E. Steinmetz, and R. F. Thompson. 1988. Classical conditioning does not occur when direct stimulation of red nucleus or cerebellar nuclei is the unconditioned stimulus. *Brain Research* 442:97–104.

Chopin, S. F. and A. A. Buerger. 1975. Graded acquisition of an instrumental avoidance response by the spinal rat. *Physiology and Behavior* 15:155–158.

Chorover, S. L. and P. H. Schiller. 1965. Short-term retrograde amnesia in rats. *Journal of Comparative and Physiological Psychology* 61:34–41.

Church, R. M. and N. D. Lerner. 1976. Does the headless roach learn to avoid? *Physiological Psychology* 3:439–442.

Churchland, P. M. and P. S. Churchland. 1990. Could a machine think? *Scientific American* 262:26–31.

Clark, G. A. and E. R. Kandel. 1984. Branch-specific heterosynaptic facilitation in *Aplysia* siphon sensory cells. *Proceedings of the National Academy of Sciences* 81:2577–2581.

Clark, G. A., D. A. McCormick, D. G. Lavond, and R. F. Thompson. 1984. Effects of lesions of cerebellar nuclei on conditioned behavioral and hippocampal neuronal responses. *Brain Research* 291:125–136.

Cogan, D. C., T. B. Posey, and J. L. Reeves. 1976. Response patterning in hippocampectomized rats. *Physiology and Behavior* 168:569–576.

Cohen, N. J. 1984. Preserved learning capacity in amnesia: Evidence for multiple memory systems. In L. R. Squire and N. Butters, eds., *Neuropsychology of Memory,* pp. 83–103. New York: Guilford Press.

Cohen, N. J. and L. R. Squire. 1981. Retrograde amnesia and remote memory impairment. *Neuropsychologia* 19:337–356.

Colavita, F. B. 1965. Dual function of the US in classical salivary conditioning. *Journal of Comparative and Physiological Psychology* 60:218–222.

Collin, N. G., A. Cowey, R. Latto, and C. Marzi. 1982. The role of frontal eye-fields and superior colliculi in visual search and non-visual search in rhesus monkeys. *Behavioural Brain Research* 4:177–193.

Collingridge, G. L., S. J. Kehl, and H. McLennan. 1983. Excitatory amino acids in synaptic transmission in the Schaffer collateral-commissural pathway of the rat hippocampus. *Journal of Physiology* 334:33–46.

Colwill, R. M., R. A. Absher, and M. L. Roberts. 1988. Context-US learning in *Aplysia californica. Journal of Neuroscience* 8:4434–4439.

Cook, D. G. and T. J. Carew. 1986. Operant conditioning of head waving in *Aplysia. Proceedings of the National Academy of Sciences* 83:1120–1124.

Corkin, S. 1984. Lasting consequences of bilateral medial temporal lobectomy: Clinical course and experimental findings in H.M. *Seminars in Neurology* 4:249–259.

Courville, J., J. R. Augustine, and P. Martel. 1977. Projections from the inferior olive to the cerebellar nuclei in the cat demonstrated by retrograde transport of horseradish peroxidase. *Brain Research* 130:405–419.

Crow, T. J. 1983. Conditioned modification of locomotion in *Hermissenda crassicornis:* Analysis of time-dependent associative and non-associative components. *Journal of Neuroscience* 3:2621–2628.

Crowne, D. P. and W. I. Riddell. 1969. Hippocampal lesions and the cardiac component of the orienting response in the rat. *Journal of Comparative and Physiological Psychology* 69:748–755.

Dale, N., E. R. Kandel, and S. Schacher. 1987. Serotonin produces long-term changes in the excitability of *Aplysia* sensory neurons in culture that depend on new protein synthesis. *Journal of Neuroscience* 7:2232–2238.

Dale, N., S. Schacher, and E. R. Kandel. 1988. Long-term facilitation in *Aplysia* involves increase in transmitter release. *Science* 239:282–285.

Davies, S. N., R. A. J. Lester, K. G. Reymann, and G. L. Collingridge. 1989. Temporally distinct pre- and post-synaptic mechanisms maintain long-term potentiation. *Nature* 338:500–503.

Davis, M. 1972. Differential retention of sensitization and habituation of the startle response in the rat. *Journal of Comparative and Physiological Psychology* 78:260–267.

Davis, M. and S. E. File. 1984. Intrinsic and extrinsic mechanisms of habituation and sensitization: Implications for the design and analysis of experiments. In H. V. S. Peeke and L. Petrinovich, eds., *Habituation, Sensitization, and Behavior*, pp. 287–323. Orlando, Fla.: Academic Press.

Davis, M., D. S. Gendelman, M. D. Tischler, and P. M. Gendelman. 1982. A primary acoustic startle cicruit: Lesion and stimulation studies. *Journal of Neuroscience* 2:791–805.

Dean, P. 1976. Effects of inferotemporal lesions on the behavior of monkeys. *Psychological Bulletin* 83:41–71.

Dember, W. N. 1956. Response by the rat to environmental change. *Journal of Comparative and Physiological Psychology* 49:93–95.

Deng, S.-Y., M. E. Goldberg, M. A. Segraves, L. G. Ungerleider, and M. Mishkin. 1986. The effect of unilateral ablation of the frontal eye fields on saccadic performance in the monkey. In E. L. Keller and D. S. Zee, eds., *Adaptive Processes in Visual and Oculomotor Systems*, pp. 201–208. Advances in the Biosciences, vol. 57. Oxford: Pergamon.

Desimone, R. and C. G. Gross. 1976. Absence of retinotopic organization in inferior temporal cortex. *Society for Neuroscience Abstracts* 2:1108.

Desmond, N. L. and W. B. Levy. 1986. Changes in the numerical density of synaptic contacts with long-term potentiation in the hippocampal dentate gyrus. *Journal of Comparative Neurology* 253:466–475.

Diamond, D. M. and N. M. Weinberger. 1984. Physiological plasticity of single neurons in auditory cortex of the cat during acquisition of the pupillary conditioned response. II. Secondary field (AII). *Behavioral Neuroscience* 98:189–210.

Dickinson, A. 1980. *Contemporary Animal Learning theory.* Cambridge University Press; Cambridge.

Dickinson, A. and N. J. Mackintosh. 1978. Classical conditioning in animals. *Annual Review of Psychology* 29:587–612.

Dietl, M. M., R. Cortés, and J. M. Palacios. 1988a. Neurotransmitter receptors in the avian brain. III. GABA-benzodiazepine receptors. *Brain Research* 439:366–371.

—— 1988b. Neurotransmitter receptors in the avian brain. II. Muscarinic cholinergic receptors. *Brain Research* 439:360–365.

Dietrichs, E., J. Bjaalie, and P. Brodal. 1983. Do pontocerebellar fibers send collaterals to the cerebellar nuclei? *Brain Research* 259:127–131.

Disterhoft, J. F., D. A. Coulter, and D. L. Alkon. 1986. Conditioning-specific membrane changes of rabbit hippocampal neurons measured *in vitro*. *Proceedings of the National Academy of Sciences* 83:2733–2737.

Downer, J. L. de C. 1961. Changes in visual gnostic functions and emotional behaviour following unilateral temporal pole damage in the "split-brain" monkey. *Nature* 191:50–51.

Dumuis, A., M. Sebben, L. Haynes, J.-P. Pin, and J. Bockaert. 1988. NMDA receptors activate the arachidonic acid cascade system in striatal neurons. *Nature* 336:68–70.

Durkovic, R. G. 1983. Classical conditioning of the flexion reflex in spinal cat: Features of the reflex circuitry. *Neuroscience Letters* 39:155–160.

—— 1986. The spinal cord: A simplified system for the study of neural mechanisms of mammalian learning and memory. In M. E. Goldberger, A. Gorio, and M. Murray, eds., *Development and Plasticity of the Mammalian Spinal Cord*. Fidia Research Series, vol. 3, pp. 149–162. Padua: Livian Press.

Durkovic, R. G. and A. R. Light. 1975. Spinal conditioning: Unconditioned stimulus intensity requirement. *Brain Research* 98:364–368.

Durkovic, R. G. and E. N. Damianopoulos. 1986. Forward and backward classical conditioning of the flexion reflex in the spinal cat. *Journal of Neuroscience* 6:2921–2925.

Eccles, J. C. 1953. *The Neurophysiological Basis of Mind*. Oxford: Clarendon Press.

—— 1977a. *The Understanding of the Brain*. 2d ed. New York: McGraw-Hill.

—— 1977b. An instruction-selection theory of learning in the cerebellar cortex. *Brain Research* 127:327–352.

Egger, M. D. 1978. Sensitization and habituation of dorsal horn cells in cats. *Journal of Physiology* 279:153–166.

Egger, M. D. and P. D. Wall. 1971. The plantar cushion reflex circuit: An oligosynaptic cutaneous reflex. *Journal of Physiology* 216:483–501.

Egger, M. D., J. W. Bishop, and C. H. Cone. 1976. Sensitization and habituation of the plantar cushion reflex in cats. *Brain Research* 103:215–228.

Eichenbaum, H., S. I. Wiener, M. L. Shapiro, and N. J. Cohen. 1989. The organization of spatial coding in the hippocampus: A study of neural ensemble activity. *Journal of Neuroscience* 9:2764–2775.

Elias, H. and D. Schwartz. 1969. Surface areas of the cerebral cortex of mammals determined by stereological methods. *Science* 166:111–113.

Erichsen, J. T., V. P. Bingman, and J. R. Krebs. 1991. The distribution of neuropeptides in the dorsomedial telencephalon of the pigeon (*Columba livia*): A basis for regional subdivisions. *Journal of Comparative Neurology* 314:478–492.

Erickson, M. T. and E. T. Walters. 1988. Differential expression of pseudoconditioning and sensitization by siphon responses in *Aplysia:* Novel response selection after training. *Journal of Neuroscience* 8:3000–3010.

Farel, P. B. 1974a. Persistent increase in synaptic efficacy following a brief tetanus in isolated frog spinal cord. *Brain Research* 66:113–120.

—— 1974b. Dual processes control response habituation across a single synapse. *Brain Research* 72:323–327.

Farel, P. B., D. L. Glanzman, and R. F. Thompson. 1973. Habituation of a monosynaptic response in the vertebrate central nervous system: Lateral column—motoneuron pathway in isolated frog spinal cord. *Journal of Neurophysiology* 36:1117–1130.

Farley, J. 1987. Contingency learning and causal detection in *Hermissenda:* 1. Behavior. *Behavioral Neuroscience* 101:13–27.

Farley, J. and D. L. Alkon. 1980. Neural organization predicts stimulus specificity for a retained associative behavioral change. *Science* 210:1373–1375.

Farley, J. and E. Schuman, E. 1991. Protein kinase C inhibitors prevent induction and continued expression of cell memory in *Hermissenda* type B photoreceptors. *Proceedings of the National Academy of Sciences* 88:2016–2020.

Farley, J., W. Richards, L. Ling, E. Liman, and D. L. Alkon. 1983. Membrane changes in a single photoreceptor during acquisition cause associative learning in *Hermissenda. Science* 221:1201–1203.

Floeter, M. K. and W. T. Greenough. 1979. Cerebellar plasticity: Modification of Purkinje cell structure by differential rearing in monkeys. *Science* 206:227–229.

Foster, T. C., C. A. Castro, and B. L. McNaughton. 1989. Spatial selectivity of rat hippocampal neurons: Dependence on preparedness for movement. *Science* 244:1580–1582.

Frazier, W. T., E. R. Kandel, I. Kupfermann, R. Waziri, and R. E. Coggeshall. 1967. Morphological and functional properties of identified neurons in the abdominal ganglion of *Aplysia californica. Journal of Neurophysiology* 30:1288–1351.

Freund, T. F. and M. Antal. 1988. GABA-containing neurons in the septum control inhibitory interneurons in the hippocampus. *Nature* 336:170–173.

Frost, W. N., G. A. Clark, and E. R. Kandel. 1988. Parallel processing of short-term memory for sensitization in *Aplysia. Journal of Neurobiology* 19:297–334.

Frost, W. N., V. Castellucci, R. D. Hawkins, and E. R. Kandel. 1985. Monosynaptic connections made by the sensory neurons of the gill- and siphon-withdrawal reflex in *Aplysia* participate in the storage of long-term memory for sensitization. *Proceedings of the National Academy of Sciences (U.S.A.)* 82:8266–8269.

Funahashi, S., C. J. Bruce, and P. S. Goldman-Rakic. 1989. Mnemonic coding of visual space in the monkey's dorsolateral frontal cortex. *Journal of Neurophysiology* 61:331–349.

Gaffan, D. 1972. Loss of recognition memory in rats with lesions of the fornix. *Neuropsychologia* 10:327–341.

—— 1974. Recognition impaired and association intact in the memory of monkeys after transection of the fornix. *Journal of Comparative and Physiological Psychology* 86:1100–1109.

Gaffan, D. and S. Harrison. 1987. Amygdalectomy and disconnection in visual learning for auditory secondary reinforcement by monkeys. *Journal of Neuroscience* 7:2285–2292.

—— 1988. Infero-temporal disconnection and fornix transection in visuomotor conditional learning by monkeys. *Behavioral Brain Research* 31:149–163.

—— 1989. Place memory and scene memory: Effects of fornix transection in the monkey. *Experimental Brain Research* 74:202–212.

Gaffan, D. and E. A. Murray. 1992. Monkeys (*Macaca fascicularis*) with rhinal cortex ablations succeed in object discrimination learning despite 24-hr intertrial intervals and fail at matching to sample despite double sample presentations. *Behavioral Neuroscience* 106:30–38.

Gaffan, D. and L. Weiskrantz. 1980. Recency effects and lesion effects in delayed non-matching to randomly baited samples by monkeys. *Brain Research* 196:373–386.

Gaffan, E. A., D. Gaffan, and S. Harrison. 1988. Disconnection of the amygdala from visual association cortex impairs visual reward-association learning in monkeys. *Journal of Neuroscience* 8:3144–3150.

Gaffan, D., R. C. Saunders, E. A. Gaffan, S. Harrison, C. Shields, and M. J. Owen. 1984. Effects of fornix transection upon associative memory in monkeys: Role of the hippocampus in learned action. *Quarterly Journal of Experimental Psychology* 36B:173–221.

Gallagher, M. and P. C. Holland. 1992. Preserved configural learning and spatial learning impairment in rats with hippocampal damage. *Hippocampus* 2:81–88.

Garrud, P., J. N. P. Rawlins, N. J. Mackintosh, G. Goodall, M. M. Cotton, and J. Feldon. 1984. Successful overshadowing and blocking in hippocampectomized rats. *Behavioural Brain Research* 12:39–53.

Glanzman, D. L. and R. F. Thompson. 1979. Evidence against conduction failure as the mechanism underlying monosynaptic habituation in frog spinal cord. *Brain Research* 174:329–332.

—— 1980. Alterations in spontaneous miniature potential activity during habituation of a vertebrate monosynaptic pathway. *Brain Research* 189:377–390.

Glanzman, D. L., E. R. Kandel, and S. Schacher. 1990. Target-dependent structural changes accompanying long-term synaptic facilitation in *Aplysia* neurons. *Science* 249:799–802.

Glanzman, D. L., S. L. Mackey, R. D. Hawkins, A. M. Dyke, P. E. Lloyd, and E. R. Kandel. 1989. Depletion of serotonin in the nervous system of *Aplysia* reduces the behavioral enhancement of gill withdrawal as well as the heterosynaptiec facilitation produced by tail shock. *Journal of Neuroscience* 9:4200–4213.

Goldberg, J. I. and K. Lukowiak. 1984. Transfer of habituation in *Aplysia:* Contribution of heterosynaptic pathways in habituation of the gill-withdrawal reflex. *Journal of Neurobiology* 15:395–411.

Goldman, P. S., H. E. Rosvold, B. Vest, and T. W. Galkin. 1971. Analysis of the delayed alternation deficit produced by dorsolateral prefrontal lesions in the rhesus monkey. *Journal of Comparative and Physiological Psychology* 77:212–220.

Goldman-Rakic, P. S. 1984. The frontal lobes: Uncharted provinces of the brain. *Trends in Neurosciences* 7:425–429.

—— 1987. Circuitry of primate prefrontal cortex and regulation of behavior by representational memory. In F. Plum, ed., *Handbook of Physiology*. Section 1, vol. 5, *Higher Functions of the Brain (Part 1)*, pp. 373–417. Bethesda, Md.: American Physiological Society.

Good, M. 1988. The role of the avian hippocampal in learning and memory. Ph.D. diss., University of York.

Good, M. and R. C. Honey. 1991. Conditioning and contextual retrieval in hippocampal rats. *Behavioral Neuroscience* 105:499–509.

Good, M. and E. M. Macphail. In preparation. Hippocampal lesions in pigeons (*Columba livia*) selectively disrupt spatial short-term memory.

Goodale, M. A. and R. H. I. Dale. 1981. Radial-maze performance in the rat following lesions of posterior neocortex. *Behavioural Brain Research* 3:273–288.

Gormezano, I. 1972. Investigations of defense and reward conditioning in the rabbit. In A. H. Black and W. F. Prokasy, eds., *Classical Conditioning II: Current Research and Theory,* pp. 151–181. New York: Appleton-Century-Crofts.

Gormezano, I., N. Schneiderman, E. Deaux, and I. Fuentes. 1962. Nictitating membrane: Classical conditioning and extinction in the albino rabbit. *Science* 138:33–34.

Grafman, J., A. Salazar, H. Weingartner, S. Vance, and D. Amin. 1986. The relationship of brain-tissue loss volume and lesion location to cognitive deficit. *Journal of Neuroscience* 6:301–307.

Grastyán, E., K. Lissak, I. Madarasz, and H. Donhoffer. 1959. Hippocampal electrical activity during the development of conditioned reflexes. *Electroencephalography and Clinical Neurophysiology* 11:409–430.

Grau, J. W. 1987. Activation of the opioid and nonopioid analgesic systems: Evidence for a memory hypothesis and against the coulometric hypothesis. *Journal of Experimental Psychology: Animal Behavior Processes* 13:215–225.

Grau, J. W., J. A. Salinas, P. A. Illich, and M. W. Meagher. 1990. Associative learning and memory for an antinociceptive response in the spinalized rat. *Behavioral Neuroscience* 104:489–494.

Gray, J. A. 1971. *The Psychology of Fear and Stress.* New York: McGraw-Hill.

Gray, J. A. and G. G. Ball. 1970. Frequency-specific relation between hippocampal theta rhythm, behavior and amobarbital action. *Science* 168:1246–1248.

Gray, J. A. and N. McNaughton. 1983. Comparison between the behavioural effects of septal and hippocampal lesions: A review. *Neuroscience and Biobehavioral Reviews* 7:119–188.

Graybiel, A. M. 1972. Some fiber pathways related to the posterior thalamic region in the cat. *Brain, Behavior, and Evolution* 6:363–393.

—— 1973. The thalamocortical projection of the co-called posterior nuclear group: A study with anterograde degeneration methods in the cat. *Brain Research* 49:229–244.

Greenberg, S. M., V. F. Castellucci, H. Bayley, and J. H. Schwartz. 1987. A molecular mechanism for long-term sensitization in *Aplysia. Nature* 329:62–65.

Gross, C. G., D. B. Bender, and G. L. Gerstein. 1979. Activity of inferior temporal neurons in behaving monkeys. *Neuropsychologia* 17:215–229.

Gross, C. G., C. E. Rocha-Miranda, and D. B. Bender. 1972. Visual properties of neurons in inferotemporal cortex of the macaque. *Journal of Neurophysiology* 35:96–111.

Grover, L. M. and J. Farley. 1987. Temporal order sensitivity of associative neural and behavioral changes in *Hermissenda. Behavioral Neuroscience* 101:658–675.

Groves, P. M. and R. F. Thompson. 1970. Habituation: A dual-process theory. *Psychological Review* 77:419–450.

Groves, P. M., D. L. Glanzman, M. M. Patterson, and R. F. Thompson. 1970. Excitability of cutaneous afferent terminals during habituation and sensitization in acute spinal cat. *Brain Research* 18:388–392.

Gustafson, J. W. and L. J. Koenig. 1979. Hippocampal function in distractibility and generalization : A behavioral investigation. *Physiology and Behavior* 22:297–303.

Hagan, J. J., J. D. Salamone, J. Simpson, S. D. Iversen, and R. G. M. Morris. 1988. Place navigation in rats is impaired by lesions of medial septum and diagonal band but not nucleus basalis magnocellularis. *Behavioural Brain Research* 27:9–20.

Haley, J. E., G. L. Wilcox, and P. F. Chapman. 1992. The role of nitric oxide in hippocampal long-term potentiation. *Neuron* 8:211–216.

Hall, G. and S. Channell. 1985. Differential effects of contextual change on latent inhibition and on the habituation of an orienting response. *Journal of Experimental Psychology: Animal Behavior Processes* 11:470–481.

Hall, J. F. 1984. Backward conditioning in Pavlovian type studies. *Pavlovian Journal of Biological Science* 19:163–168.

Hargreaves, E. L., D. P. Cain, and C. H. Vanderwolf. 1990. Learning and behavioral long-term potentiation: Importance of controlling for motor activity. *Journal of Neuroscience* 10:1472–1478.

Harris, E. W. and C. W. Cotman. 1986. Long-term potentiation of guinea pig mossy fiber responses is not blocked by N-methyl-D-aspartate antagonists. *Neuroscience Letters* 70:132–137.

Harris, E. W., A. H. Ganong, and C. W. Cotman. 1984. Long-term potentiation in the hippocampus involves activation of N-methyl-D-aspartate receptors. *Brain Research* 323:132–137.

Hawkins, R. D. 1989. Localization of potential serotonergic facilitator neurons in *Aplysia* by glyoxylic acid histofluorescence combined with retrograde fluorescent labelling. *Journal of Neuroscience* 9:4214–4226.

Hawkins, R. D. and E. R. Kandel. 1984. Is there a cell-biological alphabet for simple forms of learning? *Psychological Review* 91:375–391.

Hawkins, R. D. and S. Schacher. 1989. Identified facilitator neurons L29 and L28 are excited by cutaneous stimuli used in dishabituation, sensitization and classical conditioning of *Aplysia*. *Journal of Neuroscience* 9:4236–4245.

Hawkins, R. D., T. J. Carew, and E. R. Kandel. 1986. Effects of interstimulus interval and contingency on classical conditioning of the *Aplysia* siphon withdrawal reflex. *Journal of Neuroscience* 6:1695–1701.

Hawkins, R. D., V. Castellucci, and E. R. Kandel. 1981. Interneurons involved in mediation and modulation of gill-withdrawal reflex in *Aplysia*. II. Identified neurons produce heterosynaptic facilitation contributing to behavioral sensitization. *Journal of Neurophysiology* 45:315–326.

Hawkins, R. D., T. W. Abrams, T. J. Carew, and E. R. Kandel. 1983. A cellular mechanism of classical conditioning in *Aplysia:* Activity-dependent amplification of presynaptic facilitation. *Science* 219:400–405.

Hawkins, R. D., N. Lalevic, G. A. Clark, and E. R. Kandel. 1989. Classical conditioning of the *Aplysia* siphon-withdrawal reflex exhibits response specificity. *Proceedings of the National Academy of Sciences* 86:7620–7624.

Hebb, D. O. 1949. *Organization of Behavior.* New York: Wiley; reprint, New York: Science Editions, 1961.

Hernandez-Péon, R. 1960. Neurophysiological correlates of habituation and other manifestations of plastic inhibition. *Electroencephalographic and Clinical Neurophysiology,* Supplement 13:101–114.

Hill, A. J. 1978. First occurrence of hippocampal spatial firing in a new environment. *Experimental Neurology* 62:282–297.

Hilton, S. C. and J. R. Krebs. 1990. Spatial memory of four species of *Parus:* Performance in an open-field analogue of a radial maze. *Quarterly Journal of Experimental Psychology* 42B:345–368.

Hirsh, R. 1980. The hippocampus, conditional operations, and cognition. *Physiological Psychology* 8:175–182.

Hitch, G. J. 1983. Short-term memory processes in humans and animals. In A. R. Mayes, ed., *Memory in Animals and Humans,* pp. 177–202. Wokingham, U.K.: Van Nostrand-Reinhold.

Hochner, B., M. Klein, S. Schacher, and E. R. Kandel. 1986. Additional component in the cellular mechanism of presynaptic facilitation contributes to behavioral dishabituation in *Aplysia. Proceedings of the National Academy of Sciences* 83:8794–8798.

Hodos, W. 1961. Progressive ratio as a measure of reward strength. *Science* 134:943–944.

Hodos, W. and G. Kalman. 1963. Effects of increment size and reinforcer value on progressive ratio. *Journal of the Experimental Analysis of Behavior* 6:387–392.

Hoehler, F. K. and R. F. Thompson. 1980. Effect of interstimulus (CS-UCS) interval on hippocampal unit activity during classical conditioning of the nictitating membrane response of the rabbit. *Journal of Comparative and Physiological Psychology* 94:201–215.

Honig, W. K. 1978. Studies of working memory in the pigeon. In S. H. Hulse, H. Fowler, and W. K. Honig, eds., *Cognitive Processes in Animal Behavior,* pp. 211–248. Hillsdale, N.J.: Lawrence Erlbaum.

Honig, W. K. and R. K. R. Thompson. 1978. Retrospective and prospective processing in animal working memory. In G. H. Bower, ed., *The psychology of learning and motivation: Advances in Research and Theory,* 16:239–283. New York: Academic Press.

Hoover, J. E. and R. G. Durkovic. 1989. Retention of a backward classically conditioned reflex response in spinal cat. *Experimental Brain Research* 77:621–627.

Horn, G. 1985. *Memory, Imprinting, and the Brain.* Oxford: Clarendon Press.

Horridge, G. A. 1962. Learning of leg position by the ventral nerve cord in headless insects. *Proceedings of the Royal Society* B157:33–52.

Hubel, D. H. and T. N. Wiesel. 1962. Receptive fields, binocular interaction and functional architecture in the cat's visual cortex. *Journal of Physiology* 160:106–154.

—— 1963. Receptive fields of cells in striate cortex of very young, visually inexperienced kittens. *Journal of Neurophysiology* 26:994–1002.

—— 1970. The period of susceptibility to the physiological effects of unilateral eye closure in kittens. *Journal of Physiology* 206:419–436.

Hunter, W. S. 1930. A consideration of Lashley's theory of the equipotentiality of cerebral action. *Journal of General Psychology* 3:455–468.

Huppert, F. A. and M. Piercy. 1977. Recognition memory in amnesic patients: A defect of acquisition? *Neuropsychologia* 15:643–652.

Hyvärinen, J. 1982. Posterior parietal lobe of the primate brain. *Physiological Reviews* 62:1060–1129.

Ito, M. 1984. *The Cerebellum and Neural Control.* New York: Raven Press.

Iversen, S. D. and M. Mishkin. 1970. Perseverative interference in monkeys following selective lesions of the inferior prefrontal convexity. *Experimental Brain Research* 11:376–386.

Jacobsen, C. F., J. B. Wolfe, and T. A. Jackson. 1938. An experimental analysis of the functions of the frontal association areas in primates. *Journal of Nervous and Mental Disease* 82:1–14.

Jagielo, J. A., A. J. Nonneman, W. L. Isaac, and P. A. Jackson-Smith. 1990. Hippocampal lesions impair rats' performance of a nonspatial matching-to-sample task. *Psychobiology* 18:55–62.

James, G. O., M. J. Hardiman, and C. H. Yeo. 1987. Hippocampal lesions and trace conditioning in the rabbit. *Behavioural Brain Research* 23:109–116.

Jarrard, L. E. 1975. Role of interference in retention in rats with hippocampal lesions. *Journal of Comparative and Physiological Psychology* 89:400–408.

—— 1983. Selective hippocampal lesions and behavior: Effects of kainic acid lesions on performance of place and cue tasks. *Behavioral Neuroscience* 97:873–889.

—— 1985. Is the hippocampus really involved in memory? In B. E. Will and J. C. Dalrymple-Alford, eds., *Brain Plasticity, Learning, and Memory,* pp. 363–372. New York: Plenum.

—— 1986. Selective hippocampal lesions and behavior: Implications for current research and theorizing. In R. L. Isaacson and K. H. Pribram, eds., *The Hippocampus,* 4:93–126. New York: Plenum.

Jarrard, L. E. and J. H. Korn. 1969. Effects of hippocampal lesions on heart rate during habituation and passive avoidance. *Communications in Behavioral Biology* A3:141–150.

Jarrard, L. E., H. Okaichi, O. Steward, and R. B. Goldschmidt. 1984. On the role of hippocampal connections in the performance of place and cue tasks: Comparisons with damage to hippocampus. *Behavioral Neuroscience* 98:946–954.

Jerison, H. J. 1973. *Evolution of the Brain and Intelligence.* New York: Academic Press.

Jolly, A. 1987. Boiling down intelligence. *Behavioral and Brain Sciences* 10:671.

Jones, B. and M. Mishkin. 1972. Limbic lesions and the problem of stimulus-reinforcement associations. *Experimental Neurology* 36:362–377.

Jordan, W. P. 1989. Mesencephalic reticular formation lesions made after habituation training abolish long-term habituation of the acoustic startle response in rats. *Behavioral Neuroscience* 103:805–815.

Jordan, W. P. and R. N. Leaton. 1982a. Startle habituation in rats after lesions in the brachium of the inferior colliculus. *Physiology and Behavior* 28:253–258.

—— 1982b. Effects of mesencephalic reticular formation lesions on long- and short-term habituation of the startle and lick suppression responses in the rat. *Journal of Comparative and Physiological Psychology* 96:170–183.

—— 1983. Habituation of the acoustic startle response in rats after lesions in the mesencephalic reticular formation or in the inferior colliculus. *Behavioral Neuroscience* 97:710–724.

Källén, B. 1962. Embryogenesis of brain nuclei in the chick telencephalon. *Ergebnisse der Anatomie und Entwicklungsgeschichte Wiesbaden* 36:62–82.

Kamin, L. J. 1969. Predictability, surprise, attention and conditioning. In B. A. Campbell and R. M. Church, eds., *Punishment and aversive behavior*, pp. 279–296. New York: Appleton-Century-Crofts.

Kandel, E. R. 1976. *Cellular basis of behavior: An introduction to behavioral neurobiology*. San Francisco: W. H. Freeman.

—— 1979. *Behavioral biology of Aplysia*. San Francisco: W. H. Freeman.

Kandel, E. R. and J. H. Schwartz. 1982. Molecular biology of learn ing: Modulation of transmitter release. *Science* 218:433–443.

—— 1985. *Principles of neural science*. 2d ed. New York: Elsevier.

Kandel, E. R. and L. Tauc. 1965. Heterosynaptic facilitation in neurones of the abdominal ganglion of *Aplysia depilans*. *Journal of Physiology* 181:1–27.

Kandel, E. R., T. W. Abrams, L. Bernier, T. J. Carew, R. D. Hawkins, and J. H. Schwartz. 1983. Classical conditioning and sensitization share aspects of the same molecular cascade in *Aplysia*. *Cold Spring Harbor Symposium*, no. 48, pp. 821–830.

Kapp, B. S., R. C. Frysinger, M. Gallagher, and J. R. Haselton. 1979. Amygdala central nucleus lesions: Effect on heart rate conditioning in the rabbit. *Physiology and Behavior* 23:1109–1117.

Karten, H. J. and W. Hodos. 1967. *A Stereotaxic Atlas of the Brain of the Pigeon (Columba livia)*. Baltimore, Md.: Johns Hopkins University Press.

Kauer, J. A., R. C. Malenka, and R. A. Nicoll. 1988. A persistent postsynaptic modification mediates long-term potentiation in the hippocampus. *Neuron* 1:911–917.

Kaye, H. and J. M. Pearce. 1987. Hippocampal lesions attenuate latent inhibition and the decline of the orienting response in rats. *Quarterly Journal of Experimental Psychology* 39B:107–125.

Keith, J. R. and J. W. Rudy. 1990. Why NMDA-receptor-dependent long-term potentiation may not be a mechanism of learning and memory: Reappraisal of the NMDA-receptor blockade strategy. *Psychobiology* 18:251–257.

Kelly, T. M., C.-C. Zuo, and J. R. Bloedel. 1990. Classical conditioning of the eyeblink reflex in the decerebrate-decerebellate rabbit. *Behavioural Brain Research* 38:7–18.

Kemble, E. D., D. C. Blanchard, R. J. Blanchard, and R. Takushi. 1984. Taming in wild rats following medial amygdaloid lesions. *Physiology and Behavior* 32:131–134.

Kessler, M., M. Baudry, and G. Lynch. 1987. Use of cystine to distinguish glutamate binding from glutamate sequestration. *Neuroscience Letters* 81:221–226.

Kettner, R. E. and R. F. Thompson. 1982. Auditory signal detection and decision processes in the nervous system. *Journal of Comparative and Physiological Psychology* 96:328–331.

Kim, J. J. and M. S. Fanselow. 1992. Modality-specific retrograde amnesia of fear. *Science* 256:675–677.

Kitt, C. A. and S. E. Brauth. 1986. Telencephalic projections from midbrain and isthmal cell groups in the pigeon. I. Locus coeruleus and subcoeruleus. *Journal of Comparative Neurology* 247:69–91.

Klein, M. and E. R. Kandel. 1980. Mechanism of calcium current modulation underlying presynaptic facilitation and behavioral sensitization in *Aplysia*. *Proceedings of the National Academy of Sciences* 77:6912–6916.

Klein, M., J. Camardo, and E. R. Kandel. 1982. Serotonin modulates a specific potassium current in the sensory neurons that show presynaptic facilitation in *Aplysia*. *Proceedings of the National Academy of Sciences* 79:5713–5717.

Klein, M., E. Shapiro, and E. R. Kandel. 1980. Synaptic plasticity and the modulation of the Ca^{2+} current. *Journal of Experimental Biology* 89:117–157.

Kleinschmidt, A., M. F. Bear, and W. Singer. 1987. Blockade of "NMDA" receptors disrupts experience-dependent plasticity of kitten striate cortex. *Science* 238:355–358.

Kling, A. 1968. Effects of amygdalectomy and testosterone on sexual behavior of male juvenile macaques. *Journal of Comparative and Physiological Psychology* 65:466–471.

Klosterhalfen, W. and S. Klosterhalfen. 1985. Habituation of heart rate in functionally decorticate rats. *Behavioral Neuroscience* 99:555–563.

Kluver, H. and P.C. Bucy. 1937. "Psychic blindness" and other symptoms following bilateral temporal lobectomy in rhesus monkeys. *American Journal of Physiology* 119:352–353.

Knowlton, B. J., D. G. Lavond, and R. F. Thompson. 1988. The effect of lesions of cerebellar cortex on retention of the classically conditioned eyeblink response when stimulation of the lateral reticular nucleus is used as the conditioned stimulus. *Behavioral and Neural Biology* 49:293–301.

Kolb, B. 1986. Functions of the frontal cortex of the rat: A comparative review. *Brain Research Reviews* 8:65–98.

Konishi, M. 1985. Birdsong: From behavior to neuron. *Annual Review of Neuroscience* 8:125–170.

Konorski, J. 1967. *Integrative activity of the brain*. Chicago: University of Chicago Press.

Kornhuber, H. H., D. Bechinger, H. Jung, and E. Sauer. 1985. A quantitative relationship between the extent of localized cerebral lesions and the intellectual and behavioural deficiency in children. *European Archives of Psychiatry and Neurological Sciences* 235:129–133.

Koyano, K., K. Kuba, and S. Minota. 1985. Long-term potentiation of transmitter release induced by repetitive presynaptic activities in bullfrog (*Rana catesbeiana*) sympathetic ganglia. *Journal of Physiology* 359:219–234.

Krane, R. V., H. M. Sinnamon, and G. J. Thomas. 1976. Conditioned taste aversions and neophobia in rats with hippocampal lesions. *Journal of Comparative and Physiological Psychology* 90:680–693.

Krayniak, P. F. and A. Siegel. 1978a. Efferent connections of the hippocampus and adjacent regions in the pigeon. *Brain, Behavior, and Evolution* 15:372–388.

—— 1978b. Efferent connections of the septal area in the pigeon. *Brain, Behavior, and Evolution* 15:389–404.

Krebs, J. R. 1990. Food-storing in birds: Adaptive specialization in brain and behaviour? *Philosophical Transactions of the Royal Society* B329:153–160.

Krebs, J. R., J. T. Erichsen, and V. P. Bingman. 1991. The distribution of neurotransmitters and neurotransmitter-related enzymes in the dorsomedial telencephalon of the pigeon (*Columba livia*). *Journal of Comparative Neurology* 314:467–477.

Krebs, J. R., D. F. Sherry, S. D. Healy, V. H. Perry, and A. L. Vaccarino. 1989. Hippocampal specialization of food-storing birds. *Proceedings of the National Academy of Sciences* 86:1388–1392.

Kubie, J. L., R. U. Muller, and E. Bostock. 1990. Spatial firing properties of hippocampal theta cells. *Journal of Neuroscience* 10:8 1110–1123.

Kupfermann, I., V. Castellucci, H. M. Pinsker, and E. R. Kandel. 1970. Neuronal correlates of habituation and dishabituation of the gill-withdrawal reflex in *Aplysia*. *Science* 167:1743–1745.

Lachter, J. and T. G. Bever, 1988. The relation between linguistic structure and associative theories of language learning: A constructive critique of some connectionist learning models. *Cognition* 28:195–247.

Larsell, O. 1952. The morphogenesis and adult pattern of the lobules and fissures of the cerebellum of the white rat. *Journal of Comparative Neurology* 97:281–356.

—— 1953. The anterior lobe of the mammalian and the human cerebellum. *Anatomical Record* 115:341.

Larson, J. and G. Lynch. 1986. Induction of synaptic potentiation in hippocampus by patterned stimulation involves two events. *Science* 232:985–988.

Larson, J., D. Wong, and G. Lynch. 1986. Patterned stimulation at the theta frequency is optimal for the induction of hippocampal long-term potentiation. *Brain Research* 368:347–350.

Lashley, K. S. 1929. *Brain Mechanisms and Intelligence: A Quantitative Study of Injuries to the Brain*. Reprint, New York: Dover, 1963.

—— 1949. Persistent problems in the evolution of mind. *Quarterly Review of Biology* 24:28–42.

—— 1950. In search of the engram. *Society of Experimental Biology Symposium*, no. 4: *Mechanisms in Animal Behaviour*, pp. 478–505.

Lashley, K. S. and D. A. McCarthy. 1926. The survival of the maze habit after cerebellar injuries. *Journal of Comparative Psychology* 6:423–433.

Lavond, D. G. and J. E. Steinmetz. 1989. Acquisition of classical conditioning without cerebellar cortex. *Behavioural Brain Research* 33:113–164.

Lavond, D. G., T. L. Hembree, and R. F. Thompson. 1985. Effect of kainic acid lesions of the cerebellar interpositus nucleus on eyelid conditioning in the rabbit. *Brain Research* 326:179–182.

Lavond, D. G., J. S. Lincoln, D. A. McCormick, and R. F. Thompson. 1984. Effect of bilateral lesions of the dentate interpositus cerebellar nuclei on conditioning of heart rate and nictitating membrane/eyelid responses in the rabbit. *Brain Research* 305:323–330.

Leaton, R. N. 1981. Habituation of startle response, lick suppression, and exploratory behavior in rats with hippocampal lesions. *Journal of Comparative and Physiological Psychology* 95:813–826.

Leaton, R. N. and W. F. Supple. 1986. Cerebellar vermis: Essential for long-term habituation of the acoustic startle response. *Science* 232:513–515.

Leaton, R. N., J. V. Cassella, and G. S. Borszcz. 1985. Short-term and long-term habituation of the acoustic startle response in chronic decerebrate rats. *Behavioral Neuroscience* 99:901–912.

Lederhendler, I. and D. L. Alkon. 1986. Implicating causal relations between cellular function and learning behavior. *Behavioral Neuroscience* 100:833–838.

Lederhendler, I., S. Gart, and D. L. Alkon. 1986. Classical conditioning of *Hermissenda:* Origin of a new response. *Journal of Neuroscience* 6:1325–1331.

LeDoux, J. E., A. Sakaguchi, and D. J. Reis. 1984. Subcortical efferent projections of the medial geniculate nucleus mediate emotional responses conditioned to acoustic stimuli. *Journal of Neuroscience* 4:683–698.

Lee, K. S. 1982. Sustained enhancement of evoked potentials following brief, high-frequency stimulation of the cerebral cortex *in vitro. Brain Research* 238:617–623.

Lee, K. S., F. Schottler, M. Oliver, and G. Lynch. 1980. Brief bursts of high-frequency stimulation produce two types of structural change in rat hippocampus. *Journal of Neurophysiology* 44:247–258.

Leonard, C. M. 1969. The prefrontal cortex of the rat. Part 1: Cortical projections of the mediodorsal nucleus. Part 2: Efferent projections. *Brain Research* 12:321–343.

Leonard, J. L., J. Edstrom, and K. Lukowiak. 1989. Reexamination of the gill withdrawal reflex of *Aplysia californica* Cooper (Gastropoda; Opisthobranchia). *Behavioral Neuroscience* 103:585–604.

Leung, L.-W. S. and K. A. Desborough. 1988. APV, an N-methyl-D-aspartate receptor antagonist, blocks the hippocampal theta rhythm in behaving rats. *Brain Research* 463:148–152.

Lewis, D. and T. J. Teyler. 1986. Long-term potentiation in the goldfish optic tectum. *Brain Research* 375:246–250.

Lewis, F. T. 1923. The significance of the term *Hippocampus. Journal of Comparative Neurology* 35:213–230.

Lewis, J. L., J. J. LoTurco, and P. R. Solomon. 1987. Lesions of the middle cerebellar peduncle disrupt acquisition and retention of the rabbit's classically conditioned nictitating membrane response. *Behavioral Neuroscience* 101:151–157.

Linden, D. J. and A. Routtenberg. 1989. The role of protein kinase C in long-term potentiation: A testable model. *Brain Research Reviews* 14:279–296.

Llinás, R. R. 1975. The cortex of the cerebellum. *Scientific American* 232:56–71.

Lømo, T. 1966. Frequency potentiation of excitatory synaptic activity in the dentate area of the hippocampal formation. *Acta physiologica scandinavica* 68 (Supplement 277).

Lopiano, L., C. de'Sperati, and P. G. Montarolo. 1990. Long-term habituation of the acoustic startle response: Role of the cerebellar vermis. *Neuroscience* 35:79–84.

LoTurco, J. J., D. A. Coulter, and D. L. Alkon. 1988. Enhancement of synaptic potentials in rabbit CA1 pyramidal neurons following classical conditioning. *Proceedings of the National Academy of Sciences* 85:1672–1676.

Lovinger, D. M., K. Wong, K. Murakami, and A. Routtenberg. 1987. Protein kinase C inhibitors eliminate hippocampal long-term potentiation. *Brain Research* 436:177–183.

Lubow, R. E. 1973. Latent inhibition. *Psychological Bulletin* 79:398–407.

Lubow, R. E., B. Rifkin, and M. Alek. 1976. The context effect: The relationship between stimulus preexposure and environmental preexposure determines subsequent learning. *Journal of Experimental Psychology: Animal Behavior Processes* 2:38–47.

Lukowiak, K. and J. W. Jacklet. 1972. Habituation and dishabituation: Interactions between peripheral and central nervous systems in *Aplysia*. *Science* 178:1306–1308.

Lynch, G. 1986. *Synapses, Circuits, and the Beginnings of Memory*. Cambridge, Mass.: MIT Press.

Lynch, G. and M. Baudry. 1984. Biochemistry of memory: A new and specific hypothesis. *Science* 224:1057–1063.

Lynch, G., V. K. Gribkoff, and S. A. Deadwyler. 1976. Long-term potentiation is accompanied by a reduction in dendritic responsiveness to glutamic acid. *Nature* 263:151–153.

Lynch, G., J. Larson, S. Kelso, G. Barrionuevo, and F. Schottler. 1983. Intracellular injections of EGTA block induction of hippocampal long-term potentiation. *Nature, 305,* 719–721.

Mackey, S. L., E. R. Kandel, and R. D. Hawkins. 1989. Identified serotonergic neurons LCB1 and RCB1 in the cerebral ganglia of *Aplysia* produce presynaptic facilitation of siphon sensory neurons. *Journal of Neuroscience* 9:4227–4235.

Mackey, S. L., D. L. Glanzman, S. A. Small, A. M. Dyke, E. R. Kandel, and R. D. Hawkins. 1987. Tail shock produces inhibition as well as sensitization of the siphon-withdrawal reflex of *Aplysia:* Possible behavioral role for presynaptic inhibition mediated by the peptide Phe-Met-Arg-Phe-NH^2. *Proceedings of the National Academy of Sciences* 84:8730–8734.

Mackintosh, N. J. 1974. *The psychology of animal learning*. London: Academic Press.

—— 1975. A theory of attention: Variations in the associability of stimuli with reinforcement. *Psychological Review* 82:276–298.

—— 1983. *Conditioning and associative learning*. Oxford: Clarendon Press.

—— 1987. Neurobiology, psychology and habituation. *Behaviour Research and Therapy* 25:81–97.

Macphail, E. M. 1982. *Brain and intelligence in vertebrates*. Oxford: Clarendon Press.

—— 1985a. Ecology and intelligence. In N. M. Weinberger, J. L. McGaugh, and G.

Lynch, eds., *Memory Systems of the Brain: Animal and Human Cognitive Processes*, pp. 279–286. New York: Guilford Press.

—— 1985b. Vertebrate intelligence: The null hypothesis. *Philosophical Transactions of the Royal Society*, Series B 308:37–51.

—— 1986. Animal memory: Past, present and future. *Quarterly Journal of Experimental Psychology* 38B:349–364.

—— 1987. The comparative psychology of intelligence. *Behavioral and Brain Sciences* 10:645–695.

Macphail, E. M. and S. Reilly. 1989. Rapid acquisition of a novelty versus familiarity concept by pigeons (*Columba livia*). *Journal of Experimental Psychology: Animal Behavior Processes* 15:242–252.

Mahut, H. 1971. Spatial and object reversal learning in monkeys with partial temporal lobe ablations. *Neuropsychologia* 9:409–424.

—— 1972. A selective spatial deficit in monkeys after transection of the fornix. *Neuropsychologia* 10:65–74.

Mahut, H. and S. M. Zola. 1973. A non-modality-specific impairment in spatial learning after fornix lesions in monkeys. *Neuropsychologia* 11:244–269.

Mahut, H., M. Moss, and S. Zola-Morgan. 1981. Retention deficits after combined amygdalo-hippocampal and selective hippocampal resections in the monkey. *Neuropsychologia* 19:201–225.

Mahut, H., S. Zola-Morgan, and M. Moss. 1982. Hippocampal resections impair associative learning and recognition memory in the monkey. *Journal of Neuroscience* 9:1214–1229.

Maier, N. R. F. and T. C. Schneirla. 1935. *Principles of Animal Psychology.* New York: McGraw-Hill.

Malamut, B. L., R. C. Saunders, and M. Mishkin. 1984. Monkeys with combined amygdalo-hippocampal lesions succeed in object discrimination learning despite 24-hour intertrial intervals. *Behavioral Neuroscience* 98:759–769.

Mamounas, L. A., R. F. Thompson, and J. Madden. 1987. Cerebellar GABAergic processes: Evidence for critical involvement in a form of simple associative learning in the rabbit. *Proceedings of the National Academy of Sciences* 84:2101–2105.

Manilow, R. and R. W. Tsien. 1990. Presynaptic enhancement shown by whole-cell recordings of long-term potentiation in hippocampal slices. *Nature* 346:177–180.

Marcus, E. A., T. G. Nolen, C. H. Rankin, and T. J. Carew. 1988. Behavioral dissociation of dishabituation, sensitization, and inhibition in *Aplysia*. *Science* 241:210–213.

Markowska, A. L., D. S. Olton, E. A. Murray, and D. Gaffan. 1989. A comparative analysis of the role of the fornix and cingulate cortex in memory: Rats. *Experimental Brain Research* 74:187–201.

Marr, D. 1969. A theory of cerebellar cortex. *Journal of Physiology* 202:437–470.

—— 1971. Simple memory: A theory of archicortex. *Philosophical Transactions of the Royal Society of London* B262:23–81.

Marslen-Wilson, W. D. and H.-L. Teuber. 1975. Memory for remote events in anterograde amnesia: Recognition of public figures from news photographs. *Neuropsychologia* 13:353–364.

Matthies, H. H., H. Ruethrich, T. Ott, H. K. Matthies, and R. Matthies. 1986. Low-frequency perforant path stimulation as a conditioned stimulus demonstrates correlations between long-term potentiation and learning. *Physiology and Behavior* 36:811–821.

Matzel, L. D., B. G. Schreurs, I. Lederhendler, and D. L. Alkon. 1990. Acquisition of conditioned associations in *Hermissenda:* Additive effects of contiguity and the forward interstimulus interval. *Behavioral Neuroscience* 104:597–606.

Mauk, M. D. and R. F. Thompson. 1987. Retention of classically conditioned eyelid responses following acute decerebration. *Brain Research* 403:89–95.

Mauk, M. D., J. E. Steinmetz, and R. F. Thompson. 1986. Classical conditioning using stimulation of the inferior olive as the unconditioned stimulus. *Proceedings of the National Academy of Sciences* 83:5349–5353.

Mayes, A. R. 1988. *Human Organic Memory Disorders.* Cambridge: Cambridge University Press.

McCormick, D. A. and R. F. Thompson. 1984. Neuronal responses of the rabbit cerebellum during acquisition and performance of a classically conditioned nictitating membrane-eyelid response. *Journal of Neuroscience* 11:2811–2822.

McCormick, D. A., P. E. Guyer, and R. F. Thompson. 1982. Superior cerebellar peduncle lesions selectively abolish the ipsilateral classically conditioned nictitating membrane/eyelid response of the rabbit. *Brain Research* 244:347–350.

McCormick, D. A., J. E. Steinmetz, and R. F. Thompson. 1985. Lesions of the inferior olivary complex cause extinction of the classically conditioned eyeblink response. *Brain Research* 359:120–130.

McCormick, D. A., G. A. Clark, D. G. Lavond, and R. F. Thompson. 1982. Initial localization of the memory trace for a basic form of learning. *Proceedings of the National Academy of Sciences* 79:2731–2735.

McCormick, D. A., D. G. Lavond, G. A. Clark, R. E. Kettner, C. E. Rising, and R. F. Thompson. 1981. The engram found? Role of the cerebellum in classical conditioning of nictitating membrane and eyelid responses. *Bulletin of the Psychonomic Society* 18:103–105.

McCrea, R. A., G. A. Bishop, and S. T. Kitai. 1977. Electrophysiological and horseradish peroxidase studies of precerebellar afferents to the nucleus interpositus anterior. II. Mossy fiber system. *Brain Research* 122:215–228.

McNaughton, B. L. 1989. Neuronal mechanisms for spatial computation and information storage. In L. Nadel, L. A. Cooper, P. Culicover, and R. M. Harnish, eds., *Neural Connections, Mental Computation*, pp. 285–350. Cambridge: MIT Press.

McNaughton, B. L. and R. G. M. Morris. 1987. Hippocampal synaptic enhancement and information storage within a distributed memory system. *Trends in Neuroscience* 10:408–415.

McNaughton, B. L. and L. Nadel. 1989. Hebb-Marr networks and the neurobiological representation of action in space. In M. A. Gluck and D. E. Rumelhart, eds., *Neuroscience and Connectionist Theory*, pp. 1–63. Hillsdale, N.J.: Lawrence Erlbaum.

McNaughton, B. L., C. A. Barnes, and P. Andersen. 1981. Synaptic efficacy and

EPSP summation in granule cells of rat fascia dentata studied *in vitro. Journal of Neurophysiology* 46:952–956.

McNaughton, B. L., C. A. Barnes, J. Meltzer, and R. J. Sutherland. 1989. Hippocampal granule cells are necessary for normal spatial learning but not for spatially selective pyramidal cell discharge. *Experimental Brain Research* 76:485–496.

McNaughton, B. L., C. A. Barnes, G. Rao, J. Baldwin, and M. Rasmussen. 1986. Long-term enhancement of hippocampal synaptic transmission and the acquisition of spatial information. *Journal of Neuroscience* 6:563–571.

Meck, W. H. 1988. Hippocampal function is required for feedback control of an internal clock's criterion. *Behavioral Neuroscience* 102:54–60.

Meck, W. H., R. M. Church, and D. S. Olton. 1984. Hippocampus, time and memory. *Behavioral Neuroscience* 98:3–22.

Megela, A. L. and T. J. Teyler. 1979. Habituation amd the human-evoked potential. *Journal of Comparative and Physiological Psychology* 93:1154–1170.

Miller, C. R., R. L. Elkins, and L. J. Peacock. ,1971. Disruption of a radiation-induced preference shift by hippocampal lesions. *Physiology and Behavior* 2:283–285.

Miller, J. S., A. J. Nonneman, K. S. Kelly, J. L. Niesewander, and W. L. Isaac. 1986. Disruption of neophobia, conditioned odor aversion, and conditioned taste aversion in rats with hippocampal lesions. *Behavioral and Neural Biology* 45:240–253.

Miller, V. M. and P. J. Best. 1980. Spatial correlates of hippocampal unit activity are altered by lesions of the fornix and entorhinal cortex. *Brain Research* 194: 311–323.

Milner, B. 1965. Memory disturbance after bilateral hippocampal lesions. In P. M. Milner and S. E. Glickeman, eds., *Cognitive Processes and the Brain,* pp. 97–111. Princeton, N.J.: Van Nostrand.

Milner, B., S. Corkin, and H.-L. Teuber. 1968. Further analysis of the hippocampal amnesic syndrome; 14-year follow-up study of H.M. *Neuropsychologia* 6:215–234.

Milner, P. M. 1970. *Physiological Psychology.* New York: Holt, Rinehart, and Winston.

Mis, F. W. 1977. A midbrain–brain stem circuit for conditioned inhibition of the nictitating membrane response in the rabbit (*Oryctolagus cuniculus*). *Journal of Comparative and Physiological Psychology* 91:975–988.

Mishkin, M. 1978. Memory in monkeys severely impaired by combined but not by separate removal of amygdala and hippocampus. *Nature* 273:297–298.

—— 1982. A memory system in the monkey. *Philosophical Transactions of the Royal Society of London,* B298:85–95.

Mishkin, M. and T. Appenzeller. 1987. The anatomy of memory. *Scientific American* 256:62–71.

Mishkin, M. and J. Delacour. 1975. An analysis of short-term visual memory in the monkey. *Journal of Experimental Psychology: Animal Behavior Processes* 1:326–334.

Mishkin, M. and F. J. Manning. 1978. Non-spatial memory after selective prefrontal lesions in monkeys. *Brain Research* 143:313–323.

Mishkin, M. and K. H. Pribram. 1955. Analysis of the effects of frontal lesions in monkeys: I. Variations of delayed alternation. *Journal of Comparative and Physiological Psychology* 48:492–495.

Mishkin, M., M. E. Lewis, and L. G. Ungerleider. 1982. Equivalence of parieto-occipital subareas for visuospatial ability in monkeys. *Behavioural Brain Research* 6:41–55.

Mishkin, M., B. L. Malamut, and J. Bachevalier. 1984. Memories and habits: Two neural systems. In G. Lynch, J. L. McGaugh, and N. M. Weinberger, eds., *Neurobiology of Learning and Memory*, pp. 65–77. New York: Guilford Press.

Mishkin, M., B. J. Spiegler, R. C. Saunders, and B. L. Malamut. 1982. An animal model of global amnesia. In S. Corkin, K. L. Davis, J. H. Growdon, E. Usdin, and R. J. Wurtman, eds., *Alzheimer's Disease*, pp. 235–247. New York: Raven Press.

Misulis, K. E. and R. G. Durkovic. 1984. Conditioned stimulus intensity: Role of cutaneous fiber size in classical conditioning of the flexion reflex in the spinal cat. *Experimental Neurology* 86:81–92.

Mitchell, S. J., J. N. P. Rawlins, O. Steward, and D. S. Olton. 1982. Medial septal area lesions disrupt theta rhythm and cholinergic staining in medial entorhinal cortex and produce impaired radial arm maze behavior in rats. *Journal of Neuroscience* 3:292–302.

Monaghan, D. T. and C. W. Cotman. 1985. Distribution of N-methyl-D-aspartate sensitive L-[^{3}H]-glutamate binding sites in rat brain. *Journal of Neuroscience* 5:2909–2919.

Mondadori, C., L. Weiskrantz, H. Buerki, F. Petschke, and G. E. Fagg. 1989. NMDA receptor antagonists can enhance or impair learning performance in animals. *Experimental Brain Research* 75:449–456.

Montarolo, P. G., P. Goelet, V. Castellucci, J. Morgan, E. R. Kandel, and S. Schacher. 1986. A critical period for macromolecular synthesis in long-term heterosynaptic facilitation in *Aplysia*. *Science* 234:1249–1254.

Morris, R. G. M. 1981. Spatial localisation does not depend on the presence of local cues. *Learning and Motivation* 12:239–260.

—— 1988. Elements of a hypothesis concerning the participation of hippocampal NMDA receptors in learning. In D. Lodge, ed., *Excitatory Amino Acids in Health and Disease*, pp. 297–320. New York: Wiley.

—— 1989. Synaptic plasticity and learning: Selective impairment of learning in rats and blockade of long-term potentiation *in vivo* by the N-methyl-D-aspartate receptor antagonist AP5. *Journal of Neuroscience* 9:3040–3057.

—— 1990. It's heads they win, tails I lose! *Psychobiology* 18:261–266.

Morris, R. G. M. and J. J. Hagan. 1983. Hippocampal electrical activity and ballistic movement. In W. Seifert, ed., *Neurobiology of the hippocampus*, pp. 321–331. London: Academic Press.

Morris, R. G. M., E. Anderson, G. Lynch, and M. Baudry. 1986. Selective impairment of learning and blockade of long-term potentiation by an N-methyl-D-aspartate receptor antagonist, AP5. *Nature* 319:774–776.

Morris, R. G. M., P. Garrud, J. N. P. Rawlins, and J. O'Keefe. 1982. Place navigation impaired in rats with hippocampal lesions. *Nature* 297:681–683.

Moyer, J. R., R. A. Deyo, and J. F. Disterhoft. 1990. Hippocampectomy disrupts trace eye-blink conditioning in rabbits. *Behavioral Neuroscience* 104:243–252.

Mpitsos, G. J. and K. Lukowiak. 1985. Learning in gastropod mulluscs. In A. O. D. Willows, ed., *The Mollusca.* Vol. 8, *Neurobiology and Behavior (Part 1),* pp. 95–267. New York: Academic Press.

Muller, D. and G. Lynch. 1989. Evidence that changes in presynaptic calcium currents are not responsible for long-term potentiation in hippocampus. *Brain Research* 479:290–299.

Muller, D., M. Joly, and G. Lynch. 1988. Contributions of quisqualate and NMDA receptors to the induction and expression of LTP. *Science* 242:1694–1697.

Muller, R. U., J. L. Kubie, and J. B. Ranck. 1987. Spatial firing patterns of hippocampal complex-spike cells in a fixed environment. *Journal of Neuroscience* 7:1935–1950.

Murphy, L. R. and T. S. Brown. 1974. Hippocampal lesions and learned taste aversion. *Physiological Psychology* 2:60–64.

Murray, E. A. and M. Mishkin. 1984. Severe tactual as well as visual memory deficits follow combined removal of the amygdala and hippocampus in monkeys. *Journal of Neuroscience* 10:2565–2580.

—— 1986. Visual recognition in monkeys following rhinal cortical ablations combined with either amygdalectomy or hippocampectomy. *Journal of Neuroscience* 6:1991–2003.

Murray, E. A., M. Davidson, D. Gaffan, D. S. Olton, and S. Suomi. 1989. Effects of fornix transection and cingulate cortical ablation on spatial memory in rhesus monkeys. *Experimental Brain Research* 74:173–186.

Nachman, M. and J. H. Ashe. 1974. Effects of basolateral amygdala lesions on neophobia, learned taste aversions, and sodium appetite in rats. *Journal of Comparative and Physiological Psychology* 87:622–643.

Nauta, W. J. H. and M. Feirtag. 1986. *Fundamental Neuroanatomy.* New York: W. H. Freeman.

Nazif, F. A., J. H. Byrne, and L. J. Cleary. 1991. cAMP induces long-term morphological changes in sensory neurons of *Aplysia. Brain Research* 539:324–327.

Neary, J. T., T. Crow, and D. L. Alkon. 1981. Change in a specific phosphoprotein band following associative learning in *Hermissenda. Nature* 293:568–660.

Nelson, R. B., D. J. Linden, and A. Routtenberg. 1989. Phosphoproteins localized to presynaptic terminal linked to persistence of long-term potentiation (LTP): Quantitative analysis of two-dimensional gels. *Brain Research* 497:30–42.

Nelson, T. J., C. Collin, and D. L. Alkon. 1990. Isolation of a G protein that is modified by learning and reduces potassium currents in *Hermissenda. Science* 247:1479–1483.

Nicoll, R. A. 1988. The coupling of neurotransmitter receptors to ion channels in the brain. *Science* 241:545–551.

Nicoll, R. A., J. A. Kauer, and R. C. Malenka. 1988. The current excitement in long-term potentiation. *Neuron* 1:97–103.

Nordholm, A. F., D. G. Lavond, and R. F. Thompson. 1991. Are eyeblink responses to tone in the decerebrate, decerebellate rabbit conditioned responses? *Behavioural Brain Research* 44:27–34.

O'Keefe, J. 1976. Place units in the hippocampus of the freely moving rat. *Experimental Neurology* 51:78–109.

—— 1979. A review of the hippocampal place cells. *Progress in Neurobiology* 13:419–439.

—— 1989. Computations the hippocampus might perform. In L. Nadel, L. A. Cooper, P. Culicover, and R. M. Harnish, eds., *Neural Connections, Mental Computation,* pp. 225–284. Cambridge: MIT Press.

O'Keefe, J. and D. H. Conway. 1978. Hippocampal place units in the freely moving rat: Why they fire where they fire. *Experimental Brain Research* 31:573–590.

O'Keefe, J. and J. Dostrovsky. 1971. The hippocampus as a spatial map: Preliminary evidence from unit activity in the freely moving rat. *Brain Research* 34:171–175.

O'Keefe, J. and L. Nadel. 1978. *The Hippocampus as a Cognitive Map.* Oxford: Clarendon Press.

O'Keefe, J. and A. Speakman. 1987. Single unit activity in the rat hippocampus during a spatial memory task. *Experimental Brain Research* 68:1–27.

O'Keefe, J., L. Nadel, and J. Willner. 1979. Tuning out irrelevancy? Comments on Solomon's temporal mapping view of the hippocampus. *Psychological Bulletin* 86:1280–1289.

Ocorr, K. A., E. T. Walters, and J. H. Byrne. 1985. Associative conditioning analog selectively increases cAMP levels of tail sensory neurons in *Aplysia. Proceedings of the National Academy of Sciences* 82:2548–2552.

Oliver, M. W., M. Baudry, and G. Lynch. 1989. The protease inhibitor leupeptin interferes with the development of LTP in hippocampal slices. *Brain Research* 505:233–238.

Olton, D. S. and W. A. Feustle. 1981. Hippocampal function required for nonspatial working memory? *Experimental Brain Research* 41:380–389.

Olton, D. S. and B. C. Papas. 1979. Spatial memory and hippocampal function. *Neuropsychologia* 17:669–682.

Olton, D. S. and R. J. Samuelson. 1976. Remembrance of places passed: Spatial memory in rats. *Journal of Experimental Psychology: Animal Behavior Processes* 2:97–116.

Olton, D. S. and M. A. Werz. 1978. Hippocampal function and behavior: Spatial discrimination and response inhibition. *Physiology and Behavior* 20:597–605.

Olton, D. S., J. T. Becker, and G. E. Handelmann. 1979. Hippocampus, space and memory. *Behavioral and Brain Sciences* 2:313–365.

Olton, D. S., W. H. Meck, and R. M. Church. 1987. Separation of hippocampal and amygdaloid involvement in temporal memory dysfunctions. *Brain Research* 404:180–188.

Olton, D. S., J. A. Walker, and F. H. Gage. 1978. Hippocampal connections and spatial discrimination. *Brain Research* 139:295–308.

Onifer, S. M. and R. G. Durkovic. 1988. Evidence that the neural pathways involved in backward conditioning are different from those involved in forward conditioning. *Journal of Neuroscience* 8:502–507.

Overman, W. H., G. Ormsby, and M. Mishkin. 1990. Picture recognition vs. picture discrimination learning in monkeys with medial temporal removals. *Experimental Brain Research* 79:18–24.

Owen, M. J. and S. R. Butler. 1981. Amnesia after transection of the fornix in monkeys: Long-term memory impaired, short-term memory intact. *Behavioural Brain Research* 3:115–123.

—— 1984. Does amnesia after transection of the fornix in monkeys reflect abnormal sensitivity to proactive interference? *Behavioural Brain Research* 14:183–192.

Pandya, D. N. and B. Seltzer. 1982. Association areas of the cerebral cortex. *Trends in Neurosciences* 5:381–390.

Pandya, D. N. and E. H. Yeterian. 1984. Proposed neural circuit for spatial memory in the primate brain. *Neuropsychologia* 22:109–122.

Papez, J. W. 1937. A proposed mechanism of emotion. *Archives of Neurology and Psychiatry* 38:725–743.

Parkin, A. J. 1987. *Memory and Amnesia: An Introduction.* Oxford: Basil Blackwell.

Parkinson, J. K., E. A. Murray, and M. Mishkin. 1988. A selective mnemonic role for the hippocampus in monkeys: Memory for the location of objects. *Journal of Neuroscience* 8:4159–4167.

Passingham, R. E. 1975. Delayed matching after selective prefrontal lesions in monkeys (*Macaca mulatta*). *Brain Research* 92:89–102.

—— 1978. Information about movements in monkeys (*Macaca mulatta*). *Brain Research* 152:313–328.

—— 1985a. Memory of monkeys (*Macaca mulatta*) with lesions in prefrontal cortex. *Behavioral Neuroscience* 99:3–21.

—— 1985b. Cortical mechanisms and cues for action. *Philosophical Transactions of the Royal Society of London* B308:101–111.

Patterson, M. M. 1975. Effects of forward and backward classical conditioning procedures on a spinal cat hind-limb flexor nerve response. *Physiological Psychology* 3:86–91.

—— 1976. Mechanisms of classical conditioning and fixation in spinal mammals. In A. Riesen and R. Thompson, eds., *Advances in Psychobiology.* 3:381–436. New York: Wiley.

—— 1980. Mechanisms of classical conditioning of spinal reflexes. In R. F. Thompson, L. H. Hicks, and V. B. Shvyrkov, eds., *Neural Mechanisms of Goal-Directed Behavior and Learning,* pp. 263–272. New York: Academic Press.

Patterson, M. M., T. W. Berger, and R. F. Thompson. 1979. Hippocampal neuronal plasticity recorded from cat during classical conditioning. *Brain Research* 163:339–343.

Patterson, M. M., C. P. Cegavske, and R. F. Thompson. 1973. Effects of a classical conditioning paradigm on hind-limb flexor nerve response in immobilized spinal cats. *Journal of Comparative and Physiological Psychology* 84:88–97.

Patterson, T. A., D. B. Gilbert, and S. P. R. Rose. 1990. Pre- and post-training lesions of the intermediate medial hyperstriatum ventrale and passive avoidance learning in the chick. *Experimental Brain Research* 80:189–195.

Pearce, J. M. and G. Hall. 1980. A model for Pavlovian learning: Variations in the effectiveness of conditioned but not of unconditioned stimuli. *Psychological Review* 87:532–552.

Penick, S. and P. R. Solomon. 1991. Hippocampus, context, and conditioning. *Behavioral Neuroscience* 105:611–617.

Petrides, M. 1982. Motor conditional associative-learning after selective prefrontal lesions in the monkey. *Behavioural Brain Research* 5:407–413.

—— 1985. Deficits in non-spatial conditional associative learning after periarcuate lesions in the monkey. *Behavioural Brain Research* 16:95–101.

Phillips, R. G. and J. E. LeDoux. 1992. Differential contribution of amygdala and hippocampus to cued and contextual fear conditioning. *Behavioral Neuroscience* 106:274–285.

Phillips, R. R., B. L. Malamut, J. Bachevalier, and M. Mishkin. 1988. Dissociation of the effects of inferior temporal and limbic lesions on object discrimination learning with 24-hr intertrial intervals. *Behavioural Brain Research* 27:99–107.

Pickett, J. M. 1952. Non-equipotential cortical function in maze learning. *American Journal of Psychology* 65:177–195.

Pin, J.-P., J. Bockaert, and M. Recasesn. 1984. The Ca^{2+}/Cl- dependent L-[^{3}H] glutamate binding: A new receptor or a particular transport process? *FEBS Letters* 175:31–36.

Pinsker, H. M., W. A. Hening, T. J. Carew, and E. R. Kandel. 1973. Long-term sensitization of a defensive withdrawal reflex in *Aplysia*. *Science* 182:1039–1042.

Pinsker, H. M., I. Kupfermann, V. Castellucci, and E. R. Kandel. 1970. Habituation and dishabituation of the gill-withdrawal reflex in *Aplysia*. *Science* 167:1740–1742.

Polenchar, B. E., M. M. Patterson, D. G. Lavond, and R. F. Thompson. 1985. Cerebellar lesions abolish an avoidance response in rabbit. *Behavioral and Neural Biology* 44:221–227.

Port, R. L. and M. M. Patterson. 1984. Fimbrial lesions and sensory preconditioning. *Behavioral Neuroscience* 98:584–589.

Port, R. L., A. L. Beggs, and M. M. Patterson. 1987. Hippocampal substrate of sensory associations. *Physiology and Behavior* 39:643–647.

Port, R. L., A. A. Mikhail, and M. M. Patterson. 1985. Differential effects of hippocampectomy on classically conditioned rabbit nictitating membrane response related to interstimulus interval. *Behavioral Neuroscience* 99:200–208.

Port, R. L., A. G. Romano, and M. M. Patterson. 1986. Stimulus duration discrimination in the rabbit: Effects of hippocampectomy on discrimination and reversal learning. *Physiological Psychology* 14:124–129.

Port, R. L., A. G. Romano, J. E. Steinmetz, A. A. Mikhail, and M. M. Patterson. 1986. Retention and acquisition of classical trace conditioned responses by rabbits with hippocampal lesions. *Behavioral Neuroscience* 100:745–752.

Racine, R. J., N. W. Milgram, and S. Hafner. 1983. Long-term potentiation phenomena in the rat limbic forebrain. *Brain Research* 260:217–231.

Racine, R. J., D. A. Wilson, R. Gingell, and D. Sunderland. 1986. Long-term potentiation in the interpositus and vestibular nuclei in the rat. *Experimental Brain Research* 63:158–162.

Raffaelle, K. C. and D. S. Olton. 1988. Hippocampal and amygdaloid involvement
in working memory for nonspatial stimuli. *Behavioral Neuroscience* 102:349–
355.

Randich, A. and V. M. LoLordo. 1979. Associative and non-associative theories of
the UCS preexposure effect: Implications for Pavlovian conditioning. *Psychological Bulletin* 86:523–548.

Rankin, C. H. and T. J. Carew. 1988. Dishabituation and sensitization emerge as
separate processes during development in *Aplysia*. *Journal of Neuroscience* 8:197–
211.

Rasmussen, M., C. A. Barnes, and B. L. McNaughton. 1989. A systematic test of
cognitive mapping, working-memory, and temporal discontiguity theories of hippocampal function. *Psychobiology* 17:335–348.

Rawlins, J. N. P. 1985. Associations across time: The hippocampus as a temporary
memory store. *Behavior and Brain Sciences* 8:479–486.

Reilly, S. and M. Good. 1987. Enhanced DRL and impaired forced-choice alternation
performance following hippocampal lesions in the pigeon. *Behavioural Brain Research* 26:185–197.

—— 1989. Hippocampal lesions and associative learning in the pigeon. *Behavioral
Neuroscience* 103:731–742.

Reiner, A., B. M. Davis, N. C. Brecha, and H. J. Karten. 1984. The distribution of
enkephalinlike immunoreactivity in the telencephalon of the adult and developing
domestic chicken. *Journal of Comparative Neurology* 228:245–262.

Rescorla, R. A. 1968. Probability of shock in the presence and absence of CS in fear
conditioning. *Journal of Comparative and Physiological Psychology* 66:1–5.

—— 1969. Pavlovian conditioned inhibition. *Psychological Bulletin* 72:77–94.

——. 1973. Effect of US habituation following conditioning. *Journal of Comparative
and Physiological Psychology* 82:137–143.

—— 1974. Effect of inflation of the unconditioned stimulus value following conditioning. *Journal of Comparative and Physiological Psychology* 86:101–106.

Rescorla, R. A. and A. R. Wagner. 1972. A theory of Pavlovian conditioning: Variations in the effectiveness of reinforcement and nonreinforcement. In A. H. Black
and W. F. Prokasy, eds., *Classical Conditioning II: Current Research and Theory*,
pp. 64–99. New York: Appleton-Century-Crofts.

Richards, W. G., J. Farley, and D. L. Alkon. 1984. Extinction of associative learning
in *Hermissenda*: Behavior and neural correlates. *Behavioural Brain Research*
14:161–170.

Richmond, B. J., R. H. Wurtz, and T. Sato. 1983. Visual responses of inferior temporal neurons in awake rhesus monkey. *Journal of Neurophysiology* 50:1415–
1432.

Rickert, E. J., T. L. Bennett, P. L. Lane, and J. French. 1978. Hippocampectomy
and the attenuation of blocking. *Behavioral Biology* 22:147–160.

Rickert, E. J., J. F. Lorden, R. Dawson, and E. Smyly. 1981. Limbic lesions and the
blocking effect. *Physiology and Behavior* 26:601–606.

Rickert, E. J., J. F. Lorden, R. Dawson, E. Smyly, and M. F. Callahan. 1979. Stimulus processing and stimulus selection in rats with hippocampal lesions. *Behavioral and Neural Biology* 27:454–465.

Riddell, W. I., L. A. Rothblat, and W. A. Wilson. 1969. Auditory and visual distraction in hippocampectomized rats. *Journal of Comparative and Physiological Psychology* 67:216–219.

Ringo, J. L. 1988. Seemingly discrepant data from hippocampectomized macaques are reconciled by detectability analysis. *Behavioral Neuroscience* 102:173–177.

Roberts, W. A. and D. S. Grant. 1976. Studies of short-term memory in the pigeon using the delayed matching to sample procedure. In D. L. Medin, W. A. Roberts, and R. T. Davis, eds., *Processes of Animal Memory*, pp. 79–112. Hillsdale, N.J.: Lawrence Erlbaum.

Roberts, W. A. and N. van Veldhuizen. 1985. Spatial memory in pigeons on the radial arm maze. *Journal of Experimental Psychology: Animal Behavior Processes* 11:241–259.

Roberts, W. A., K. Cheng, and J. S. Cohen. 1989. Timing light and tone signals in pigeons. *Journal of Experimental Psychology: Animal Behavior Processes* 15:23–35.

Rockel, A. J., R. W. Hiorns, and T. P. S. Powell. 1980. The basic uniformity in structure of the neocortex. *Brain* 103:221–244.

Rogers, H. R. and W. B. Levy. 1978. The effects of Ca^{2+} and Mg^{2+} on the habituating LC-VR reflex of the frog spinal cord. *Brain Research* 139:183–189.

Rolls, E. T. 1989. Parallel distributed processing in the brain: Implications of the functional architecture of neuronal networks in the hippocampus. In R. G. M. Morris, ed., *Parallel Distributed Processing: Implications for Psychology and Neurobiology*, pp. 286–388. Oxford: Clarendon Press.

Rosene, D. L. and G. W. van Hoesen. 1987. The hippocampal formation of the primate brain: A review of some comparative aspects of cytoarchitecture and connections. In E. G. Jones and A. Peters, eds., *Cerebral Cortex*, 8:345–456. New York: Plenum.

Rosenfield, M. E. and J. W. Moore. 1983. Red nucleus lesions disrupt the classically conditioned nictitating membrane response in rabbits. *Behavioural Brain Research* 10:393–398.

Rosenkilde, C. E., H. E. Rosvold, and M. Mishkin. 1980. Time discrimination with positional responses after selective prefrontal lesions in monkeys. *Brain Research* 210:129–144.

Rosenstock, J., T. D. Field, and E. Greene. 1977. The role of mammillary bodies in spatial memory. *Experimental Neurology* 55:340–352.

Rothblat, L. A. and L. F. Kromer. 1991. Object recognition memory in the rat: The role of the hippocampus. *Behavioural Brain Research* 42:25–32.

Routtenberg, A. 1985. Protein kinase C activation leading to protein F1 phosphorylation may regulate synaptic plasticity by presynaptic terminal growth. *Behavioral and Neural Biology* 44:186–200.

Routtenberg, A., D. M. Lovinger, and O. Steward. 1985. Selective increase in phosphorylation of a 47-kDa protein (F1 directly related to long-term potentiation. *Behavioral and Neural Biology* 43:3–11.

Rudy, J. W. and R. J. Sutherland. 1989. The hippocampal formation is necessary for rats to learn and remember configural associations. *Behavioural Brain Research* 34:97–109.

Rumelhart, D. E., J. L. McLelland, and the PDP Research Group. 1986. *Parallel Distributed Processing: Explorations in the Microstructure of Cognition.* 2 vols. Cambridge: MIT Press.

Rupniak, N. M. J. and D. Gaffan. 1987. Monkey hippocampus and learning about spatially directed movements. *Journal of Neuroscience* 7:2331–2337.

Russell, W. R. and P. W. Nathan. 1946. Traumatic amnesia. *Brain* 69:280–300.

Sacktor, T. C. and J. H. Schwartz. 1990. Sensitizing stimuli cause translocation of protein kinase C in *Aplysia* sensory neurons. *Proceedings of the National Academy of Sciences* 87:2036–2039.

Sahgal, A. 1984. Hippocampal lesions disrupt recognition memory in pigeons. *Behavioural Brain Research* 11:47–58.

Sahley, C., J. W. Rudy, and A. Gelperin. 1981. An analysis of associative learning in a terrestrial mollusc. 1. Higher-order conditioning, blocking and a transient US pre-exposure effect. *Journal of Comparative Physiology* A144:1–8.

Salmon, D. P., S. Zola-Morgan, and L. R. Squire. 1987. Retrograde amnesia following combined hippocampus-amygdala lesions in monkeys. *Psychobiology* 15:37–47.

Sarter, M. and H. J. Markowitsch. 1985. Involvement of the amygdala in learning and memory: A critical review, with emphasis on anatomical relations. *Behavioral Neuroscience* 99:342–380.

Saunders, R. C. and L. Weiskrantz. 1989. The effects of fornix transection and combined fornix transection, mammillary body lesions and hippocampal ablations on object-pair association memory. *Behavioural Brain Research* 35:85–94.

Schacher, S., V. F. Castellucci, and E. R. Kandel. 1988. cAMP evokes long-term facilitation in *Aplysia* sensory neurons that requires new protein synthesis. *Science* 240:1667–1669.

Schmajuk, N. A., N. E. Spear, and R. L. Isaacson. 1983. Absence of overshadowing in rats with hippocampal lesions. *Physiological Psychology* 11:59–62.

Schneider, A. M., B. Kapp, C. Aron, and M. E. Jarvik. 1969. Retroactive effects of transcorneal and transpinnate ECS on step-through latencies of mice and rats. *Journal of Comparative and Physiological Psychology* 69:505–509.

Schneiderman, N. 1972. Response system divergences in aversive classical conditioning. In A. H. Black and W. H. Prokasy, eds., *Classical Conditioning.* Vol. 2: *Current Theory and Research,* pp. 341–376. New York: Appleton-Century-Crofts.

Scholz, K. P. and J. H. Byrne. 1987. Long-term sensitization in *Aplysia:* Biophysical correlates in tail sensory neurons. *Science* 235:685–687.

—— 1988. Intracellular injection of cAMP induces a long-term reduction of neuronal K^+ currents. *Science* 240:1664–1666.

Schreiner, L. H. and A. Kling. 1953. Behavioral changes following rhinencephalic injury in cat. *Journal of Neurophysiology* 16:643–659.

Schuman, E. M. and D. V. Madison. 1991. A requirement for the intercellular messenger nitric oxide in long-term potentiation. *Science* 254:1503–1506.

Schwartzkroin, P. A. and J. S. Taube. 1986. Mechanisms underlying long-term potentiation. In D. L. Alkon and C. D. Woody, eds., *Neural Mechanisms of Conditioning*, pp. 319–329. New York: Plenum Press.

Scoville, W. B. and B. Milner. 1957. Loss of recent memory after bi lateral hippocampal lesion. *Journal of Neurology, Neurosurgery and Psychiatry* 20:11–21.

Searle, J. R. 1990. Is the brain's mind a computer program? *Scientific American* 262:20–25.

Sears, L. L. and J. E. Steinmetz. 1991. Dorsal accessory olive activity diminishes during acquisition of the rabbit classically conditioned eyelid response. *Brain Research* 545:112–122.

Seubert, P., J. Larson, M. Oliver, M. W. Jung, M. Baudry, and G. Lynch. 1988. Stimulation of NMDA receptors induces proteolysis of spectrin in hippocampus. *Brain Research* 460:189–194.

Sharp, P. E., B. L. McNaughton, and C. A. Barnes. 1985. Enhancement of hippocampal field potentials in rats exposed to a novel, complex environment. *Brain Research* 339:361–365.

Sharp, P. E., C. A. Barnes, and B. L. McNaughton. 1987. Effects of aging on environmental modulation of hippocampal evoked responses. *Behavioral Neuroscience* 101:170–178.

Sharpless, S. and H. Jasper. 1956. Habituation of the arousal reaction. *Brain* 79:655–680.

Sherman, B. S., F. K. Hoehler, and A. A. Buerger. 1982. Instrumental avoidance conditioning of increased leg lowering in the spinal rat. *Physiology and Behavior* 25:123–128.

Sherry, D. F. 1984. What food-storing birds remember. *Canadian Journal of Psychology* 38:304–321.

Sherry, D. F. and D. Schacter. 1987. The evolution of multiple learning systems. *Psychological Review* 94:439–454.

Sherry, D. F. and A. L. Vaccarino. 1989. Hippocampus and memory for food caches in black-capped chickadees. *Behavioral Neuroscience* 103:308–313.

Sherry, D. F., A. L. Vaccarino, K. Buckenham, and R. S. Herz. 1989. The hippocampal complex of food-storing birds. *Brain, Behavior, and Evolution* 34:308–317.

Shimamura, A. P. and L. R. Squire. 1986. Korsakoff's syndrome: A study of the relation between anterograde amnesia and remote memory impairment. *Behavioral Neuroscience* 100:165–170.

Sidman, M., L. T. Stoddard, and J. P. Mohr. 1968. Some additional quantitative observations of immediate memory in a patient with bilateral hippocampal lesions. *Neuropsychologia* 6:245–254.

Siegelbaum, S. A., J. Camardo, and E. R. Kandel. 1982. Serotonin and cyclic AMP close single K$^+$ channels in *Aplysia* sensory neurons. *Nature* 299:413–417.

Singer, W. 1987. Activity-dependent self-organization of synaptic connections as a substrate for learning. In J. P. Changeux and M. Konishi, eds., *The neural and molecular bases of learning*, pp. 301–336. Chichester: Wiley.

Skelton, R. W. 1988. Bilateral cerebellar lesions disrupt conditioned eyelid responses in unrestrained rats. *Behavioral Neuroscience* 102:586–590.

Skelton, R. W., M. D. Mauk, and R. F. Thompson. 1988. Cerebellar nucleus lesions dissociate alpha conditioning from alpha responses in rabbits. *Psychobiology* 16:126–134.

Skelton, R. W., J. J. Miller, and A. G. Phillips. 1985. Long-term potentiation facilitates behavioral responding to single-pulse stimulation of the perforant path. *Behavioral Neuroscience* 99:603–620.

Sokolov, E. N. 1960. Neuronal models and the orienting reflex. In M. A. B. Brazier, ed., *The Central Nervous System and Behaviour,* pp. 187–276. Transactions of the third conference, Josiah Macy Foundation. Madison, N.J.: Madison Printing Company.

Solomon, P. R. 1977. Role of the hippocampus in blocking and conditioned inhibition of the rabbit's nictitating membrane response. *Journal of Comparative and Physiological Psychology* 91:407–417.

—— 1979. Temporal versus spatial information processing theories of hippocampal function. *Psychological Bulletin* 86:1272–1279.

Solomon, P. R. and J. W. Moore. 1975. Latent inhibition and stimulus generalization of the classically conditioned nictitating membrane response in rabbits following dorsal hippocampal ablation. *Journal of Comparative and Physiological Psychology* 89:1192–1203.

Solomon, P. R., G. T. Stowe, and W. M. Pendlbeury. 1989. Disrupted eyelid conditioning in a patient with damage to cerebellar afferents. *Behavioral Neuroscience* 103:898–902.

Solomon, P. R., E. R. Vander Schaaf, R. F. Thompson, and D. J. Weisz. 1986. Hippocampus and trace conditioning of the rabbit's conditioned nictitating membrane response. *Behavioral Neuroscience* 100:729–744.

Spencer, W. A., R. F. Thompson, and D. R. Neilson. 1966. Decrement of ventral root electrotonus and intracellularly recorded post-synaptic potentials produced by iterated cutaneous afferent volleys. *Journal of Neurophysiology* 29:253–274.

Sperry, R. W. 1969. A modified concept of consciousness. *Psychological Review* 79:532–536.

Spetch, M. L. and C. A. Edwards. 1986. Spatial memory in pigeons (*Columba livia*) in an open-field environment. *Journal of Comparative Psychology* 100:266–278.

Spetch, M. L., D. M. Wilkie, and J. P. J. Pinel. 1981. Backward conditioning: A reevaluation of the empirical evidence. *Psychological Bulletin* 89:163–175.

Spiegler, B. J. and M. Mishkin. 1981. Evidence for the sequential participation of inferior temporal cortex and amygdala in the acquisition of stimulus-reward associations. *Behavioural Brain Research* 3:303–317.

Squire, L. R. 1987. *Memory and Brain.* New York: Oxford University Press.

—— 1992. Memory and the hippocampus: A synthesis from findings with rats, monkeys, and humans. *Psychological Review* 99:195–231.

Squire, L. R. and N. J. Cohen. 1979. Memory and amnesia: Resistance to disruption develops for years after learning. *Behavioral and Neural Biology* 25:115–125.

—— 1984. Human memory and amnesia. In G. Lynch, J. L. McGaugh, and N. M. Weinberger, eds., *Neurobiology of Learning and Memory,* pp. 3–64. New York: Guilford Press.

Squire, L. R. and C. W. Spanis. 1984. Long gradient of retrograde amnesia in mice: Continuity with the findings in humans. *Behavioral Neuroscience* 98:345–348.

Squire, L. R. and S. Zola-Morgan. 1983. The neurology of memory: The case for correspondence between the findings in man and non-human primate. In J. A. Deutsch, ed., *The Physiological Basis of Memory*, pp. 199–268. 2d ed. New York: Academic Press.

Squire, L. R., N. J. Cohen, and L. Nadel. 1984. The medial temporal region and memory consolidation: A new hypothesis. In H. Weingartner and E. Parker, eds., *Memory Consolidation*, pp. 185–210. Hillsdale, N.J.: Lawrence Erlbaum.

Squire, L. R., A. P. Shimamura, and P. Graf. 1985. Independence of recognition memory and priming effects: A neuropsychological analysis. *Journal of Experimental Psychology: Learning, Memory and Cognition* 11:37–44.

Squire, L. R., S. Zola-Morgan, and K. S. Chen. 1988. Human amnesia and animal models of amnesia: Performance of amnesic patients on tests designed for the monkey. *Behavioral Neuroscience* 102:210–221.

Stanton, P. K. and T. J. Sejnowski. 1989. Associative long-term depression in the hippocampus induced by hebbian covariance. *Nature* 339:215–218.

Staubli, U. and G. Lynch. 1987. Stable hippocampal long-term potentiation elicited by "theta" pattern stimulation. *Brain Research* 435:227–234.

Staubli, U., M. Baudry, and G. Lynch. 1984. Leupeptin, a thiol protease inhibitor, causes a selective impairment of spatial maze performance in rats. *Behavioral and Neural Biology* 40:58–69.

—— 1985. Olfactory discrimination learning is blocked by leupeptin, a thiol protease inhibitor. *Brain Research* 337:333–336.

Staubli, U., G. Ivy, and G. Lynch. 1984. Hippocampal denervation causes rapid forgetting of olfactory information in rats. *Proceedings of the National Academy of Sciences* 81:5885–5887.

Steinmetz, J. E., D. J. Rosen, P. F. Chapman, D. G. Lavond, and R. F. Thompson. 1986. Classical conditioning of the rabbit eyelid response with a mossy-fiber stimulation CS: I. Pontine nuclei and middle cerebellar peduncle stimulation. *Behavioral Neuroscience* 100:878–887.

Steinmetz, J. E., C. G. Logan, D. J. Rosen, J. K. Thompson, D. G. Lavond, and R. F. Thompson. 1987. Initial localization of the acoustic conditioned stimulus projection system to the cerebellum essential for classical eyelid conditioning. *Proceedings of the National Academy of Sciences* 84:3531–3535.

Stent, G. S. 1973. A physiological mechanism for Hebb's postulate of learning. *Proceedings of the National Academy of Sciences* 70:997–1001.

Stephan, H. and J. Manolescu. 1980. Comparative investigations on hippocampus in insectivores and primates. *Z. mikrosk.-anat. Forsch.* 94:1025–1050.

Supple, W. F. and R. N. Leaton. 1990. Cerebellar vermis: Essential for classically conditioned bradycardia in the rat. *Brain Research* 509:17–23.

Supple, W. F., J. Cranney, and R. N. Leaton. 1988. Effects of lesions of the cerebellar vermis on VMH lesion-induced hyperdefensiveness, spontaneous mouse-killing, and freezing in rats. *Physiology and Behavior* 42:145–153.

Susswein, A. J., M. Schwartz, and E. Feldman. 1986. Learned changes of feeding behavior in *Aplysia* in response to edible and inedible foods. *Journal of Neuroscience* 6:1513–1527.

Sutherland, N. S. and N. J. Mackintosh. 1971. *Mechanisms of Animal Discrimination Learning*. London: Academic Press.

Sutherland, R. J. and R. J. McDonald. 1990. Hippocampus, amygdala, and memory deficits in rats. *Behavioural Brain Research* 37:57–79.

Sutherland, R. J. and J. W. Rudy. 1988. Place learning in the Morris place navigation task is impaired by damage to the hippocampal formation even if the temporal demands are reduced. *Psychobiology* 16:157–163.

—— 1989. Configural association theory: The role of the hippocampal formation in learning, memory, and amnesia. *Psychobiology* 17:129–144.

Sutherland, R. J., I. Q. Whishaw, and B. Kolb. 1988. Contributions of cingulate cortex to two forms of spatial learning and memory. *Journal of Neuroscience* 8:1863–1872.

Sweatt, J. D. and E. R. Kandel. 1989. Persistent and transcriptionally dependent increase in protein phosphorylation in long-term facilitation of *Aplysia* sensory neurons. *Nature* 339:51–54.

Taube, J. S., R. U. Muller, and J. B. Ranck. 1990. Head-direction cells recorded from the postsubiculum in freely moving rats. 1. Description and quantitative analysis. *Journal of Neuroscience* 10:420–435.

Teuber, H. L. and S. Weinstein. 1956. Ability to find hidden figures after cerebral lesions. *Archives of Neurology and Psychiatry* 76:369–379.

Thompson, L. T. and P. J. Best. 1989. Place cells and silent cells in the hippocampus of freely behaving rats. *Journal of Neuroscience* 9:2382–2390.

—— 1990. Long-term stability of the place-field activity of single units recorded from the dorsal hippocampus of freely behaving rats. *Brain Research* 509:299–308.

Thompson, R. F. 1986. The neurobiology of learning and memory. *Science* 233:941–947.

—— 1988. The neural basis of associative learning of discrete behavioral responses. *Trends in Neuroscience* 11:152–155.

Thompson, R. F. and N. H. Donegan. 1986. The search for the engram. In J. L. Martinez and R. P. Kesner, eds., *Learning and Memory: A Biological View*, pp. 3–52. Orlando, Fla.: Academic Press.

Thompson, R. F. and D. L. Glanzman. 1976. Neural and behavioral mechanisms of habituation and sensitization. In T. J. Tighe and R. N. Leaton, eds., *Habituation: Perspectives from Child Development, Animal Behavior and Neurophysiology*, pp. 49–93. Hillsdale, N.J.: Lawrence Erlbaum.

Thompson, R. F. and W. A. Spencer. 1966. Habituation: A model phenomenon for the study of neuronal substrates of behavior. *Psychological Review* 173:16–43.

Thompson, R. F. and W. I. Welker. 1963. Role of auditory cortex in reflex head orientation by cats to auditory stimuli. *Journal of Comparative and Physiological Psychology* 56:996–1002.

Thompson, R. F., T. W. Berger, S. D. Berry, F. K. Hoehler, R. E. Kettner, and D. J. Weisz. 1980. Hippocampal substrate of classical conditioning. *Physiological Psychology* 8:262–279.

Thompson, R. F., G. A. Clark, N. H. Donegan, D. G. Lavond, J. Madden, L. A. Mamounas, M. D. Mauk, and D. A. McCormick. 1984. Neuronal substrates of basic associative learning. In L. R. Squire and N. Butters, eds., *Neuropsychology of Memory*, pp. 424–442. New York: Guilford Press.

Thompson, R. F., N. H. Donegan, G. A. Clark, D. G. Lavond, J. S. Lincoln, J. Madden, L. A. Mamounas, M. D. Mauk, and D. A. McCormick. 1987. Neuronal substrates of discrete, defensive conditioned reflexes, conditioned fear states, and their interactions in the rabbit. In Í. Gormezano, W. F. Prokasy, and R. F. Thompson, eds., *Classical Conditioning*, pp. 371–399. 3d ed. Hillsdale. N.J.: Lawrence Erlbaum.

Thompson, R. F., G. A. Clark, N. H. Donegan, D. G. Lavond, J. S. Lincoln, J. Madden, L. A. Mamounas, M. D. Mauk, D. A. McCormick, and J. K. Thompson. 1984. Neuronal substrates of learning and memory: A "multiple-trace" view. In G. Lynch, J. L. McGaugh, and N. M. Weinberger, eds., *Neurobiology of Learning and Memory*, pp. 137–164. New York: Guilford Press.

Tilson, H. A., G. J. Harry, R. L. McLamb, N. J. Peterson, B. C. Rodgers, P. Pediaditakis, and S. F. Ali. 1988. Role of dentate gyrus cells in retention of a radial arm maze task and sensitivity of rats to cholinergic drugs. *Behavioral Neuroscience* 102:835–842.

Tonkiss, J., R. G. M. Morris, and J. N. P. Rawlins. 1988. Intra-ventricular infusion of the NMDA antagonist AP5 impairs performance on a non-spatial operant DRL task in the rat. *Experimental Brain Research* 73:181–188.

Turner, R. W., K. G. Baimbridge, and J. J. Miller. 1982. Calcium-induced long-term potentiation in the hippocampus. *Neuroscience* 7:1411–1416.

Valenstein, E. S. 1973. *Brain Control: A Critical Examination of Brain Stimulation and Psychosurgery.* New York: Wiley.

Vanderwolf, C. H. 1969. Hippocampal electrical activity and voluntary movement in the rat. *Electroencephalography and Clinical Neurophysiology* 26:407–418.

Vinogradova, O. S. 1970. Registration of information and the limbic system. In G. Horn and R. A. Hinde, eds., *Short-Term Changes in Neural Activity and Behaviour*, pp. 95–148. Cambridge: Cambridge University Press.

—— 1975. The hippocampus and the orienting reflex. In E. N. Sokolov and O. S. Vinogradova, eds., *Neuronal Mechanisms of the Orienting Reflex*, pp. 128–154. Hillsdale, N.J.: Lawrence Erlbaum.

Von Neumann, J. 1958. *The Computer and the Brain.* New Haven: Yale University Press.

Wagner, A. R. 1976. Priming in STM: An information-processing mechanism for self-generated or retrieval-generated depression in performance. In T. J. Tighe and R. N. Leaton, eds., *Habituation: Perspectives from Child Development, Animal Behavior and Neurophysiology*, pp. 95–128. Hillsdale, N.J.: Lawrence Erlbaum.

—— 1981. SOP: A model of automatic memory processing in animal behavior. In N. E. Spear and R. R. Miller, eds., *Information Processing in Animals: Memory Mechanisms*, pp. 5–47. Hillsdale, N.J.: Lawrence Erlbaum.

Wagner, A. R. and N. H. Donegan, 1989. Some relationships between a computational model (SOP) and a neural circuit for Pavlovian (rabbit eyeblink) conditioning. In R. D. Hawkins and G. H. Bower, eds., *Computational Models of Learning in Simple Neural Systems,* pp. 157–203. *The Psychology of Learning and Motivation: Advances in Research and Theory* series, vol. 23,

Wagner, A. R. and R. A. Rescorla. 1972. Inhibition in Pavlovian conditioning: Application of a theory. In R. A. Boakes and M. S. Halliday, eds., *Inhibition and Learning,* pp. 301–336. London: Academic Press.

Wagner, A. R., J. W. Rudy, and J. W. Whitlow. 1973. Rehearsal in animal conditioning. *Journal of Experimental Psychology* 97:407–426.

Wagner, A. R., F. A. Logan, K. Haberlandt, and T. Price. 1968. Stimulus selection in animal discrimination learning. *Journal of Experimental Psychology* 76:171–180.

Walker, J. A. and D. S. Olton. 1979. Spatial memory deficit following fimbria-fornix lesions: Independent of time for stimulus processing. *Physiology and Behavior* 23:11–15.

Walters, E. T. 1989. Transformation of siphon responses during conditioning of *Aplysia* suggests a model of primitive stimulus-response association. *Proceedings of the National Academy of Sciences* 86:7616–7619.

Walters, E. T. and J. H. Byrne. 1983. Associative conditioning of single sensory neurons suggests a cellular mechanism for learning. *Science* 219:405–408.

Walters, E. T. and M. T. Erickson. 1986. Directional control and the functional organization of defensive responses in *Aplysia. Journal of Comparative Physiology* A159:339–351.

Walters, E. T., T. J. Carew, and E. R. Kandel. 1981. Associative learning in *Aplysia:* Evidence for conditioned fear in an in vertebrate. *Science* 211:504–506.

Watson, P. J. 1978. Nonmotor functions of the cerebellum. *Psychological Bulletin* 85:944–967.

Waxler, M. and H. E. Rosvold. 1970. Delayed alternation in monkeys after removal of the hippocampus. *Neuropsychologia* 8:137–146.

Weinberger, N. M. and D. M. Diamond. 1987. Physiological plasticity in auditory cortex: Rapid induction by learning. *Progress in Neurobiology* 29:1–55.

Weinstein, S. and H. L. Teuber. 1957. Effects of penetrating brain injury on intelligence test scores. *Science* 125:1036–1037.

Weiskrantz, L. 1956. Behavioral changes associated with ablation of the amygdaloid complex in monkeys. *Journal of Comparative and Physiological Psychology* 49:381–391.

Weiskrantz, L. and R. C. Saunders. 1984. Impairments of visual object transforms in monkeys. *Brain* 107:1033–1072.

Weiskrantz, L. and E. K. Warrington. 1979. Conditioning in amnesic patients. *Neuropsychologia* 17:187–194.

Weisz, D. J., G. A. Clark, and R. F. Thompson. 1984. Increased responsivity of dentate granule cells during nictitating membrane response conditioning in rabbit. *Behavioural Brain Research* 12:145–154.

Welsh, J. P. and J. A. Harvey. 1989. Cerebellar lesions and the nictitating membrane reflex: Performance deficits of the conditioned and unconditioned response. *Journal of Neuroscience* 9:299–311.

—— 1991. Pavlovian conditioning in the rabbit during inactivation of the interpositus nucleus. *Journal of Physiology* 444:459–480.

West, A., E. Barnes, and D. L. Alkon. 1982. Primary changes of voltage responses during retention of associative learning. *Journal of Neurophysiology* 48:1243–1255.

Whishaw, I. Q. and J. Tomie. 1991. Simple, conditional, and configural learning using tactile and olfactory cues is spared in hippocampal rats: Implications for hippocampal function. *Behavioral Neuroscience* 105:787–797.

Whishaw, I. Q. and C. H. Vanderwolf. 1971. Hippocampal EEG and behavior: Effects of variation in body temperature and relation of EEG to vibrissae movement, swimming and shivering. *Physiology and Behavior* 6:391–397.

Whitlow, J. W. 1975. Short-term memory in habituation and dishabituation. *Journal of Experimental Psychology: Animal Behavior Processes* 1:189–206.

Wible, C. G., R. L. Findling, M. Shapiro, E. J. Lang, S. Crane, and D. S. Olton. 1986. Mnemonic correlates of unit activity in the hippocampus. *Brain Research* 399:97–110.

Wickelgren, B. G. 1967. Habituation of spinal interneurons. *Journal of Neurophysiology* 30:1424–1438.

Wiener, S. I., C. A. Paul, and H. Eichenbaum. 1989. Spatial and behavioral correlates of hippocampal neuronal activity. *Journal of Neuroscience* 9:2737–2763.

Wieraszko, A. and G. F. Ball. 1991. Long-term enhancement of synaptic responses in the songbird hippocampus. *Brain Research* 538:102–102.

Williams, J. H., M. L. Errington, M. A. Lynch, and T. V. P. Bliss. 1989. Arachidonic acid induces a long-term activity-dependent enhancement of synaptic transmission in the hippocampus. *Nature* 341:739–742.

Willner, J., M. Gallagher, P. W. Graham, and G. B. Crooks. 1992. N-methyl-D-aspartate receptor antagonist D-APV selectively disrupts taste-potentiated odor aversion learning. *Behavioral Neuroscience* 106:315–323.

Willott, J. F., A. Schnerson, and G. P. Urban. 1979. Sensitivity of the acoustic startle response and neurons in the subnuclei of the mouse inferior colliculus to stimulus parameters. *Experimental Neurology* 65:625–644.

Wilson, D. A. and R. J. Racine. 1983. The postnatal development of post-activation potentiation in the rat neocortex. *Developmental Brain Research* 7:271–276.

Winfield, D. A., K. C. Gatter, and T. P. S. Powell. 1980. An electron microscopic study of the types and proportions of neurons in the cortex of the motor and visual areas of the cat and rat. *Brain* 103:245–258.

Winocur, G. 1990. Anterograde and retrograde amnesia in rats with dorsal hippocampal or dorsomedial thalamic lesions. *Behavioural Brain Research* 38:145–154.

Winocur, G. and M. Gilbert. 1984. The hippocampus, context and information processing. *Behavioral and Neural Biology* 40:27–43.

Winocur, G. and M. Moscovitch. 1990. Hippocampal and prefrontal cortex contributions to learning and memory: Analysis of lesion and aging effects on maze learning in rats. *Behavioral Neuroscience* 104:544–551.

Winocur, G. and J. Olds. 1978. Effects of context manipulation on memory and reversal learning in rats with hippocampal lesions. *Journal of Comparative and Physiological Psychology* 92:312–321.

Woodruff-Pak, D. S., D. G. Lavond, and R. F. Thompson. 1985. Trace conditioning: Abolished by cerebellar nuclear lesions but not by lateral cerebellar cortex aspirations. *Brain Research* 348:249–260.

Wyss, J. M. 1981. An autoradiographic study of the efferent connections of the entorhinal cortex in the rat. *Journal of Comparative Neurology* 199:495–512.

Yeo, A. G. and D. A. Oakley. 1983. Habituation of distraction to a tone in the absence of neocortex in rats. *Behavioural Brain Research* 8:403–409.

Yeo, C. H., M. J. Hardiman, and M. Glickstein. 1984. Discrete lesions of the cerebellar cortex abolish the classically conditioned nictitating membrane response of the rabbit. *Behavioural Brain Research* 13:261–266.

—— 1985a. Classical conditioning of the nictitating membrane response of the rabbit. I. Lesions of the cerebellar nuclei. *Experimental Brain Research* 60:87–98.

—— 1985b. Classical conditioning of the nictitating membrane response of the rabbit. II. Lesions of the cerebellar cortex. *Experimental Brain Research* 60:99–113.

—— 1986. Classical conditioning of the nictitating membrane response of the rabbit. IV. Lesions of the inferior olive. *Experimental Brain Research* 63:81–92.

Young, A. B. and G. E. Fagg. 1990. Excitatory amino acid receptors in the brain: Membrane binding and receptor autoradiographic approaches. *Trends in Pharmacological Science* 11:126–133.

Zalutsky, R. A. and R. A. Nicoll. 1990. Comparison of two forms of long—term potentiation in single hippocampal neurons. *Science* 248:1619–1624.

Zangwill, O. L. 1961. Lashley's concept of cerebral mass action. In W. H. Thorpe and O. L. Zangwill, eds., *Current Problems in Animal Behaviour*, pp. 59–86. Cambridge: Cambridge University Press.

Zeki, S. M. 1978. Uniformity and diversity of structure and function in rhesus monkey prestriate visual cortex. *Journal of Physiology* 277:273–290.

Zola, S. M. and H. Mahut. 1973. Paradoxical facilitation of object reversal learning after transection of the fornix in monkeys. *Neuropsychologia* 11:271–284.

Zola-Morgan, S. and L. R. Squire. 1984. Preserved learning in monkeys with medial temporal lesions: Sparing of motor and cognitive skills. *Journal of Neuroscience* 4:1072–1085.

—— 1985. Medial temporal lesions in monkeys impair memory in a variety of tasks sensitive to amnesia. *Behavioral Neuroscience* 99:22–34.

—— 1986. Memory impairment in monkeys following lesions limited to the hippocampus. *Behavioral Neuroscience* 100:155–160.

—— 1990. The primate hippocampal formation: Evidence for a time-limited role in memory storage. *Science* 250:288–290.

Zola-Morgan, S., L. R. Squire, and D. G. Amaral. 1986. Human amnesia and the medial temporal region: Enduring memory impairment following a bilateral lesion limited to field CA1 of the hippocampus. *Journal of Neuroscience* 6:2950–2967.

—— 1989. Lesions of the amygdala that spare adjacent cortical regions do not impair memory or exacerbate the impairment following lesions of the hippocampal formation. *Journal of Neuroscience* 9:1922–1936.

Zola-Morgan, S., L. R. Squire, and M. Mishkin. 1982. The neuroanatomy of amnesia: Amygdala-hippocampus versus temporal stem. *Science* 218:1337–1339

Zola-Morgan, S., L. R. Squire, D. G. Amaral, and W. A. Suzuki. 1989. Lesions of the perirhinal and parahippocampal cortex that spare the amygdala and hippocampal formation produce severe memory impairment. *Journal of Neuroscience* 9:4355–4370.

Author Index

Subject Index